NUCLEAR CARDIOLOGY

TECHNICAL APPLICATIONS

NUCLEAR CARDIOLOGY

TECHNICAL APPLICATIONS

Gary V. Heller, MD, PhD

Associate Director, Cardiology
Director, Nuclear Cardiology
Director, Cardiovascular Fellowship Program
Professor of Medicine and Nuclear Medicine
University of Connecticut School of Medicine
Hartford Hospital
Hartford, Connecticut

April Mann, BA, CNMT, NCT, RT(N)

Manager, Non-Invasive Cardiology
Hartford Hospital
Hartford, Connecticut

Robert C. Hendel, MD, FACC, FAHA, FASNC

Midwest Heart Specialists
Winfield, Illinois

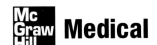

New York Chicago San Francisco Lisbon London
Madrid Mexico City Milan New Delhi San Juan
Seoul Singapore Sydney Toronto

Nuclear Cardiology: Technical Applications

1 2 3 4 5 6 7 8 9 0   DOC/DOC   12 11 10 9 8

ISBN   978-0-07-146475-8
MHID 0-07-146475-1

This book was set in Galliard by Aptara® Inc.
The editors were Ruth W. Weinberg and Kim J. Davis.
The production supervisor was Sherri Souffrance.
The cover designer was Aimee Davis.
Project management was provided by Sandhya Joshi, Aptara® Inc.
R.R. Donnelley was the printer and binder.

The background cover image is an X-ray of a human heart (David Bassett/Photo Researchers, Inc.). The smaller cover images (left to right) are a color enhanced scanning electron micrograph of cardiac muscle tissue (Asa Thoresen/Photo Researchers, Inc.), stenosis of the coronary artery (Gondelon/Photo Researchers, Inc.), a computer illustration of a wire-frame model of a healthy human heart (Alfred Pasieka/Photo Researchers, Inc.), a colored scanning electron micrograph (SEM) of the heart's chordae tendineae (Steve Gschmeissner/Photo Researchers, Inc.), and a colored angiogram (X-ray) of the coronary (heart) arteries of a patient with heart disease (Zephyr/Photo Researchers, Inc.).

This book was printed on acid-free paper.

Library of Congress Cataloging-in-Publication Data

Nuclear cardiology : technical applications / [edited by] Gary V. Heller, April Mann, Robert C. Hendel.
    p.   ;   cm.
  Includes bibliographical references and index.
  ISBN-13: 978-0-07-146475-8 (hardcover : alk. paper)
  ISBN-10: 0-07-146475-1 (hardcover : alk. paper)
  1. Heart—Radionuclide imaging.   I. Heller, Gary V.   II. Mann, April.   III. Hendel, Robert.
  [DNLM: 1. Heart—radionuclide imaging.   2. Cardiovascular Diseases—radionuclide imaging.
3. Nuclear Medicine—methods.   4. Radiopharmaceuticals—pharmacology.   5. Tomography,
Emission-Computed,   Single-Photon. WG 141.5.R3 N9642 2009]
  RC683.5.R33N835   2009
  616.1′207575—dc22

                                                              2008009015

DEDICATION

To Susan, who has affected me in more ways than can be imagined, all positive.

G.V.H.

To my loving and supportive family (you all know who you are) without whom everything I have accomplished would not have been possible.

A.M.

To the man who in his 10th decade is still teaching myself and others the **technical** *(and loving)* **applications** *of life—my father, Stan Hendel.*

R.C.H.

Contents

Contributors

Brian G. Abbott, MD

Assistant Professor of Medicine,
Department of Cardiology,
Brown Medical School;
Staff Cardiologist,
Rhode Island Hospital,
East Greenwich, Rhode Island

James A. Arrighi, MD

Associate Professor of Medicine,
Division of Biology and Medicine,
Brown Medical School;
Director, Nuclear Cardiology,
Rhode Island Hospital,
Providence, Rhode Island

Haris Athar, MD

Hartford Hospital,
Central Connecticut
Cardiologists, LLC,
Hartford, Connecticut

John Babich, PhD

Molecular Insight Pharmaceuticals, Inc.,
Cambridge, Massachusetts

Timothy M. Bateman, MD

Professor of Medicine,
University of Missouri
School of Medicine;
Co-Director Cardiovascular
Radiologic Imaging,
Cardiovascular Consultants, PC,
Kansas City, Missouri

Rob S. B. Beanlands, MD

Professor, Medicine, Radiology,
Cellular and Molecular Medicine,
University of Ottawa;
Chief Cardiac Imaging,
Director, Cardiovascular PET
Molecular Imaging Program,
National Cardiac Pet Center,
Ottawa, Ontario, Canada

James A. Case, PhD

CV Imaging Technologies, LLC,
Kansas City, Missouri

James R. Corbett, MD

Professor of Radiology and
Internal Medicine,
Director of Cardiovascular
Nuclear Medicine,
Division of Nuclear Medicine,
Department of Radiology,
Department of Cardiology,
University of Michigan Medical Center,
Ann Arbor, Michigan

S. James Cullom, PhD

Director, Research and
Development, Cardiovascular
Imaging Technologies, Inc.,
Kansas City, Missouri

Edouard Daher, MD

Harper Hospital,
Detroit, Michigan

Robert A. deKemp, PhD

Associate Professor,
Medicine and Engineering,
University of Ottawa;
Head Imaging Physicist,
Cardiac Imaging,
University of Ottawa Heart Institute,
Ottawa, Ontario, Canada

Marcelo F. DiCarli, MD

Division of Nuclear Medicine/PET,
Department of Radiology,
Brigham and Women's Hospital,
Boston, Massachusetts

Rami Doukky, MD

Assistant Professor of Medicine,
Rush Medical College;
Director, Nuclear Cardiology &
Stress Testing Laboratories,
Rush University Medical Center,
Chicago, Illinois

Edward P. Ficaro, PhD

Research Assistant Professor,
Division of Nuclear Medicine,
Department of Radiology,
University of Michigan Medical Center,
Ann Arbor, Michigan

Russell D. Folks, BS, CNMT, RT(N)

Senior Associate in Radiology,
Emory University School of Medicine,
Atlanta, Georgia

Gary V. Heller, MD, PhD

Associate Director, Cardiology;
Director, Nuclear Cardiology;
Director, Cardiovascular Fellowship Program
Professor of Medicine and Nuclear Medicine,
University of Connecticut School of
Medicine; Hartford Hospital,
Hartford, Connecticut

Robert C. Hendel, MD, FACC

Midwest Heart Specialists,
Winfield, Illinois

Bai-Ling Hsu, PhD

Director, Advance Physics,
Cardiovascular Imaging Technologies, LLC,
Kansas City, Missouri

James N. Kritzman, BS, CNMT

Whitmore Lake, Michigan

April Mann, BA, CNMT, NCT, RT(N)

Manager, Non-Invasive Cardiology,
Hartford Hospital,
Hartford, Connecticut

Gavin Noble, MD

Division of Cardiology,
Bend Memorial Clinic,
Bend, Oregon

Christopher Pastore, MD

Tufts University School of Medicine,
Division of Cardiology,
Tufts-New England Medical Center,
Boston, Massachusetts

Jennifer Prekeges, MS, CNMT

Program Chair, Nuclear Medicine
   Technology,
Bellevue Community College,
Bellevue, Washington

Mark I. Travin, MD

Professor of Clinical Nuclear
Medicine and Clinical Medicine,
Albert Einstein College of Medicine;
Director of Cardiovascular Nuclear
Medicine, Montefiore Medical
Center-Moses Division,
Bronx, New York

James E. Udelson, MD

Associate Professor of Medicine
and Radiology, Tufts University
School of Medicine;
Acting Chief, Division of Cardiology,
Tufts Medical Center,
Boston, Massachusetts

Frans J. Th. Wackers, MD

Professor Emeritus of Diagnositic
Radiology and Medicine (Cardiology),
Senior Research Scientist;
Yale University School of Medicine,
Attending Physician,
Yale-New Haven Hospital,
Cardiovascular Nuclear Imaging Laboratory,
New Haven, Connecticut

R. Glenn Wells, PhD, FCCPM

Assistant Professor,
Department of Medicine,
University of Ottawa, Medical Imaging
    Physicist,
Department of Cardiac Imaging,
University of Ottawa Heart Institute,
Ottawa, Ontario, Canada

Kim A. Williams, MD

Professor of Medicine and Radiology,
Director of Nuclear Cardiology,
Sections of Cardiology
and Nuclear Medicine,
University of Chicago,
Chicago, Illinois

Preface

Nuclear cardiology procedures have become essential components in the evaluation of patients with known or suspected cardiovascular disease. The success of our modality has, in large part, been due to advanced technology that continues to improve and expand the field. This has included the evolution of SPECT technologies, development of PET techniques, new radiopharmaceuticals, and cardiovascular CT.

The past few years have seen a virtual explosion of technical development. While exciting, understanding and using these complex technologies is critical for the creation of accurate data for interpretation and clinical use. Knowledge of these technologies is important for physicians and technologists performing and interpreting the studies, as well as health care providers who refer patients and then incorporate imaging results into clinical practice. Our goal in producing *Nuclear Cardiology: Technical Applications* was to provide a single, concise volume which would address the complex technological aspects of SPECT, PET, and cardiovascular CT. We also sought to provide technical information regarding stress procedures and imaging agents, as well as acquisition and processing protocols related to nuclear cardiology and cardiovascular CT.

This book is divided into eight sections. The first section comprises a review of instrumentation for both single photon emission computerized tomography (SPECT) and positron emission tomography (PET). Section 2 discusses key aspects of radiopharmaceuticals presently in widespread use, as well as newer agents. Sections 3 and 4 deal with the nuts and bolts of daily nuclear cardiology imaging including the technical aspects of stress testing, image acquisition, processing, and quantitation. The remainder of this book includes other nuclear cardiology procedures including PET and PET/CT, imaging ventricular function, and also touches on key regulatory issues.

It has been a pleasure to work on this project with our dedicated and learned contributors. We hope that this book will provide you, the reader, with information necessary to perform or utilize the highest-quality nuclear cardiology and cardiovascular CT data.

SECTION 1

CAMERA AND INSTRUMENTATION

CHAPTER 1

SPECT Instrumentation

James Kritzman

Single photon emission computed tomography (SPECT) allows for multiplane display of myocardial perfusion images (Figure 1-1). A simplified layman's explanation of SPECT imaging is as follows: The camera contains a crystal that detects the photons coming out of the body from the administered radiopharmaceutical. Each photon that hits the crystal creates a flash of light, which is converted to a digital signal and transferred to the acquisition station (Figure 1-2). The composite of these signals creates an image. The images are taken from multiple angles. A three-dimensional (3D) image is created from the sum of these images. This image volume can be re-sliced from multiple angles to allow the interpreting physician to look inside the target organ for abnormalities. If the patient moves during the acquisition, the images may not be reconstructed properly, creating or obscuring abnormalities. Although adequate for patient instruction and compliance, a more comprehensive understanding of the defi-

nition of SPECT imaging and reconstruction is necessary for clinicians.

HISTORY

SPECT is dependent on photon detection/localization and multiplane image acquisition and reconstruction. Dr. Harold Anger paved the way for SPECT imaging through the introduction of scintillation or Anger camera in the 1950s. The basic physics of the Anger camera allows for photon detection and estimation of the photon origination for planar imaging. The essential components of photon detection and localization for imaging include the crystal, photomultiplier tube (PMT), electronics, and collimator. The foundation of modern myocardial perfusion SPECT imaging was completed when the Anger camera was combined with the pioneering work performed by Dr. David Kuhl in the 1960s, applying emission computed tomography to nuclear

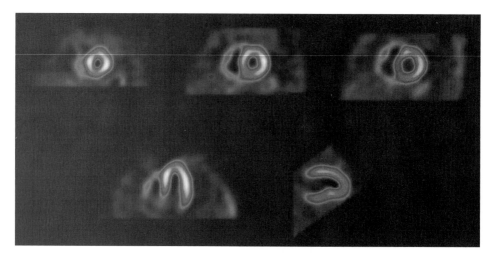

Figure 1-1.   Representative slices of a myocardial perfusion SPECT examination. (See color insert.)

medicine imaging for the first time. Emission computed tomography allowed for data acquisition from multiple angles around an object and multiplane reconstruction. The imaging equipment must, in addition to photon detection and localization, acquire data from multiple angles around the object of interest and combine the resulting images through robust computer algorithms to meet the requirements for SPECT imaging. When applied to the myocardium, SPECT imaging provides the ability to evaluate perfusion, shape, and, if gated, function.[1]

CRYSTAL

The crystal is constructed of a material that scintillates or "lights up" when struck by a photon. The scintillation is created when a photon deposits all of its energy in the crystal through the photoelectric effect. Compton scattering also occurs, but to a much lesser degree. The brightness or degree of scintillation created is directly proportional to the energy of the photon deposited. The scintillation generated allows for measurement by a PMT to determine the characteristics

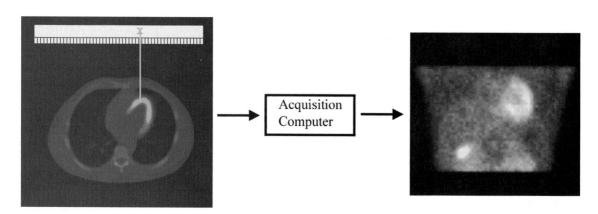

Figure 1-2.   Simplified schematic of image formation. (See color insert.)

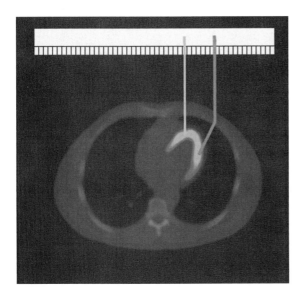

Figure 1-3. An ideal photon detection is indicated by the green path in the cross section of a collimator and crystal. The red path represents a "scattered" photon whose path has been altered by bone. (See color insert.)

of the photon, including energy level and estimation of origin. Desired photons for image reconstruction match the characteristic energy level (i.e., 140 keV for technetium 99m (Tc-99m)) of the isotope/radiopharmaceutical administered to the patient. Photons of reduced energy are typically "scattered" into the crystal from a secondary locations, not the photon origination (Figure 1-3). Scattered photons may degrade image reconstruction, creating or obscuring clinically relevant perfusion defects in myocardial SPECT perfusion imaging.

Specific properties of the crystal include density, thickness, and overall dimensions. The density of the crystal will determine useful energy range and resolution that can be detected. Sodium io-

dide crystals (NaI) activated with nonradioactive thallium have provided the best sensitivity for isotopes with energy levels between 50 and 150 keV, those typically used in nuclear cardiology (Tc-99m and thallium 201 (Tl-201)). Other media have been proposed, but the imaging characteristics are less optimal than NaI in the desired energy range for standard gamma camera imaging. Crystal sensitivity and resolution are affected by crystal thickness. Current sensitivity for most commercially available systems, when collimated, is approximately 3% for a 3/8-inch thick crystal. Sensitivity increases with crystal thickness, especially for higher-energy isotopes, as there are more media to react with incoming photons. A large fraction of high-energy photons simply passes through thin crystals without being detected. However, the increased sensitivity of thicker crystals comes at the cost of image resolution. As thickness increases, a single scintillation or event is observed by a larger area of the crystal. Increasing thickness reduces the ability of the PMT to accurately localize the scintillation coordinates within the crystal, reducing resolution (Figure 1-4). A crystal thickness of 3/8 inch is optimal for current Tc-99m myocardial SPECT procedures. As new molecular imaging agents using a wide array of isotopes are developed, tailored to hot spot imaging of particular disease processes, a more sensitive (thicker) crystal may be desired. Sodium iodide crystals are fragile and hygroscopic, so they must be sealed, typically with aluminum, to prevent incidental damage and hydration of the crystal from the environment. Although sealed, care must still be taken to avoid mechanical damage to the crystal surface.

PHOTOMULTIPLIER TUBE

The PMTs are arranged in an array covering the entire crystal. Hexagonal shaping allows for tight

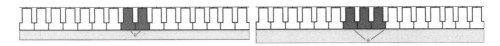

Figure 1-4. The black tubes illustrate scintillation dispersion in crystals of varying thickness. (This image is licensed under the GNU Free Documentation License. It uses material modified from the Wikipedia article "Gamma Camera.").

spacing of the PMTs. Large field-of-view (FOV) SPECT systems may employ large numbers of PMTs (>50) to cover the entire FOV. The PMTs measure the specific properties of scintillations in the crystal. These include the spatial X and Y coordinates of the event and the Z pulse or energy level of the event. Events are typically observed by multiple PMTs, with greatest intensity at the origination of the scintillation. Only one event will be registered, although observed by multiple PMTs. Weighted averages of the output from the PMTs are used to determine the most precise localization of the scintillation (Figure 1-5).

In analog detectors, the ability of multiple PMTs to observe the event and the use of weighted spatial average allow for more accurate determination of the X and Y coordinates of the event. This is facilitated through the use of a "light pipe" between the crystals and the PMTs. The light pipe is composed of an optically coupled thin sheet of glass. The PMTs adhere to the light pipe with the use of coupling gel. More current "digital" detectors have an analog-to-digital converter (ADC) on each PMT to digitize the signal and allow improved photon localization. The ability to localize discrete scintillation events dictates the intrinsic spatial resolution of the system (typically ~3.5 mm).

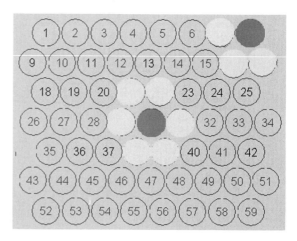

Figure 1-5. Red PMTs represent primary locations of scintillation. Adjacent tubes (yellow) also observe the event. (See color insert.)

The Z pulse (energy) or scintillation intensity must match the isotope window or energy spectrum defined for the isotope being used to be considered a valid data point (Figure 1-6). Although the primary energy for Tc-99m is 140 keV, a range or window of 15% centered at 140 keV is typically used for imaging to capture the majority of the useful photopeak, improving statistics and reducing imaging time. The range exists because of

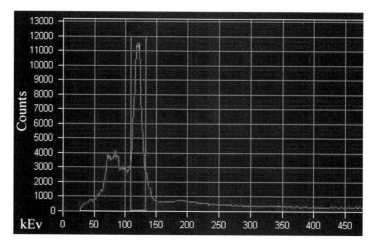

Figure 1-6. The energy spectrum displayed by the analyzer for Co-57 illustrates the photopeak of the isotope and the window set for imaging.

low-angle scatter of the emission isotope and inherent variations in the PMTs and crystal. The full width at half maximum (FWHM) of the photopeak determines the energy resolution or ability to distinguish photons of different energy levels. As the isotope window is narrowed, the amount of scattered photons is reduced, as energy of the photon reduces with increasing scattering angle.[2] Photons with energy levels falling outside of the window are ignored.

There is a physical limit to the number of simultaneous events that can be detected by the imaging system. The PMT has a finite recovery time (dead time) after an event is detected, when it is unable to detect another event. As the number of detected events increases, the recovery time or "dead time" increases. Dead time is typically displayed in the analyzer settings of modern gamma cameras. If the dead time is too high, typically >10%, counts may be preferentially collected over the center of the PMT. If this occurs during quality control, an erroneous nonuniform image may be acquired. (For this reason, system calibration, quality control, and patient imaging should occur within a proper dead time range, typically less than 10%.) Specific methodology for dead time measurement is available in National Electrical Manufacturers Association (NEMA) publications.[3] Observed count rates of most systems will not reach a 10% dead time level for recommended patient radioisotope administrations. If the system is collecting data with an incorrect energy window (i.e., off-peak or drift after prolonged system downtime), data may be collected preferentially near the edges or centers of the tube, depending on the direction of peak shift. With the routine use of multidetector imaging systems, count rate capabilities, sensitivity, and dead time must be comparable between detectors to avoid potential image artifacts.

ELECTRONICS

Proper performance of the electronic components of the detector is integral to quality image formation. The signal from the PMT passes through a preamplifier and amplifier, along with pulse arithmetic analyzers to determine the X and Y coordinates for photon origination. The pulse height analyzer (PHA) measures the energy or Z pulse of the scintillation. Once the X and Y coordinates and Z pulse are verified for a valid event, the photon or "count" is digitized and added to the appropriate digital pixel location in the image array (Figure 1-7). The signal from the photomultiplier travels through a preamplifier and an amplifier in order to be registered as a valid event. At this point, the analog signal can be converted to digital and transferred to the acquisition computer.

COLLIMATION

The collimator performs as a "camera lens," affecting sensitivity and resolution. Several types have commonly been used in myocardial perfusion imaging including low-energy high resolution (LEHR), low-energy general purpose (LEGP), and fan beam. The basic physical configuration is a sheet of lead covering the crystal with an arrangement of holes. The collimator defines the FOV because only photons that are theoretically perpendicular to the acceptance angles of the collimator holes are accepted (Figure 1-8). The best resolution is obtained at the surface of the collimator. As distance between the collimator and photon source increases, the photon dispersion increases, allowing for an increase in scattered photons degrading resolution and contrast (Figure 1-9). Patient to collimator distance should be minimized for optimal image resolution. The detection of events perpendicular to the acceptance angles is a vital function of the collimator, as this reduces the collection of scattered photons, those not originating from the target object. This property is also the weakest link in the SPECT imaging system as ~99% of emitted photons are blocked by the collimator, reducing sensitivity.

Collimator-specific properties include thickness (depth) and width (bore) of the collimator holes and angulation (diverging/converging collimation). The width and length of the holes determine the photon acceptance path. A wider bore allows for more sensitivity by opening the

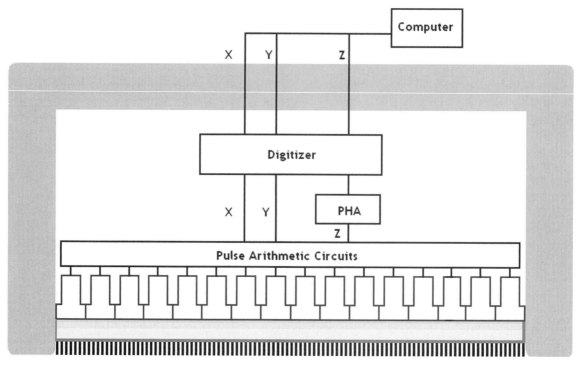

Figure 1-7. Electronic schematics of a gamma camera detector. (This image is licensed under the GNU Free Documentation License. It uses material modified from the Wikipedia article "Gamma Camera.")

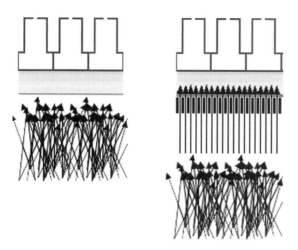

Figure 1-8. All photons, including scatter, are registered by a noncollimated crystal. Photons originating perpendicular to the crystal are collected with collimation. (This image is licensed under the GNU Free Documentation License. It uses material modified from the Wikipedia article "Gamma Camera.")

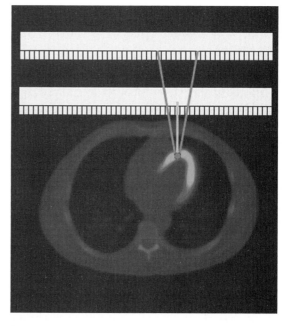

Figure 1-9. Photon dispersion increases as a function of distance. (See color insert.)

acceptance angles; however, more scattered photons will be accepted reducing resolution. The depth of the holes also affects the acceptance angles. Increasing depth reduces the acceptance angle, increasing resolution and decreasing sensitivity. The thickness of the septa also minimizes septal penetration of scattered photons in the appropriate energy range, improving resolution.[4]

Collimator selection depends on the isotope selected and the dose injected. If low-dose injections, i.e., Tl-201, are routinely used, LEGP collimation may be desirable to increase imaging statistics, as the holes are larger, increasing photon acceptance. Most nuclear cardiology examinations are performed with LEHR collimation to optimize image resolution. Image statistics for low-dose studies can be increased by increasing imaging time for LEHR collimation. Fan beam collimators have been implemented in the past to focus on the myocardium, in an effort to increase image resolution. However, image acquisition with fan beam collimation typically required offset in orbits to avoid data truncation of the myocardium in many patients. The resulting orbits were problematic, causing collision errors with a wider range of body habitus than nonoffset orbits with LEHR/LEGP collimation.

Within recent years, cameras utilizing multicrystal solid-state technology for photon detection have been introduced. The design of solid-state detectors allows for higher photon sensitivity and increased resolution through the use of semiconductor crystal materials such as cadmium zinc telluride (CZT).[5] Semiconductor materials convert incoming photons directly to digital signals. With no PMTs and their associated electronics, a thin panel serves as the detector. The detectors are made using an array of individual single pixel blocks of crystal material, allowing for precise localization of the detected photons. The cost of productions has kept current solid-state technology limited to small FOV SPECT systems. An attractive feature of these systems is service. If a detector block is not performing, it can simply be unplugged and replaced without the downtime associated with standard gamma camera technology.

Multiple panels can be arranged to cover larger portions of the acquisition orbit, reducing imaging time. At the time of this publication, no large-scale clinical trials comparing solid-state technology versus standard gamma camera techniques have been completed.

SPECT SYSTEMS

Orbit

In conventional SPECT imaging, the detector(s) acquires a series of static images over a 360-degree orbit around the patient. This can be accomplished using a single- or a multidetector system. The advantage of using a multidetector system is increased throughput as multiple projections are simultaneously obtained. A dual-head imaging system with the detectors fixed at 90 degrees is the current industry standard for myocardial SPECT imaging. This allows for the same information density as a single detector system in half of the time. Myocardial SPECT images are typically acquired over 180 degrees from right anterior oblique (−45 degrees) to left posterior oblique (135 degrees).[6] Data acquired over 180 degrees, which include a centered myocardium in its line of sight, are sufficient to reconstruct high-quality images (Figure 1-10). Innovative camera designs further reducing imaging time are currently undergoing clinical trials. These designs include upright imaging, 180-degree rings of detector material, and new approaches to collimation.

A standard 180-degree orbit assumes the position of the heart to be relatively uniform in all subjects. This will optimize image results for the anterior wall of the heart by discarding the more highly attenuated data where the heart is furthest from the camera and body surface posteriorly. Patients imaged with dextrocardia or cytus inversus using a 180-degree orbit will require an orbit adjusted for myocardial position. A 360-degree orbit may be preferred in these cases, as the reconstruction range can be defined postacquisition by most vendors. Acquiring data over 360 degrees can increase sensitivity over the inferior aspect of the heart at

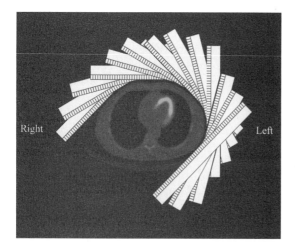

Figure 1-10. Acquisition projection range for myocardial perfusion SPECT imaging. (See color insert.)

the cost of reduced sensitivity in the anterior wall. This is a function of distance as projection data from the posterior aspects with a larger scatter component and increasing distance will decrease the resolution of the anterior wall, while improving the inferior portions. Using an orbit larger than 180 degrees may help improve image quality on subjects with atypical cardiac orientation (COPD, post TXP), as image reconstruction with standard RAO-LPO data may be insufficient.[7]

Either circular or body-contouring orbits can be implemented on modern systems. Circular orbits may prevent image distortion in patients with extreme body habitus, as the distance between the detector and myocardium may vary widely with a body-contouring orbit in this population.[8] Body-contouring orbits allow the detector to remain close to the patient for increased image resolution in typical subjects. Many current systems automatically contour to the patient. Care must be taken to avoid artifactual extremes in the orbit caused by extraneous materials such as IV lines and blankets. These extremes may cause image degradation as a result of varying distance and resolution.

The number of images or projections over the orbit also relates to the overall resolution that can

be derived from the images. A typical myocardial SPECT study contains 64 projections over 180 degrees. An image is acquired approximately every 3 degrees over the orbit. If too few projection angles are acquired, image resolution is reduced.[9] Current conventional cardiac SPECT imaging is typically performed using a dual detector system. This allows for a 50% reduction in total imaging time, as the number of camera stops is reduced by a factor of 2 over the required 180-degree orbit.

Information density of the myocardial perfusion images directly affects diagnostic quality. Acquisition time and administered dose are two components of information density. Current guidelines recommend 20 to 25 seconds of acquisition time per projection for nongated and gated acquisitions, respectively. Administered dosages of radiopharmaceuticals for myocardial perfusion imaging should be adjusted based on patient weight.[6] This allows for more uniform information density in patients of varying body masses. If dose adjustment is not feasible, information density can be more uniform across subjects with varying body masses by increasing the time acquired per projection. ASNC imaging guidelines are a valuable resource in establishing clinical imaging parameters and radiopharmaceutical dosing. Current myocardial imaging guidelines can be found at www.ASNC.org.

Pixel Size/Matrix

Pixel size also affects the quality of SPECT imaging. A pixel is the smallest discrete unit in an image matrix (Figure 1-11). Cardiac imaging can employ 64×64 or 128×128 matrices, depending on the count statistics and acquisition/reconstruction parameters employed. The number of pixels in a 128×128 matrix is exponentially larger than in a 64×64 matrix (128^2 vs. 64^2) (Figure 1-12). Doubling the matrix size over the same FOV will decrease the pixel size by a factor of 2. More counts are required for equivalent image quality when using a larger matrix to avoid increased noise, as the data are distributed over a larger number of image elements. Pixel size is also controlled by hardware

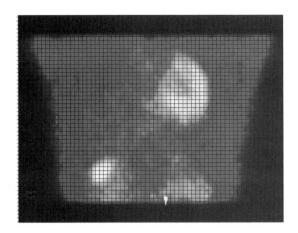

Figure 1-11. A standard projection image displayed in a 64 × 64 matrix. (See color insert.)

and software zooms. At the time of this publication, ASNC guidelines state acquisition parameters of a 64 × 64 matrix and a pixel size of 6.4 ± 0.4 mm for myocardial perfusion SPECT. Image quality for iterative techniques with resolution recovery and/or attenuation correction may provide improved image quality when acquired in a finer matrix and smaller pixel size, i.e., 128 × 128 matrix with a pixel size of 4.8 mm. Pixel size is directly

related to the acquisition matrix and hardware/software zooms implemented. Most large FOV imaging systems have a native pixel size of 9.6 mm when the acquisition matrix is 64 × 64 with a zoom of 1. To meet imaging guidelines, a hardware zoom of 1.45 is employed to yield a pixel size of approximately 6.5 mm. If no zoom were applied, the 9.6-mm pixel size would have been approximately the thickness of the myocardium. Such a pixel size is far too coarse to resolve mild/moderate perfusion defects. Numerous publications have cited overestimation of ejection fractions in subjects with small hearts (<100 mL end diastolic volume). Larger matrices like 128 × 128 and/or smaller pixel dimensions can be advantageous for estimation of ejection fraction in this population where large pixel dimensions may be too coarse to adequately estimate differences between end-diastolic and end-systolic images. If a zoom is to be employed, it should preferentially be at the time of acquisition (hardware zoom). Software zoom (pixel manipulation postacquisition) can help but will not recover resolution to the extent of a study acquired with an acquisition zoom. Physical properties of the SPECT system should also dictate the zoom selection. The acquisition

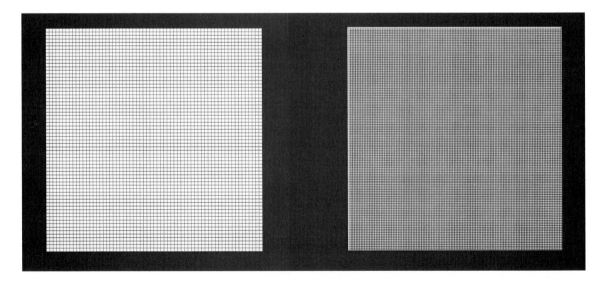

Figure 1-12. A 64 × 64 matrix compared with a 128 × 128 matrix.

matrix and hardware zoom could be set to 1 mm; however, the resulting images will not have true 1-mm resolution. It is not possible for images from conventional SPECT acquisitions to exceed the physical intrinsic resolution (∼3.5 mm) of the camera. Increased noise, especially with low-dose acquisitions when using small pixel dimensions, may negate resolution benefits if oversmoothing of count poor data is performed. If the ventricular chamber is not visualized (blurred out) at end systole in gated reconstructions, software algorithms that calculate the volumes will not have adequate statistical information and may provide erroneous results.

IMAGE RECONSTRUCTION

Filtered Back Projection

Conventional SPECT has employed back projection for reconstruction since inception. Back projection is quick and simple on current computer workstations with reconstruction times less than 5 seconds. Each projection acquired during the SPECT acquisition is simply back projected to create multiple transaxial slices, each being one pixel thick. Two-dimensional pixels that now have a depth of one pixel are referred to as voxels. The slices are stacked to create a 3D volumetric image comprised of cubic voxels (3D), not pixels (2D) (Figure 1-13).

The addition of artifactual blurring is inherent to back projection, as reprojected data overlap. This effect is called $1/r$ blurring (Figure 1-14). A ramp filter is necessary to SPECT reconstruction and is automatically applied to reduce blurring during back projection, thus the name filtered back projection.[10] Unfortunately, the ramp filter, while reducing blurring, also degrades image quality by the addition of high-frequency noise. Noise-suppression filters are used to remove noise and optimize the visual quality of SPECT data. The data must be transformed into frequency space to apply a filter. This is done through Fourier transformation. As data undergo Fourier transformation, these are broken into discrete frequencies.

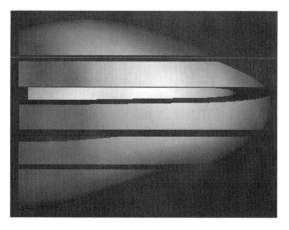

Figure 1-13. Example of 3D-rendered stacked transaxial images of the left ventricle. (See color insert)

The frequency concept can be visualized through a nonclinical image example. A SPECT acquisition performed on a cobalt 57 (Co-57) sheet source of uniform activity will serve as a model. An ideal true projection of data through the uniform sheet source would yield a count profile starting at zero,

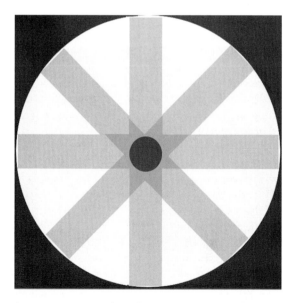

Figure 1-14. Overlap of projection data from individual rays results in $1/R$ blurring.

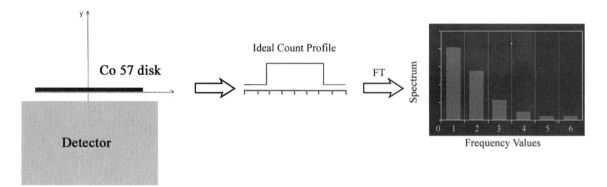

Figure 1-15. Ideal count profile of a uniform sheet source and frequency spectrum components post Fourier transformation.

with a vertical increase in activity at the edge. The count profile would be horizontal across the main body sheet source, with a vertical drop to no activity at the edge of the source. Fourier transformation of the data yields specific frequencies of the data (Figure 1-15).

The majority of an image object is comprised of low-frequency data. High-frequency data represent the sharp edges of the object and image noise. There is a trade-off between noise reduction and image resolution, as both are in the high-frequency domain. All events or counts collected are represented in the frequency graphics. Applying a low-pass filter to the collected data will remove high-frequency data, reducing noise and image resolution (Figure 1-16). The low-frequency data will have a higher weighting factor, and the resulting image will be too smooth, lacking high-resolution details. High-pass filtering, similar to the application of the ramp filter, reduces blur in the image by retaining high-frequency data. This is at the cost of added noise and a loss of the main bulk of the data.

Filters are mathematical functions weighting the data from each frequency, so that the area under the curve always equals the total number of counts. Variations in filter settings do not reduce the number of total counts in the reconstruction, although variation may occur in individual pixels and slices. A variety of filters, including Hanning, Parzen, Gaussian, and Butterworth to name a few,

have been used in nuclear imaging. Each filter type has specific properties such as cutoff frequency and order. Filter selection is typically based on image density. If the high-frequency data comprising the edges of our data are weighted too low, the resulting image is blurred because of high weighting of the low-frequency data. Conversely, if one applied a high-pass filter, cutting off the bulk of the low-frequency data, the remaining image retains sharp edges, while losing information density and exhibiting increasing noise (Figure 1-16).

The Butterworth or low-pass filter is most commonly used in reconstruction of MPI images. Order and cutoff frequency are specific properties of this filter type. The cutoff frequency is the point above which all frequencies are weighted by a factor of 0. Adjusting the cutoff frequency of the low-pass or Butterworth filter makes dramatic changes in image appearance, as frequencies below the cutoff are weighted higher and those above the cutoff are multiplied by 0 and eliminated (Figure 1-17). Adjusting the order changes the slope of the filter curve, resulting in minimal change to the area under the curve and image appearance. Order can be thought of as a fine-tuning mechanism (Figure 1-18). Typical reconstruction parameters use an order between 5 and 7, with little need for adjustment. Filter cutoff frequencies will vary between vendors as frequency may be measured in Nyquist frequency (cycles per centimeter) or cycles per pixel. Thus, a filter setting on one imaging

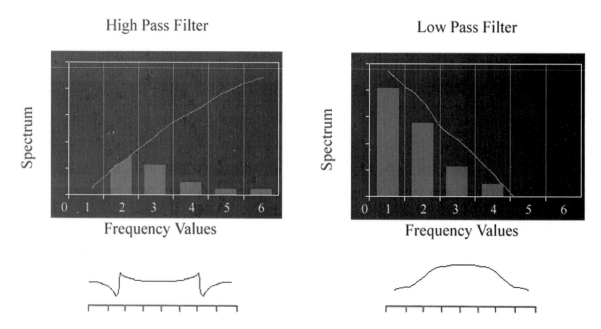

Figure 1-16. Note the loss of resolution (blurred edge profile) when high-frequency values are excluded by the low-pass filter. The high-pass filter preserves the sharp edges of the object at the cost of additive noise (baseline increases outside of image profile) and a loss of image data.

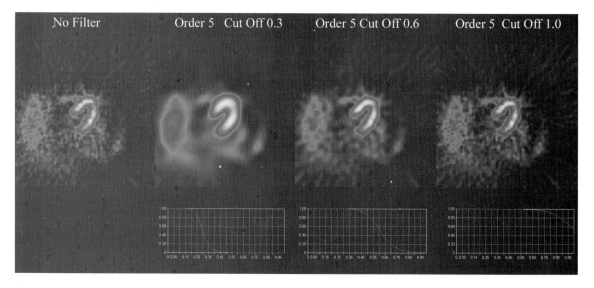

Figure 1-17. Small changes in cutoff frequency (end point of the filter function curve) using a low-pass filter create obvious changes in image appearance as the area under the filter function curve is significantly changed.

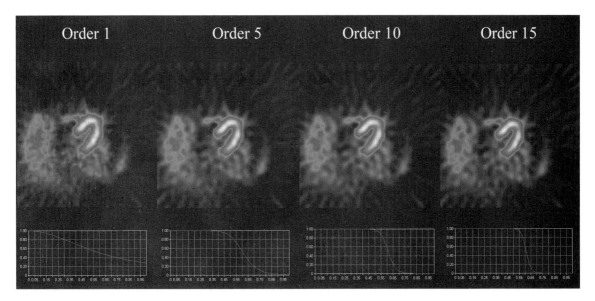

Figure 1-18. Large changes in the order or "slope" of a low-pass filter have minimal effect on reconstructed image quality. At extremes, as illustrated with an order of 1, image quality begins to change as more high-frequency scatter is included.

system may not yield the same results on another vendors system. If 4.8-mm pixel data were reconstructed using a cutoff of 0.6 cycles per centimeter (10 mm), the equivalent cutoff in cycles per pixel would be approximately 0.3. This distinction may not be apparent on the system in use. If the acquisition matrix changes from 64×64 to 128×128, roughly equivalent filter settings can be obtained by reducing the prior cutoff values by a factor of 2. The use of a weight-based dose regimen, as recommended by imaging guidelines, reduces variability in information density between patients and less variation in image quality.[6]

Iterative Reconstructions

Iterative reconstruction techniques are being more routinely employed in SPECT reconstruction, especially with the use of sealed source and CT-based attenuation correction. Iterative techniques allow the implementation of additional data into the reconstruction not possible with simple filtered back projection. This can include scatter correction, at-

tenuation correction, resolution recovery, and collimator response functions. These reconstruction algorithms are computationally complex, requiring more time and robust computer hardware. A simple analogy would be that of a golfer putting on the edge of a green. The same club or algorithm is used for each putt along with the same directional path. The first putt places the ball closer to the hole. Each successive putt places the ball closer to the desired location, eventually in the hole. A poor golfer or algorithm with instabilities could allow the ball to miss the cup or desired result, introducing error in the form of image noise.

A more technical analogy to iterative reconstruction is using Newton's method to approximate the zeroes of a function in calculus. An initial "guesstimate" is made for the solution based on the appearance of the curve or data (in the case of nuclear medicine attenuation-corrected images, a first-order Chang mathematical attenuation-corrected image could be used). The results are then run through the equation for the second iteration to get a better approximation. This cycle continues until the desired result is reached (as observed by minimized differences between successive iterations). In image reconstructions, the desired number of iterations varies between vendors and algorithms. Each successive iteration is closer to the "true" image. As iterations continue, the difference between successive iterations is smaller and eventually indistinguishable. In a robust algorithm, one cannot "overiterate" the image. An infinite number of iterations could be performed on a stable algorithm converging on the correct result. Algorithms with insufficiencies may introduce noise to the displayed images if excessive iterations are used or if data are statistically insufficient.

Iterative algorithms may be 2D or 3D in their approach to beam modeling. Beam modeling is used in characterizing photon origination within an object. Unlike filtered back projection, which assumes photon origination as a single point perpendicular to the collimator surface, 2D and 3D algorithms weight the theoretical distribution of photon origination. Two-dimensional methods weight photon origination over a given row. Three-dimensional algorithms typically use radial distance from the patient and collimator response function to approximate a conical distribution of potential photon origination points (Figure 1-19). This conical distribution is reminiscent of performing intrinsic uniformity quality control, as a point source five fields away from the crystal provides a uniform saturation of counts. This property allows for improved image count recovery, resolution, and reduction or elimination of star artifact caused by areas of intense activity in filtered back projection. Three-dimensional beam modeling uses the entire volume of data to improve image quality, while maintaining the integrity of the organ of interest (Figure 1-20).

SPECT QUALITY CONTROL

Quality control is an integral component of high-quality myocardial SPECT imaging. Insufficiencies in QC protocols can directly affect the clinical integrity of SPECT images. Quality-control proce-

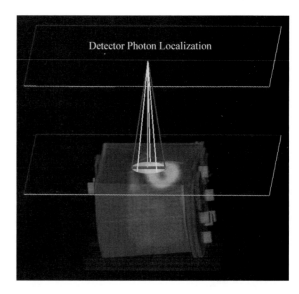

Figure 1-19. Representation of FBP (green) and 2D (blue) and 3D (yellow) beam modeling techniques, illustrating theoretical photon origination distributions. (See color insert.)

dures can be categorized into two categories (intrinsic/extrinsic) that are performed at specified intervals—initial and/or service, daily, quarterly, and annually in the case of certain accreditation protocols. Certain procedures and subsequent analyses require advanced training and equipment, which should be performed by a qualified diagnostic medical physicist to meet NEMA specifications for operation.

Intrinsic quality-control procedures are performed with no collimator on the camera. These procedures specifically test the crystal and electronics of the system. Intrinsic quality-control procedures include intrinsic resolution, pixel sizing, intrinsic uniformity, intrinsic spatial resolution and distortion (bar phantom), maximum count rate capabilities, count rate curve analysis, multiple window spatial registration, and energy resolution.

Extrinsic quality-control procedures are performed with the collimator in place and test the entire system. Examples of extrinsic quality control include system resolution, system sensitivity, total SPECT performance (Jaszczak) phantom

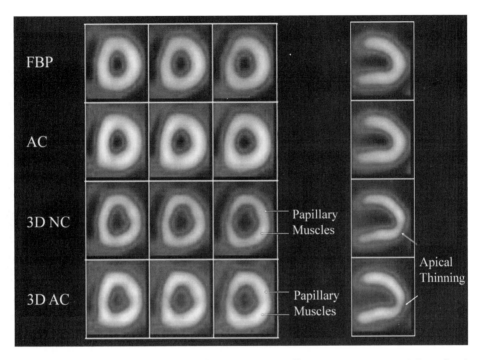

Figure 1-20.   Three-dimensional beam-modeled reconstructions illustrate more "anatomic" cardiac images, including papillary musculature and anatomic apical thinning not apparent using standard reconstruction techniques. (See color insert.)

measurements including contrast and resolution, SPECT versus planar resolution, center of rotation (COR) verification, and collimator hole angulation testing.

Initial

Upon installation of a SPECT system, the installation team verifies the intrinsic (no collimation) functionality of the SPECT system. This includes verification of PMT operation in the correct voltage range. Although all PMTs may be operating correctly, inherent variations in the crystal and electronic components will yield a nonuniform image from a uniform photon emitter. The system must stabilize (powered on) for at least 24 hours prior to this verification. Earlier attempts may result in voltage drift and incorrect peak identification for subsequent imaging procedures. The service engineer performs energy correction, spatial linearity correction, and high-count uniformity correction. The high-count uniformity correction image will be analyzed by the system to detect and compensate for areas of decreased count saturation (Figure 1-21).

Subsequent noncalibration intrinsic uniformity measurements will use these corrections to create a uniform quality-control flood image if the system is operating properly. These results will also be applied to all clinical images unless the correction is turned off. This high-count uniformity calibration should not need to be routinely repeated unless quality-control flood images begin to degrade with no other obvious cause or at vendor-specified frequency. Also, the intrinsic high-count uniformity calibration must contain more counts than any SPECT study to be corrected. Most vendors recommend 200 million counts for the intrinsic flood correction table flood for use with Tc-99m imaging. Extrinsic uniformity should also be

Figure 1-21.   The image for the high-count uniformity *correction* is not expected to be completely uniform.

verified. If applicable, the service engineer will also load high-count extrinsic uniformity calibrations for each collimator set to be used. In the case of cardiac imaging with a large FOV LEHR collimator, this flood should contain at least 120 million counts. COR calibrations should also be performed by the service engineer at the time of installation.

ACCEPTANCE TESTING

Although the flood images may be pristine when the imaging system is released by the service engineer, any SPECT system when newly installed or nonmobile SPECT system that has changed in physical location should have acceptance testing performed within 4 to 6 weeks. Acceptance testing involves a comprehensive set of quality-control procedures to verify proper functionality of the SPECT system.[11] Acceptance testing is typically performed by a qualified medical physicist. The physicist should perform all of the aforementioned QC procedures and provide a detailed report of the results and a comparison with the vendors' specifications for any discrepancies. These results should be used in obtaining corrective action for any system deficiencies.

Daily

Daily quality control should be performed and reviewed prior to clinical use. Most vendors recommend intrinsically peaking the camera as the first step in daily quality control. Peaking verifies that the correct energy window will be used for optimal photon detection. An off-peak system will result in low-resolution images with a high percentage of scatter and/or noisy count poor data. Vendor procedures must be followed when peaking the camera. Systems intended for intrinsic peaking must not be peaked extrinsically, as peak values will be reduced by collimation and scattered photons. A low-activity point source is exposed to the crystal, and the proper keV is verified/recalibrated. The source must not be too hot, or excessive dead time (>10%) may affect the peak values. If the peak value is changing/drifting, additional QC measures or service may be necessary. After peak verification, either intrinsic uniformity or extrinsic system uniformity should be performed to vendor specifications.

Daily intrinsic quality control (collimator off) is performed with a low-activity point source (Tc-99m or Co-57) for a "low-count" planar flood image (typically 15 million counts). For a single detector system, the point source should be five times the FOV away from the center of the detector to provide a uniform spread of photons across the surface. If the point source is too close, the flood will display a hot center and high variability in quantitative flood uniformity analysis. Certain dual detector systems have a fixed geometry and cannot image a point source at five FOVs. These systems have built-in geometric response or curvature corrections that allow both detectors to simultaneously acquire an intrinsic flood at a closer distance, typically centered between the detectors. If source activity is too high (<10%), erroneous flood images will be acquired, most likely with visualization of a portion the PMT array (Figure 1-22). Once acquired, the image should be visually and quantitatively analyzed. Visual evaluation should assess for any areas of nonuniformities, degradation, and/or change. Defective PMTs may

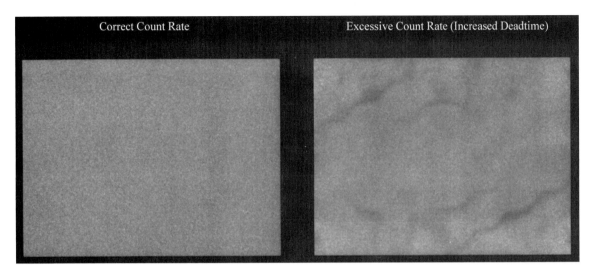

Figure 1-22.   Excessive dead time can lead to visualization of the PMT arraysince counts will be preferentially collected over the center of the PMTs. (Image courtesy of Medical Physics Consultants Inc., Ann Arbor, MI.)

be identified by circular areas of reduced or absent activity (Figure 1-23).

Physical damage to the crystal may be identified by the appearance of dark lines/cracks in the flood image. "Measling" artifacts or discrete dark spots caused by hydration of the crystal may also

Figure 1-23.   Defective PMTs are represented by circular areas of reduced or absent activity. (Image courtesy of Medical Physics Consultants Inc., Ann Arbor, MI)

be present and will degrade image quality (physical contamination of the crystal may also yield this type of artifact). Measling is a more common artifact in older imaging systems. Modern gamma cameras typically do not suffer from measling, as the crystals are sealed. Quantitative analysis is typically performed with a vendor-supplied uniformity analysis program and calculates the integral and differential uniformities of the flood image for the central field of view (CFOV) and useful field of view (UFOV). Integral uniformity is defined as the maximum absolute difference in pixel values across the entire area analyzed. Differential uniformity is the absolute maximum difference for any five adjacent pixels in a row. Therefore, the integral uniformity values will be greater than or equal to the differential values, as greater extremes would be reached over the entire image than in a given row. The uniformity calculations for low-count flood images are typically not sufficient to generate NEMA uniformity values; however, they are adequate for daily quality control. The daily uniformity values should be recorded and used to trend the performance of the system (Figure 1-24). If the values begin to rise, additional QC (tuning or new flood corrections) or service may be necessary.

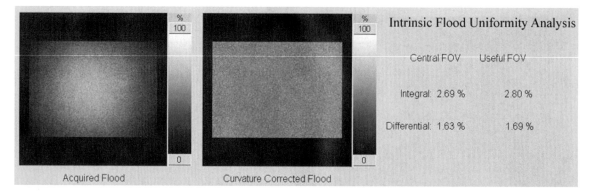

Figure 1-24.   A "hot center" raw flood image from one detector of a dual-headed system (both heads simultaneously acquired <5 FOVs). Application of curvature correction and adequate uniformity analysis results are illustrated for a single detector.

Most properly calibrated modern SPECT systems should have integral uniformity values of less than 5% and differential uniformity values less than 3% for both CFOV and UFOV. The UFOV values tend to be slightly higher than CFOV values as a result of variations at the edge of the detector.

Extrinsic (collimator on) daily quality control consists of a planar low-count (3 million for small FOV detectors and 5 million for large FOV detectors) image obtained with a Co-57 sheet source or refillable Tc-99m source on the surface of the detector. For large FOV cameras, it may be preferable to use a Co-57 sheet source, as refillable floods of this size are difficult to manipulate for uniform activity. The extrinsic flood should be visually assessed for areas of nonuniformity and compared to prior flood images for change. Collimator damage can be verified by the appearance of focal cold defects in the flood image. The cold defects result from physical damage to the septa in the collimator, obstructing photons from reaching the crystal. Slight damage may be corrected through the acquisition of new extrinsic flood correction tables; however, images should be assessed and collimators replaced as necessary for optimal clinical imaging. Uniformity analysis calculating the integral and differential uniformity of the extrinsic flood image for the CFOV and UFOV should be performed, recorded, and compared to prior values.

Daily QC, including peaking, should also be repeated anytime the camera is powered down for a prolonged amount of time. A service engineer's rule of thumb is that the system should be allowed to stabilize for 1 hour (maximum 24 hours), for each hour the power was interrupted prior to QC and clinical imaging. If not, peak values may drift as the PMTs warm up, resulting in off-peak imaging (Figure 1-25).

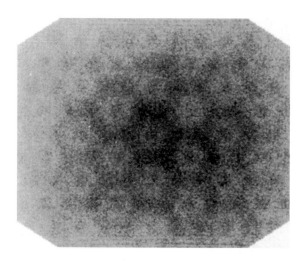

Figure 1-25.   Off-peak flood image owing to peak drift. (Image courtesy of Medical Physics Consultants Inc., Ann Arbor, MI)

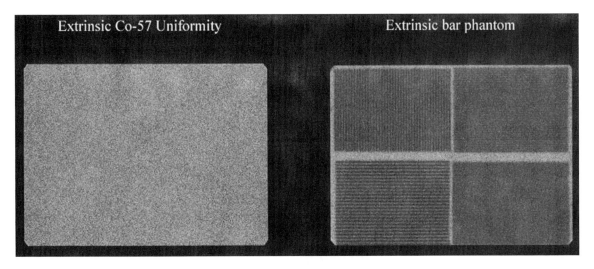

Figure 1-26. Extrinsic uniformity and bar phantom images. Note that the third quadrant of the phantom is difficult to visualize because of reduced resolution from a collimated acquisition. Intrinsic acquisition will yield optimal bar phantom resolution.

Weekly

Spatial resolution and distortion testing using a four-quadrant bar phantom should be performed weekly. This may be done intrinsically (better resolution) or extrinsically, according to vendor specifications. Bar phantom images allow the user to assess nonlinearities (bars must appear as straight lines) and loss of resolution (number of quadrants visualized). The quadrants should appear perpendicular to one another. A properly selected bar phantom will test the resolution limits of the system, with three of the four quadrants visualized clearly. The smallest-sized bar is typically 2.0 mm for intrinsic measurements or 2.5 mm for extrinsic imaging (Figure 1-26). The resulting image should be compared to prior results. If possible, the bar phantom should be rotated each week to test the resolution limits and linearity of each quadrant of the detector.

COR calibration/recalibration should be performed according to vendor specification as a minimum. Anytime a COR error is suspected or a hardware adjustment is made to the physical position/angulation of the detectors by the ser-vice engineer, the COR should be verified or recalibrated. Many systems simply recalibrate the COR and will provide the X, Y, and Z shifts applied after correction. The recalibration will have a specific protocol from each manufacturer and usually involves a SPECT scan of fixed radius using multiple point sources. A quick assessment of the system can be obtained by simply performing a SPECT scan of a low-activity point source using a clinical orbit. This will also verify if there is a problem with previously acquired data. The reconstructed image should look like a dot. If it has the appearance of a ring, there is a COR error. The ring is produced during image reconstruction, as each projection of the off-centered point is reprojected with a uniform shift (Figure 1-27). COR errors can be difficult to identify in clinical images, especially with multiple readers in a busy practice potentially unaware of consecutive similar image defects. It should be noted that dual detector systems typically have a separate COR calibration for images acquired with the detectors at 90 and 180 degrees. Verification of both configurations may be necessary depending on imaging studies performed.

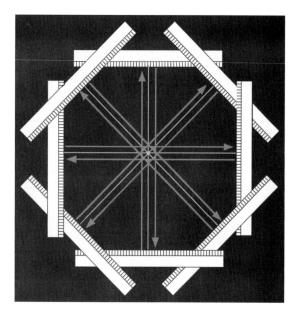

Figure 1-27. The solid rays represent the correct center location of a point source. The arrows represent a COR error. The error is propagated to all projections, and, when the point is reprojected with a shift, the resulting image is a ring, not a discrete point.

Quarterly

Acquisition of the Jaszczak total performance SPECT phantom allows the user to assess SPECT resolution, contrast, and uniformity in a single scan. The Jaszczak SPECT phantom contains a series of rods ranging in size from 6.4 to 16 mm and spheres ranging in size from 12.7 to 38.1 mm. The Deluxe Jaszczak SPECT phantom contains a smaller-diameter series of rods ranging in size from 4.6 to 12.7 mm and spheres ranging in size from 9.5 to 38.1 mm (Figure 1-28).

Camera testing using the Deluxe Jaszczak SPECT phantom is required for sites obtaining American College of Radiology (ACR) certification.[12] The Jaszczak phantom should be acquired and processed according the ACR guidelines. The phantom is filled with water and 10 to 15 mCi Tc-99m (desired count rate = 10–25 kcps). Acquisition parameters include using a 15% to 20% Tc-99m window, 128 × 128 matrix, 128 projections over 360 degrees, a zoom of 1.45 for large FOV cameras, and a radius as close to 20 cm as mechanically possible. The time per

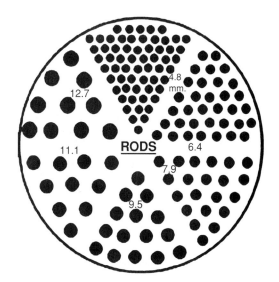

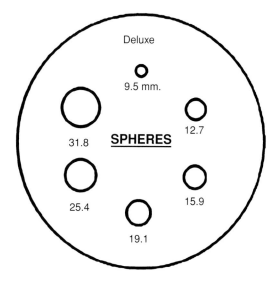

Figure 1-28.   Cross sections of the rods and spheres of the Deluxe Jaszczak total performance SPECT phantom.

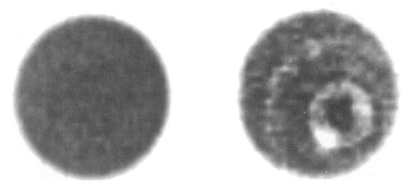

Figure 1-29.   A uniform Jaszczak image contrasts the ring artifacts created by flood field nonuniformities in SPECT reconstruction. (Image courtesy of Medical Physics Consultants Inc., Ann Arbor, MI.)

projection is determined by the following equation based on the desired total counts acquired (24 million): 24,000,000/count rate (kcps) × 128 (number of steps) = time per step. Image reconstruction and image display should also follow ACR guidelines: filter—vendor specific; apply Chang's attenuation correction coefficient: 0.11 to 0.12; display slice thickness: spheres—2 pixels, uniformity—6 pixels, and rods—16 pixels. Visual assessment of spheres for contrast and rods for linearity should be consistent with initial images acquired at the time of acceptance testing. Uniformity is assessed in reconstructed transverse images where no rods or spheres are present. The

system performance should remain constant. All transverse images should be assessed for the presence of ring artifact, which would be caused by nonuniformities.[12] Ring artifacts are caused by areas of nonuniformities in the detector, which create a band or ring of decreased activity when reprojected in SPECT reconstruction (Figure 1-29). COR errors in a Jaszczak phantom could present as shifted/blurred rods and spheres.

Any significant variations from initial acceptance test evaluations would be the cause for additional QC recalibrations (flood tables) or service. In addition to contrast, resolution, and uniformity, the Jaszczak phantom can also be used to test

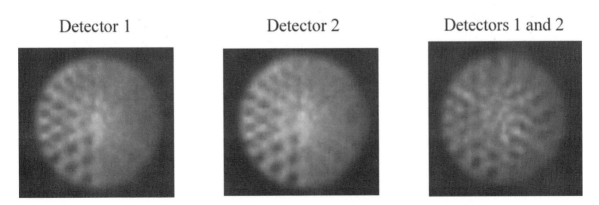

Detector 1   Detector 2   Detectors 1 and 2

Figure 1-30.   Comparable results for the individual detectors. Misregistration error degradation of the combined acquisition. (Image courtesy of Medical Physics Consultants Inc., Ann Arbor, MI.)

multidetector registration. The current industry standard for myocardial perfusion imaging is through dual detector imaging. Both detectors must be within the same operational limits. The Jaszczak phantom can be acquired over 360 degrees for each detector. The results for each detector should be independently reconstructed to assess for nonuniformities. An additional SPECT acquisition and reconstruction should be performed, with each detector covering 180 degrees of the orbit. The results of this combined SPECT should match those of the individual detectors for proper performance. Misregistration between the detectors will result in image degradation (Figure 1-30).

ANNUAL QUALITY CONTROL

Laboratory accrediting bodies have different requirements for annual recertification, which include a variety of the aforementioned QC procedures. Depending on the certification sought, a medical physicist may be required to perform/supervise the camera testing.[13] The guidelines from the accrediting body should be referenced for the particular data that are required.[14,15]

A thorough understanding of SPECT and a strong quality-control regimen are mandatory for high-quality diagnostic SPECT imaging. Quality-control images should be reviewed by the performing technologist and the interpreting physician for optimal utility. It is far easier to correct for camera nonuniformities, COR errors, and equipment malfunctions than to interpret artifact-compromised images.

REFERENCES

1. DePasquale EE, Nody AC, DePuey EG, et al. Quantitative rotational thallium-210 tomography for identifying and localizing coronary artery disease. *Circulation*. 1988;77:316–327.
2. Sorenson JA, Phelps ME. *Physics in Nuclear Medicine*. Philadelphia: WB Saunders; 1987.
3. NEMA. *Performance Measurements of Scintillation Cameras*. NEMA publication no. 1–1994. Washington, DC: National Electronic Manufacturers Association; 1994.
4. Anger, HO. Scintillation camera with multichannel collimators. *J Nucl Med*. 1964;5:515.
5. Mueller B, O'Connor MK, Phillips SW, et al. Evaluation of a small cadmium zinc telluride detector for scintimammography. *J Nucl Med*. 2003;44(4):602–609.
6. ASNC. Imaging guidelines for nuclear cardiology procedures. *J Nucl Cardiol*. 2006;13:e21–e171.
7. O'Connor MK, Hruska CB. Effect of tomographic orbit and type of rotation on apparent myocardial activity. *Nucl Med Commun*. 2005;26(1):25–30.
8. Maniawski PJ, Morgan HT, Whackers FJTH. Orbit-related variation in spatial resolution as a source of artefactual defects in thallium-210 SPECT. *J Nucl Med*. 1991;32(5):871–875.
9. Bieszk JA, Hawman EG. Evaluation of SPECT angular sampling effects: Continuous versus STEP-and-shoot acquisition. *J Nucl Med*. 1987;28:1308–1314.
10. Parker, JA. *Image Reconstruction in Radiology*. Boca Raton: CRC Press; 1990.
11. AAPM. *Scintillation Camera Acceptance Testing and Performance Evaluation*. AAPM Report No. 6. New York, NY: American Institute of Physics; 1980.
12. ACR. *Site Scanning Instructions for Use of the Nuclear Medicine Phantom for the ACR*. Reston, VA: American College of Radiology; 2006.
13. MacFarlane CR. ACR accreditation of nuclear medicine and PET imaging departments. *J Nucl Med Technol*. 2006;34(1):18–24.
14. ICANL. *2007 Standards for Nuclear Cardiology, Nuclear Medicine and PET Accreditation*. Columbia, MD: The Intersocietal Commission of Nuclear Medicine Laboratories; 2007.
15. ACR. *Nuclear Medicine/PET Accreditation Program Requirements*. Reston, VA: American College of Radiology; 2007.

CHAPTER 2

Positron Emission Tomography Instrumentation

R. Glenn Wells
Robert A. deKemp
Rob S.B. Beanlands

INTRODUCTION

Positron emission tomography (PET), as its name implies, is a three-dimensional (3D) medical imaging technology based on the detection of positrons. The positron is an elementary particle that is identical to an electron but possessing a positive charge. The existence of the positron was postulated by Paul Dirac in 1928 and later seen experimentally by Carl Anderson in a cloud chamber in 1932. Dirac and Anderson both received Nobel Prizes in 1933 and 1936, respectively, for their work. Anderson's positrons were created naturally by cosmic-ray irradiation, but Irene Curie and Frederick Joliet showed in 1934 that positron-emitting radionuclides could be produced artificially. The creation of man-made radioisotopes was facilitated by the development of the cyclotron by Ernest Lawrence and colleagues at Berkley in the 1930s. The cyclotron is a charged-particle accelerator that can produce many of the radioactive isotopes used in PET imaging, such as O-15, N-13, C-11, and F-18.

Interest in positron-emitting radiotracers faded after WWII with the discovery of much longer-lived radioisotopes like C-14 and I-131 that could be produced using nuclear reactors. It was reborn in 1950s through the construction of the first positron scanner by Brownell and Sweet in 1953[1] and Ter-Pogossian's interest in cyclotron-produced O-15, which he used to study such things as the kinetics of oxygen in respiration.[2] This work led to the first installation of a cyclotron in a medical facility: the unit installed at Hammersmith Hospital in London in 1955. Stationary, scintillation-based, multidetector arrays were first developed in the 1960s at Brookhaven National Labs by Rankowitz et al.[3] These arrays were built either as a hemispherical design for brain imaging, sometimes affectionately referred as the "hair-dryer" design, or as a ring of detectors. The ring configuration is the one

Table 2-1

Common Cardiac PET Radiotracers

	Full Name	Primary Use in Cardiology
F-18-FDG	Fluorodeoxyglucose	Glucose uptake and viability
C-11-acetate	Acetate	Oxidative metabolism
C-11-palmitate	Palmitate	Fatty-acid metabolism
C-11-HED	Hydroxyephedrine	Sympathetic innervation
N-13-NH$_3$	Ammonia	Blood flow
O-15-H$_2$0	Water	Blood flow
Rb-82	Rubidium	Blood flow

still used today in modern scanners. The images produced by these multidetector arrays were of poor quality because the reconstruction methods available were still quite primitive. In 1972 this changed because Godfrey Hounsfield produced his first clinical X-ray CT image, reconstructing the image with filtered backprojection (FBP). In 1975, Ter-Pogossian et al. described a ring-based PET instrument that reconstructed images using FBP,[4] ushering in the modern era of PET imaging technology.

PET RADIOTRACERS

PET images are based on the detection of a tracer that is typically injected into the body. By comparing the distribution of the tracer in a patient to normal templates, a physician is able to evaluate how well different organs and systems in the body are functioning. The tracer consists of two components: a pharmaceutical and a radioactive label. The radiopharmaceutical is given in very low concentrations, usually on the order of nano- to picomolar (10^{-9}–0^{-12} mol/L), so that there is typically no pharmacological effect; that is, the tracer does not disturb the physiology that it is measuring. The pharmaceutical component determines where the tracer goes in the body and how it behaves. Hence, it determines the organ or process that will be measured by the PET scan. For example, glucose is one of the fuels used by the heart. F-18-fluorodeoxyglucose (FDG) is an analog of glucose and so is taken up by the heart tissues in the

same way that glucose is, and images of FDG distribution provide a picture that reflects this uptake. Images from C-11-palmitate, on the other hand, provide a measure of free-fatty-acid metabolism in the heart. Some of the more common tracers used in cardiac imaging are given in Table 2-1 and will be discussed in greater detail in later chapters.

The signal measured by PET is generated when the radioactive label attached to the pharmaceutical decays and emits a positron (Figure 2-1). Positrons are antimatter particles that have all of the same properties as an electron, except that the charge on the particle is positive instead of negative. The positrons interact with the patient tissues, gradually losing energy and slowing down

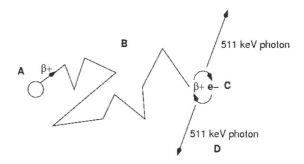

Figure 2-1. Positron decay. (**A**) A proton-rich nucleus emits a positron. (**B**) The positron interacts with surrounding tissues, gradually losing its kinetic energy. (**C**) Once it has slowed down enough, the positron combines with an electron and annihilates producing (**D**) two 511-keV gamma-ray photons.

until their speed is low enough that they can be captured by an electron. The electron–positron pair combines to form a transitory molecule called positronium. Positronium is like hydrogen, but with a positron taking the place of the proton. Positronium is very unstable and exists only for approximately 10^{-10} seconds before the positron and the electron mutually annihilate, generating two gamma rays (annihilation photons). Each annihilation photon has exactly 511 keV, the energy equivalent to the rest mass of an electron, as dictated by Einstein's famous equation: $E = mc^2$, where m is the electron mass. To conserve momentum, the two photons travel away from the site of annihilation in almost exactly opposite directions.

The most common radioisotopes used in PET are F-18, C-11, N-13, O-15, and Rb-82. The properties of these isotopes are given in Table 2-2. All of these tracers have fairly short half-lives, ranging from just more than a minute to just less than 2 hours. The very short half-lives of C-11, N-13, and O-15 mean that it is only practical to use pharmaceuticals labeled with these isotopes if there are cyclotron and radiochemistry facilities on-site that permit local production. On the other hand, F-18-labelled compounds, with an almost 2-hour half-life, decay slowly enough that they can be distributed a short distance, a fact that greatly facilitates the use of PET imaging. Rb-82 can also be distributed as it can be produced via an Sr-82 generator system, which has a half-life of 25 days and a practical lifetime of 1 to 2 months.

Another important property of PET radioisotopes is the positron range. The range refers to the distance that the positron travels before it slows down enough to annihilate with an electron. It is dependent on the kinetic energy of the positron. As positron decay entails the emission of both a positron and a neutrino (a particle that is not detected), the kinetic energy of the positron is not fixed but, instead, takes on a distribution of values up to some maximum. The maximum kinetic energy depends on the radioisotope. In addition, the path of the positron away from the site of decay is a tortuous one. Like the electron, the positron is very light and so can undergo large changes in direction when it scatters off the nuclei of surrounding tissues. The mixture of initial energies and the tortuous path of travel mean that the straight-line distance traveled by the positron from the site of decay is best described as a distribution.

The range of the positron is thus a statistical measure of the distance traveled by all positrons emitted by a particular isotope and is often quoted as the root-mean-squared (RMS) distance. The largest impact that the positron range has on PET imaging is as a reduction in spatial resolution. However, for most of the isotopes used in cardiac imaging, the range is small enough that the loss in resolution for human imaging is very small. The exception to this is Rb-82 whose range is of the same order as the other components of scanner resolution and so significantly degrades the image resolution. The factors that influence spatial

Table 2-2

Properties of Common PET Radioisotopes

	Half-Life (min)	Maximum Energy (keV)	RMS Range in Water[a] (mm)	Produced
F-18	110	635	0.23	Cyclotron
C-11	20	960	0.42	Cyclotron
N-13	10	1190	0.57	Cyclotron
O-15	2.05	1720	1.02	Cyclotron
Rb-82	1.25	3350	2.60	Sr-82 Generator

[a]The ranges given here correspond to the root-mean-squared distance traveled by the positron from the site of decay.
Data from Lecomte.[9]

resolution in PET will be discussed in more detail later on in this chapter.

PET DETECTORS

Coincidence Detection

The PET camera records positron decay events by detecting the two annihilation photons that are emitted. Both photons must be detected before an event is recorded. To distinguish between annihilation photons and photons detected from background sources, the camera accepts only those photons that arrive at close to the same time—this is referred to as *coincidence detection* (Figure 2-2).

The maximum amount of time apart that two photons can be detected and still be considered to have come from the same annihilation is determined by the coincidence timing window. The coincidence window is typically 5 to 10 ns and takes into account the time the photons take to travel to the detector from the site of annihilation and the variability in the time required to measure the photon's time of arrival.

Scintillation Crystals

Annihilation photons are detected using scintillation crystals, similar to how photons are detected

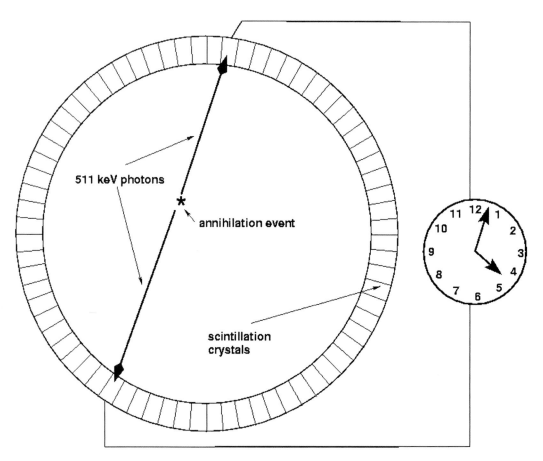

Figure 2-2. Coincidence detection. An event is recorded in PET only if the two annihilation photons are both detected by the camera within a short time interval called the coincidence timing window.

Table 2-3

Properties of Common PET Detector Crystals

Crystal	Name	Chemical Formula	Density (g/cm^3)	μ at 511 keV (cm^{-1})	Relative Light Output (% of NaI)	Decay Time (ns)
NaI	Sodium iodide	NaI	3.67	0.34	100	230
BGO	Bismuth germanate	$Bi_4Ge_3O_{12}$	7.13	0.95	21	300
LSO	Lutetium oxyorthosilicate	Lu_2SiO_5	7.4	0.88	68	40
LYSO	Lutetium yttrium oxyorthosilicate	$Lu_{1.8}Y_{.2}SiO_5$	7.1	0.83	75	41
GSO	Gadolinium oxyorthosilicate	Gd_2SiO_5	6.71	0.70	36	60

μ, linear attenuation coefficient.
Data from Melcher,[12] Saint-Gobain Crystals,[13] and Cherry et al.[14]

by the gamma camera. The 511-keV gamma ray interacts with the crystal, exciting many of the electrons in the crystal into a higher-energy state. As the electrons fall back to their ground state, they emit a photon of visible or near-ultraviolet light. There are many electrons excited by each gamma ray and so each gamma ray generates a shower of light photons. The photon shower is detected by a photomultiplier tube (PMT), which converts the light into an electrical signal and amplifies it. The amplified electrical signal can then be processed and recorded in a computer.

Although NaI is used in some PET cameras, most systems use crystals that have a much greater stopping power. One measure of stopping power is the linear attenuation coefficient ("μ"). The properties of some of the crystals more commonly used in PET are given in Table 2-3. Greater stopping power is needed to stop and thence detect the relatively high-energy gamma rays that are emitted by PET tracers. It is possible to obtain good stopping efficiency with lower-density materials by simply using a thicker amount of crystal. However, as the crystal material gets thicker, the spatial resolution is degraded through the depth-of-interaction (DOI) effect (explained in detail later on in this chapter) and the timing resolution (coincidence window) is poorer, as there is more variability in the distance between the PMTs and the point at which the gamma ray interacts with the crystal. BGO, with a much higher stopping power than NaI, was the detector of choice for many years de-spite its relatively poor light output. As the measured signal is based on the number of light photons detected, a reduction in light output leads to a reduction in the accuracy of the timing and energy measurements. More recently, new crystals such as LSO, LYSO, and GSO have become available, which combine good light output (and thus improved timing and energy resolution) with good stopping power. Additionally, these new crystals also have shorter decay times—the time required for all of the light photons to be emitted from the crystal—and this reduces the time required to measure an event and thereby reduces the detection deadtime.

Block Detector

Unlike the gamma camera, which uses a single large scintillation crystal, the detector in a PET camera is made up of a large number of small distinct crystals. Each crystal element is a few millimeters wide (typically 4–6 mm) and 2 to 3 cm in length. The crystals are then coupled to a PMT array that collects and amplifies the signal from the crystals. The exact configuration of crystals and PMTs varies between manufacturers, and one illustrative example is given in Figure 2-3. In this case, the scintillation crystals are arranged in blocks of 8×8 elements, with each block coupled to a 2×2 array of PMTs. When a gamma ray interacts with the detector, its position is localized only to the nearest crystal element. Finer positioning

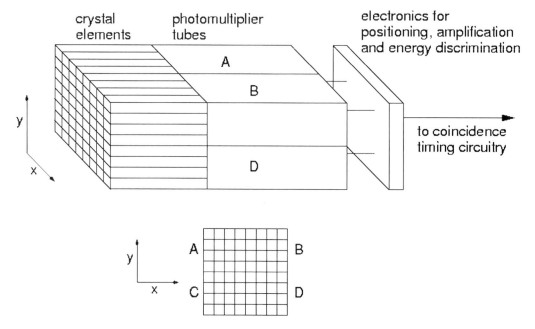

Figure 2-3. Example block detector configuration. An 8 × 8 array of scintillation crystals is backed by a 2 × 2 set of photomultiplier tubes (PMT). The PMT outputs are used to position the event within the crystal array and determine its energy.

within the element is not determined. The position is measured by comparing the relative strength of the signal emitted from each of the four PMTs as given by Eq. (2.1) in which A, B, C, and D refer to the signal strength from the corresponding PMT in Figure 2-3.

$$X = \frac{B + D - (A + C)}{A + B + C + D} \quad Y = \frac{A + B - (C + D)}{A + B + C + D}$$

$$(2.1)$$

The energy of the incident photon is related to the total number of light photons produced in the light shower. Each excitation requires a particular amount of energy and so the total energy of the gamma ray is proportional to the total number of light photons it produces in a scintillation crystal. The measured energy is used to reject those photons that have scattered in the patient or the camera before being recorded. The accuracy with which this can be done is related to the energy resolution of the system. The energy resolution depends on the number of light photons produced and consequently on the energy of the gamma ray and the type of scintillation crystal used (its light output).

TYPES OF EVENTS

The signals collected with a PET camera can be categorized into one of several types.

A *single* refers to the detection of a photon whose measured energy falls within the photopeak energy window. The photopeak energy window is wide compared to single-photon imaging, typically 400 to 600 keV. The width is caused by the generally poorer energy resolution of the PET scintillation crystals, the higher energy of the photons detected, and a desire to maximize the sensitivity of the system. The purpose of the energy window is to exclude scattered photons, and photons from other background radiation sources, based on their energy.

A *prompt* event is recorded when two singles are detected within the coincidence timing window. In the positron–electron annihilation, both photons are created simultaneously, but they may not be detected simultaneously. The site of annihilation within the scanner may be closer to one side than the other, and thus, as both photons travel at the same speed, one may arrive at the detectors before the other. The speed of light is very fast (30 cm/ns), but a bore diameter of 90 cm means that the difference in arrival times can be as large as 3 nanoseconds. Also, there are statistical fluctuations in the detection process of the gamma ray, and this leads to an additional uncertainty in the measurement of the arrival time. In total, the coincidence timing window is usually set to be 5 to 10 ns. The width of the coincidence window is set large enough to include any two photons that are truly from the same annihilation event—a so-called *true* event. The coincidence window cannot be set too large, however, as this will increase the number of *random* events. Because of the ring geometry of

the PET scanner, it can happen that one photon from the annihilation pair passes out of the top or bottom of the ring and escapes detection. Additionally, one of the photon pair may be scattered and so may miss the detector ring or be reduced in energy such that it falls outside of the photopeak energy window. These situations can lead to a single event without a corresponding true event. If two single events happen by chance to be detected within the coincidence timing window, the scanner cannot distinguish this from a true event and the 'event' is recorded. This is called a *random* coincidence event and produces a background signal unique to PET imaging (Figure 2-4). Finally, it is possible that one or both of the annihilation photons will be Compton scattered (either in the patient or in the camera itself) and yet both photons will still be detected within the photopeak energy window and the coincidence timing window. This circumstance is referred to as a *scatter* event. The total prompt event rate is the sum of the true, random, and scatter event rates.

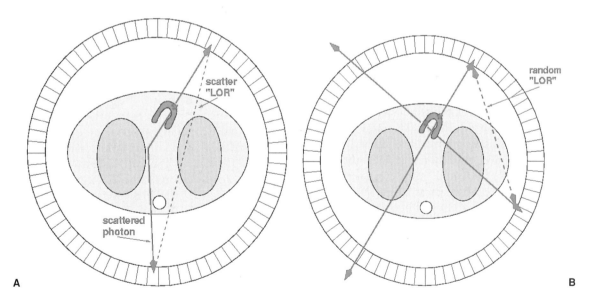

Figure 2-4.   Scattered and random coincidences. A scattered coincidence (**A**) can occur when one or both of the annihilation photons are scattered in the patient or the camera prior to detection. A random coincidence (**B**) can occur when two annihilation photons from two different positron decays are detected within the coincidence timing window. Misinterpretation of either of these events as a true event would result in an erroneous line of response or "LOR" (discussed below) that did not pass through the site of annihilation.

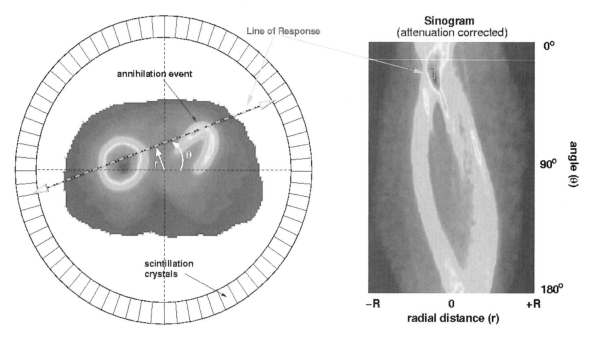

Figure 2-5.   Binning the PET signal. The two detection points of the annihilation photons form the ends of the line of response (LOR). The LOR is characterized by its axial position (z), the radial distance from the center of the scanner (r), and the angle that the LOR makes with the x-axis (θ). LOR data can be binned into a sinogram, with each point in the sinogram corresponding to the number of events detected along the LOR at (r, θ). (See color insert.)

Line of Response

When a true coincidence event is detected, we know that the two annihilation photons were traveling in opposite directions. Therefore, the two points at which they intersect the PET ring define their line of travel, and this line is called the *line of response (LOR)*. The annihilation event is assumed to have occurred somewhere along this line. All of the crystal elements can act in coincidence with all of the others, and thus all possible LORs are sampled simultaneously. The LOR (Figure 2-5) is characterized by its perpendicular distance (r) from the center of the field of view (FOV), i.e., the center of the detector ring, and by its angle of rotation (θ) with respect to the horizontal x-axis. Each plane of data acquired with the PET scanner can be histogrammed into a sinogram, with the signal along each LOR represented by the value at a given point (r, θ).

TEMPORAL SORTING OF DATA

PET sinogram data are built up over time by counting the number of events that occur along each LOR. Obtaining more counts lowers the noise in the data and leads to a clearer image of the tracer distribution. Thus, PET data are typically obtained for several minutes to an hour depending on the tracer used. However, it is sometimes helpful to consider how the tracer distribution is changing during the time of acquisition, and this has led to several different modes of acquisition that differ in how they sort the acquired data with respect to time.

Static

The simplest mode is just to acquire a *static* image. In this case, all of the data acquired during the imaging session are binned into a single-time bin, creating one sinogram for each transaxial plane. This mode would be used to obtain, for example, an uptake image of Rb-82 perfusion or F-18-FDG viability and evaluate the relative distribution of tracer in the heart.

Gated

Further functional information can be obtained through *gated* acquisition (Figure 2-6). In this mode, an ECG signal from the patient is obtained and used to generate a trigger event. Usually this event marks a particular point in the ECG trace such as the R wave that indicates the start of ventricular contraction. Because the ECG signal is periodic, a trigger event is generated every time an R wave occurs. For example, if the patient has a heart rate of 70 bpm, there will be 70 triggers generated per minute. The data recorded by the PET scanner are then sorted into different sinograms based on how much time has passed since the last triggering event. This sorts the data into phases of the cardiac cycle and adds the data from the equivalent phases of different cycles together to reduce the noise in the images. The images for each phase are reconstructed separately and can then be played back in a cine-loop for the physician, providing a movie of the cardiac contractile motion. In addition, other information such as left-ventricular ejection fraction, end-diastolic volume, and wall thickening can also be measured. These additional measures have been shown to provide incremental benefit in assessing heart disease.[5–7]

Dynamic

One advantage that PET has over SPECT imaging is that the PET scanner consists of an entire ring of detectors, and, thus, all possible LORs are collected simultaneously. This makes it possible to collect enough data to reconstruct an image in a very short period of time. By acquiring a series of images over time, it is possible to track the radiotracer immediately after injection, observing where and how fast it distributes in the body. Analysis of the temporal behavior of the tracer provides quantitatively accurate measures of physiological parameters such as blood flow (mL/min/g) or

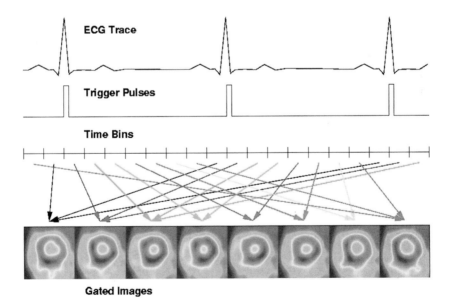

Figure 2-6.   Gated acquisition (Rb-82 perfusion imaging). Triggering can be used to sort PET data into physiologic phases. For example, cardiac gating based on a trigger from the ECG signal is used to generate images for each phase of the cardiac cycle from end diastole through end systole and back again.

neuroreceptor density (pmol/mL). Following injection, the tracer distribution changes very rapidly at first, reflecting rapid dilution throughout the blood volume and initial uptake by the tissues from a high blood concentration of tracer, but then its dynamics slow, reflecting the combination of uptake from the lower blood-pool concentrations, tracer clearance from tissue, and/or tracer retention in tissue. Therefore, a *dynamic* acquisition series (Figure 2-7) usually begins with several

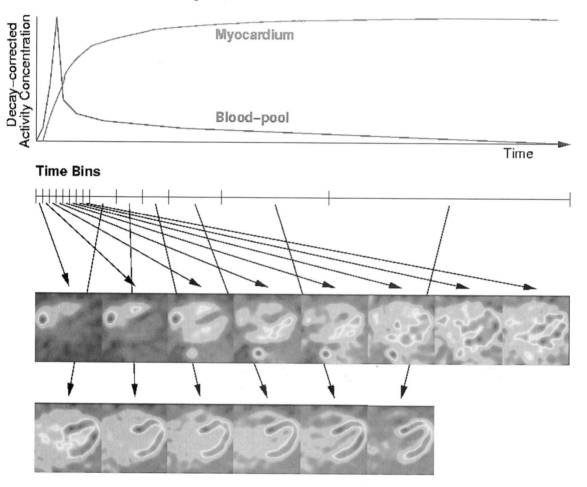

Figure 2-7.   Dynamic acquisition. PET data can be acquired in a series of images with variable duration in order to capture the changing temporal behavior of the tracer. Dynamic imaging is important because it allows absolute quantitative measurement of physiological parameters such as blood flow and receptor density. In these Rb-perfusion images, the injected tracer is seen first in the right chambers of the heart, followed by the left chambers of the heart and the descending aorta, and finally accumulates in the myocardium and clears from the blood pool. (See color insert.)

images of very short duration, followed by longer acquisition frames during the later periods. The longer acquisitions allow better count statistics to be obtained during the period that the tracer distribution is stable. Longer acquisition frames are particularly important with short-lived radioisotopes such as Rb-82, O-15, and N-13 because the amount of radioactivity in the patient is rapidly decaying during the course of the scan. The total length of the imaging series will depend on the physiological process being measured (e.g., how fast the tissue or receptor takes up the tracer) and the half-life of the radioisotope. As an example, a dynamic acquisition protocol for measuring perfusion with Rb-82 is to acquire $9 \times 10s$ frames, $3 \times 30s$, $1 \times 60s$, $1 \times 120s$, and $1 \times 240s$ for a total of 10 minutes of data acquisition. An example of C-11-HED receptor binding study would have a dynamic acquisition protocol of $9 \times 10s$, $3 \times 30s$, $2 \times 60s$, and $7 \times 300s$ for a total acquisition time of 40 minutes.

Listmode

A final acquisition mode that has recently become commercially available for clinical use is listmode. With a *listmode* acquisition, the annihilation events collected by the PET scanner are not binned immediately into sinograms as they are with static, gated, and dynamic acquisitions. Instead, each event is individually recorded as they occur, generating a long list of coincidence events. Each event record includes information about the location of the event, i.e., the location of the two ends of the LOR, the energy of the event, the times at which the photons were detected, and any other information about the event that you wish to keep track of. In addition, other types of information can be inserted into the list, information such as the trigger signal from an ECG-gating or respiratory-monitoring device. The disadvantage of this mode of acquisition is that it requires a large amount of hard-drive space to store the data set. The advantage, however, is that the event list can be reprocessed after the end of scan in whatever manner is desired. For example, from a single list of data, it

is possible to rebin just the last 5 minutes of the list into a static acquisition sinogram. It is also possible to take that same 5 minutes of list data and reprocess it into a set of cardiac-gated images and also to reprocess the entire data set into a dynamic series for quantitative analysis. In short, listmode requires more computer storage space to retain but provides a large degree of flexibility in how the data are processed and analyzed.

AXIAL DATA
Multiple Detector Rings

A single ring of detectors would only measure one thin slice of the patient at a time. To improve axial coverage, a modern PET scanner is made up of multiple rings of detector blocks stacked one on top of the other. This also opens up the possibility of further increasing sensitivity by measuring axially oblique LORs for which the two annihilation photons are detected with different rings of the scanner. A problem with accepting oblique LORs, however, is that the axial position of the annihilation event is ambiguous. Because the position of the annihilation along the LOR is unknown, it could have occurred anywhere along the LOR and hence anywhere between the two rings on which the photons were detected. One way to resolve this ambiguity is to assign the LOR to be at the average axial position of the two end points. This approach is called single-slice rebinning (SSRB). This leads to two types of acquisition planes: direct planes and cross planes (Figure 2-8). Direct planes refer to those planes positioned in the middle of a crystal element. For example, the blue arrow in Figure 2-8 between the z2 and z2 crystals ($z2 \leftrightarrow z2$) forms a direct plane. Cross planes refer to those planes positioned in between two crystal elements. For example ($z8 \leftrightarrow z9$) and ($z9 \leftrightarrow z8$) both average to an axial position midway between crystal planes z8 and z9. The greater the radial distance of the actual site of annihilation from the central axis of the scanner, the greater the error introduced in the axial repositioning of the event with SSRB. To minimize these errors, the ring difference of

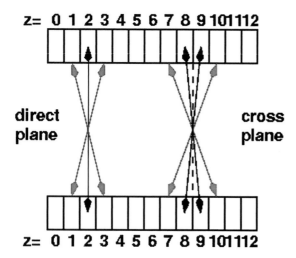

Figure 2-8.   Direct vs. cross planes. The black arrows represent the highest-resolution configuration. Sensitivity is added at the expense of resolution by including additional pairs of detectors (gray arrows) whose average axial position is in the plane as the black arrows.

accepted LORs is restricted. For example, a ring difference of 1 allows only the blue LORs in Figure 2-8, but a ring difference of 3 allows both the blue and the red LORs. LORs detected outside this range are rejected.

2D vs. 3D Acquisition

Acquiring oblique LORs with a multiring configuration greatly increases the sensitivity of the scanner, that is, the fraction of the prompt events that it is capable of detecting. Unfortunately, it also greatly increases the number of random events detected (because the randoms rate increases as the square of the singles rate) and the amount of scatter that is detected. With a single ring, any photon that is scattered out of the plane of the detectors is lost, greatly reducing the fraction of scatter collected. With a multiring scanner, this is no longer the case. A compromise solution to this problem is to insert thin absorbing tungsten septa between the crystal planes (Figure 2-9). Scanners configured with interplane septa acquire data in

what is referred to as a *2D acquisition* mode. The length of the septa and the axial width of the crystal planes determine the maximum accepted angle of the LOR and hence the maximum possible ring difference. The ring difference might be further restricted by electronically rejecting those LORs with larger-than-desired ring differences. In 2D imaging, the maximum ring difference is typically three or four rings.

An alternative solution is *3D acquisition* for which the septa are not used and any ring difference is possible (Figure 2-9). With 3D acquisitions, one relies on software to accurately compensate for the large amount of scatter and random events in the data. While there is no physical restriction on the axial acceptance angle, it is still possible to restrict the accepted ring differences electronically. Likewise, SSRB can still be used to sort all of the LORs into average axial planes as they are acquired, but one also has the option of retaining the information about the axial position of both photons and thereby increasing the dimensionality of the acquired data from 3 (r, θ, z) to 4 (r, θ, $z1$, $z2$).* Storing the raw data in this manner (r, θ, $z1$, $z2$) greatly increases the memory requirements of the camera and also greatly increases the flexibility one has in postprocessing and image reconstruction. Intermediate approaches, where data are averaged in segments of similar ring differences, are also possible.

IMAGE RECONSTRUCTION

As with acquisition, PET reconstruction can also be divided into either 2D or 3D reconstruction. With a 2D reconstruction approach, each plane of data is treated independently and a single transaxial plane is reconstructed at a time. The most common method of reconstruction remains the FBP algorithm, although other iterative algorithms such as OSEM and RAMLA are also

---

* While it is possible to retain the two end points of the LOR in 2D acquisition mode, this is not typically done.

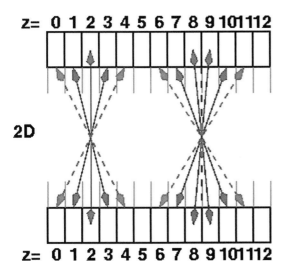
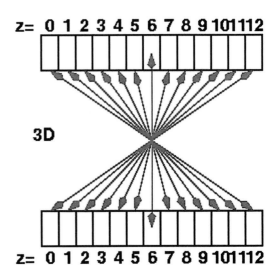

Figure 2-9. 2D vs. 3D acquisition. In 2D acquisition, septa made of an absorbing material like tungsten are placed between the crystal elements of the detectors (shown in green). This restricts the axial span of the LOR to those along which the photons do not intersect the septa (blue) and removes those that do intersect septa (red). In 3D acquisition mode, the septa are removed and much larger axial angles are still accepted. (See color insert.)

now clinically available. In a 3D approach, the entire volume of the data is used to reconstruct the image, and interactions between planes, such as cross-plane scatter, are considered. 2D reconstruction tends to be much faster than 3D, and so often, even if a 3D acquisition is used, the data will be reprocessed into 2D sinograms and then reconstructed using a 2D algorithm. The simplest method of resorting 3D data into a set of 2D sinograms is the SSRB method mentioned earlier. The advantage of acquiring the data in 3D and waiting until the end of the scan to resort the data into 2D sinograms is that one can use more sophisticated rebinning algorithms that reduce the axial blurring introduced by SSRB. One such example is Fourier rebinning (FORE), which more accurately reinterpolates the data in the Fourier domain. Fully 3D methods, such as a 3D reprojection version of FBP and iterative techniques, are also available, which reconstruct the image volume directly from a 4D data set (e.g., of the form $(r, \theta, z1, z2)$). For the interested reader, a more complete discussion of image reconstruction can be found in the text by Bailey et al.[8]

CORRECTIONS

The magnitude of the signal measured by the PET scanner can be influenced by many factors related to both the interaction of the annihilation photons with the patient and the response and configuration of the detector components of the scanner. Images that accurately depict the tracer distribution require, therefore, correction for all of these factors.

Block Uniformity and Gain

Block uniformity corrections compensate for differences in the sensitivity of the block detector from element to element. As a result of changes in the sensitivity of the PMT across its front face and reduced sensitivity in the gaps between the PMTs, not all elements respond equally to incident radiation. The variable sensitivity can be corrected by obtaining a uniformity map of the detector block (Figure 2-10) with a flood source or distant point source and electronically correcting for the differences in sensitivity. Similarly, the

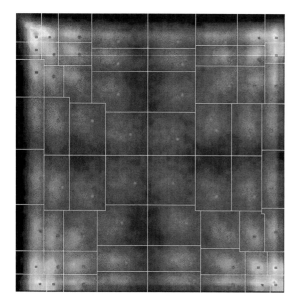

Figure 2-10. Block uniformity map. The uniformity map is segmented into areas corresponding to each crystal element in the block (indicated by the white lines). Red dots mark the computer's identification of each crystal element. The grid pattern is distorted as a result of the differences in sensitivity and amplification between the edge and the center of the PMTs. (See color insert.)

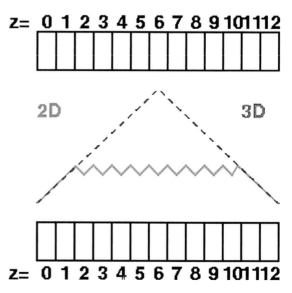

Figure 2-11. Axial sensitivity profiles for 2D (green) and 3D (blue) acquisitions. (See color insert.)

differences in gain between detector blocks can also be normalized using a weak normalization source with a negligible randoms rate.

Geometry

The sensitivity of the scanner varies from plane to plane through the axial FOV of the scanner (Figure 2-11). This effect is caused by the different number of accepted lines of response that are available to contribute to any given plane. For example, at the edge of the FOV, only the edge detector elements can contribute, whereas, in the center of the scanner, elements on either side of the plane can also be used. Even in the central FOV, the direct plane is created from photon pairs with z-position of say: $(0,0)$, $(-1, +1)$, $(+1, -1)$, whereas the cross-plane is generated with pairs $(-1, 0)$, $(0, -1)$, $(-2, +1)$, and $(+1, -2)$, a ratio of $4{:}3$. The variation in sensitivity can be corrected

by measuring a uniform cylinder or line source and then using this data to compute the relative sensitivity of each plane and rescale appropriately.

Deadtime

As the activity in the FOV of the scanner increases, the rate of annihilation photons incident on the detectors scales linearly and hence so too does the rate at which events must be processed to determine those that fall within the energy and timing windows. Eventually, the detectors and electronics are unable to keep up, and counts are lost. This is particularly true in dynamic PET imaging, where high levels of activity are present at the start of the scan and must be accurately measured to provide suitable time–activity curves. By measuring in advance the response of the camera to higher and higher activities, it is possible to determine what the deadtime losses are, and this, in turn, allows compensation for this effect when imaging.

Randoms

Random events cannot be avoided, but one can compensate for them in one of two ways. The first

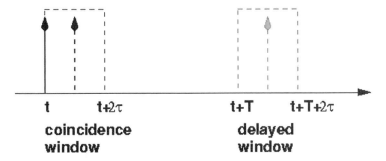

Figure 2-12. Delayed-window randoms correction. When an initial event (solid black arrow) is detected, a coincidence window of length 2τ is immediately opened and a second delayed window is also opened at a much later time T. The number of random coincidences detected in the delayed window (dashed gray arrow) is the same as the number detected in the coincidence window (dashed black arrow).

is to use a delayed window measurement. In this approach, a second coincidence window is used, similar in width to the first but offset by a large period of time (Figure 2-12). Photons in coincidence via this second window cannot have come from the same annihilation event and so provide a direct measurement of the random coincidence rate. This measurement can then be subtracted from the signal measured in the first coincidence window to compensate for randoms therein. A second approach uses a calculation of the randoms rate. The number of randoms detected by a pair of crystals is related to their singles detection rate.

$$R_{12} = 2\tau S_1 S_2 \qquad (2.2)$$

where R is the randoms rate, τ is the timing resolution (2τ is the coincidence window width), and S_1 and S_2 refer to the singles rates of the two detector elements.

Therefore, by measuring the singles rate at each crystal, it is possible to compute the randoms rate in any pair of crystals and then subtract an appropriate number of events from the corresponding sinogram element (LOR).

Scatter

Scatter events are also unavoidable in clinical PET. The scatter fraction indicates the number of scattered events divided by the sum of the true and scattered events. In 2D PET acquisitions, the scat-

ter fraction is typically on the order of 15%, but, in 3D acquisition, the fraction can be 40% or more. Techniques that correct for scatter consist of two components: a way to estimate scatter and a means of removing it. The removal is generally done by subtracting the scatter estimate from the sinogram, reconstructing the scatter data as a scatter image and then subtracting that from the reconstructed image, or, finally, in the case of iterative reconstruction, including the scatter estimate directly into the reconstruction algorithm itself. This last approach is the most accurate, but also the most complex, and hence requires the largest amount of computing power.

Estimation of the scatter is the more difficult component of the correction, and many methods of estimation have been developed. Some common approaches are energy-window-based methods, estimation of scatter from the sinograms, and calculation of scatter based on an estimate of the activity distribution. Energy-based approaches use the fact that scattered photons have less energy than unscattered ones. By setting another energy window below the photopeak, a second image can be generated based on primarily scattered photons. The scatter-window image is used as an estimate of the scatter, and a scaled version is subtracted from the photopeak image to compensate for scatter. A second approach is to estimate the scatter from the information in the sinograms. Data acquired from LORs that do not pass through the patient, i.e., those at the edge of the FOV, must be caused by scatter. Scattered photons form a smooth distribution and so can be approximated with simple functions like Gaussian curves. By fitting the scatter at the edge of the FOV to the tails of the Gaussian curves, it is possible to estimate the scatter in the central portion of the image. A third approach is to calculate the distribution of scattered photons using analytical or Monte Carlo techniques based on an estimate of the unscattered activity distribution (usually provided by first reconstructing the image without scatter correction). Calculation of scatter in this manner can be the most accurate method, but has the trade-off of also requiring the largest amount of computing time. A detailed discussion of scatter is beyond the scope of this text, but the interested reader can find further details in the text by Bailey et al.[8]

Attenuation

Attenuation correction is a major problem in PET imaging. The half-value thickness of 511-keV photons in soft tissues is approximately 7 cm. Furthermore, both annihilation photons must be detected to generate an LOR, and so attenuation can reduce the strength of the PET signal by factors of $20\times$ or more. Accurate attenuation correction requires a measurement of the distribution of tissue densities within the patient. This measurement can be obtained via a transmission scan with radioactive sources like Cs-137 or Ge/Ga-68 or through a coregistered CT scan. A further discussion of attenuation correction is given in Chapter 15.

Isotope Decay

In the case of dynamic imaging, it is also necessary to account for the physical decay of the radioisotope. Because each image in the series is acquired at a different (later) time point, the signal from radioisotopes with short half-lives like Rb-82 or O-15 can decay significantly, altering the appearance of the images and mimicking physiological changes. This is normally compensated for after reconstruction by decay-correcting the image values back to the time of the start of the acquisition.

Absolute Calibration

Lastly, an absolute calibration is needed to translate the number of counts observed in the FOV into the amount of activity present in the FOV. This is done by acquiring an image of a cylinder of water with a known, uniform amount of activity inside of it and thereby deriving an appropriate scaling factor.

NOISE-EQUIVALENT COUNT RATE

All of these methods of correction can reduce the bias in the PET image but do not remove the associated noise. For example, a calculated randoms correction can remove the mean number of detected random events, but the actual number of detected randoms varies statistically about that mean according to the Poisson distribution. Therefore, the noise in the measured signal because of the detected randoms remains, even after the randoms correction. If the correction is based on a measured value, then the uncertainty in that measurement is also added into the data. The result of this is that the uncertainty in the corrected PET data is no longer easily related to the mean of the raw data, and signal-to-noise ratio of two acquisitions can be different, even when the mean values of the corrected data are the same. To facilitate comparisons of the quality of the acquired data between different PET scanners and between different methods of acquisition and correction, the noise-equivalent count rate (NECR) is used (Figure 2-13).

As its name implies, this measure is an expression of the count rate required to obtain a given level of noise (uncertainty) in the corrected data. The NECR is given by Eq. (2.3):

$$NECR = \frac{T^2}{(T + S + kfR)} \qquad (2.3)$$

where T refers to the true count rate, S to the scatter rate, R to the randoms rate, and f to the fraction of the FOV occupied by the patient or object containing the radioactive source, and k is 1 or 2 depending on the method of randoms

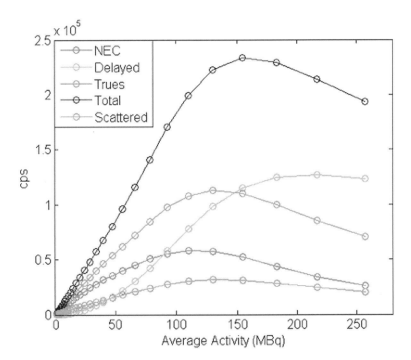

Figure 2-13. Noise-equivalent count rate. This example shows the contributions to the total number of prompts (black) detected in a PET scanner as the amount of activity in the scanner increases. The true (red) and scattered (purple) event rates initially increase in proportion to the singles rate (activity), but the randoms or delayed rate (green) increases with the square of the singles rate. Deadtime in processing events leads to a peak in the measured count rate (here at 130 MBq for the true rate and 150 MBq for the total rate). The noise-equivalent count rate (blue) peaks even earlier at approximately 110 MBq. (See color insert.)

correction (calculated from singles or measured via a delayed window).

FACTORS AFFECTING SPATIAL RESOLUTION

One of the advantages of PET over single-photon imaging is its resolution. The resolution in PET is determined by a combination of factors.

Crystal Size

The first is crystal element size. As the point of interaction of the gamma ray is only localized to within an element, the accuracy of the localization is limited by the dimensions of the crystal. Most human scanners have crystal faces of 4 to 5 mm on a side, but the need for higher resolution in mouse imaging has driven the crystal size in small-animal scanners down to 2 mm or less. The resolution loss caused by crystal size is least in the center (half of the crystal size) and degrades as the point of annihilation gets closer to the crystal face itself whereat the uncertainty becomes equal to the crystal size. For a crystal size of 4 mm, this introduces an error of 2 mm at the center of the scanner. The crystals in PET scanner are often not the same size in the axial and transaxial directions, leading to different resolutions in plane and out of plane.

Depth of Interaction

An additional factor that significantly degrades resolution is an effect called *depth of interaction*

(DOI). Not all annihilation photons strike the face of the scanner crystals perpendicularly. If a photon strikes a crystal element obliquely, it only has to traverse the width of the crystal before exiting again. The efficiency of stopping a 511-keV photon in 2 cm of crystal is quite high (85% for BGO), but probability of it stopping in 4 mm is much less (32% for BGO). When an event is detected in a crystal, the DOI is not known and so it is assumed that the photon entered the detector ring in the same crystal in which it was detected. The point of interaction, which determines one end of the LOR, is thus placed at the surface of the incorrect crystal, leading to a mispositioning of the LOR (Figure 2-14). This effect gets worse as one moves toward the edge of the FOV because more of the possible LORs are at angles other than 90 degrees to the scanner ring. DOI effects are often viewed as a distortion of the crystal size that increases as the radial position of the annihilation event increases. For a typical PET scanner with $4 \times 4 \times 30$ mm crystal elements and a detector ring diameter of

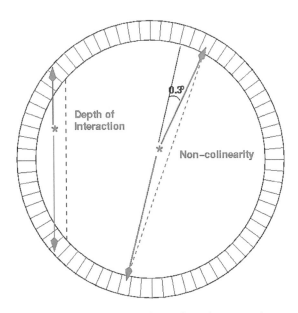

Figure 2-14. Spatial resolution loses because of depth of interaction and non-colinearity. The true photon paths are shown in the solid lines, but the LOR is processed as corresponding to the dashed line.

80 cm, DOI results in an effective increase in the crystal size by approximately 40% at 10 cm from the center of the scanner.

Non-colinearity

The next most important factor in determining resolution in a PET scanner is the bore size. When the electron and positron annihilate, the positron may retain some residual momentum. To conserve momentum, the two annihilation photons may, thus, be not quite at 180 degrees to each other. They deviate on average ±0.25 degrees from 180 degrees.

This effect is termed *non-colinearity* (Figure 2-14). For an annihilation in the center of the camera, the error in the position of the event is approximately $0.0022 \times D$, where D is the diameter of the bore. A typical bore size for a PET scanner is 80 cm, leading to an error of 1.75 mm.

Positron Range

A final factor that can affect cardiac imaging in PET is positron range. As described earlier in this chapter, the positron range is a statistical measure of how far the positron travels from the atom before it annihilates. The range is different for different isotopes. The resolution loss as a result of positron range (R_{range}) is roughly equal to 2.35 times the RMS range.[9] Therefore, for an isotope like F-18 with an RMS range of 0.23 mm, the impact on the spatial resolution of the scanner is minimal. However, Rb-82 positrons have a much higher maximum energy and their RMS range is 2.6 mm, significantly degrading the resolution of images of myocardial perfusion.

System Resolution

The system resolution of the PET scanner is because of the combination of all of these effects. As the effects are independent of one another, the uncertainties of each component add as independent errors.

$$R_{\text{system}} = \sqrt{R_{\text{detector}}^2 + R_{\text{non-collinear}}^2 + R_{\text{range}}^2}$$
$$(2.4)$$

where R_x corresponds to the resolution contribution from factor x. The DOI effects are included in this equation as a modification of the detector element size and hence of R_{detector}.

All of the component effects have a dependence on the radial distance from the center of the scanner, and so resolution changes with radial position. The typical resolution of a modern PET scanner is 5 mm at the center, degrading to 7 mm toward the edge of the FOV. Correcting for these resolution losses is difficult and is usually not done when reconstructing images with algorithms like FBP. Techniques for performing this type of resolution recovery are, nevertheless, under development. For example, one approach is to measure the radially dependent resolution and incorporate these measurements into the reconstruction algorithm.[10] These and other compensation methods have promise and may soon be available for clinical use.

PARTIAL VOLUME EFFECTS

The *partial volume effect* is simply that the counts in a nuclear medicine image are spread over a volume defined by the resolution of the system. If that volume is larger than one voxel, it means that the apparent activity of a source is distributed over several voxels and the measured activity concentration is decreased (Figure 2-15). Resolution impacts on cardiac imaging with PET, as it effectively applies a smoothing filter to the image and blurs the observed distribution of activity. This reduces contrast in regions of decreased tracer uptake, making it more difficult to distinguish small defects. It also spreads the apparent activity over a larger volume, decreasing the activity in each pixel element and thereby increasing the percentage noise in the acquired data. To compensate for the noise, smoothing filters are often applied during reconstruction, which further aggravates the partial volume effects. A rule of thumb is that, to recover the true concentration of activity, the object measured must be greater than twice the resolution FWHM. This is important in cardiac imaging because the myocardial wall thickness is on the order of 1 cm and the typical resolution of a PET scanner is 5 mm or more. This means that the measurement of the maximum activity concentration in the myocardial wall, such as is done when generating a polar plot, can be diminished by partial volume effects.

SUMMARY

Coincidence detection is the key to the success of PET imaging. Measuring a pair of annihilation photons removes the need for physical absorbing collimators, such as are used in SPECT, and thereby greatly increases the sensitivity of the scanner and its resolution. In addition, positron-emitting radioisotopes exist for atoms, such as carbon and oxygen, which are present in organic molecules, allowing us to create small, biologically relevant tracers for PET imaging. These features make PET an important tool for diagnosis, direction of treatment, and research of heart disease.

We have provided a brief introduction to the instrumentation behind PET imaging as it is today. The field is, however, continually evolving with new modifications in camera design, signal processing, and image reconstruction occurring on a regular basis. One example is the growth of multimodal platforms where PET has been combined with CT, and more recently MRI, to provide coregistered anatomical and functional information. Both CT and MRI are important tools for cardiac assessment in their own rights, and coregistration of this information with the functional data available from PET is increasing in popularity. New developments in instrumentation open up new avenues of exploration and application and make the future of cardiac PET one that is full of exciting possibilities. We have not covered specific imaging protocols for cardiac evaluation; these can be found in the American Society of Nuclear Cardiology's guidelines,[11] and many are discussed in greater detail in later chapters.

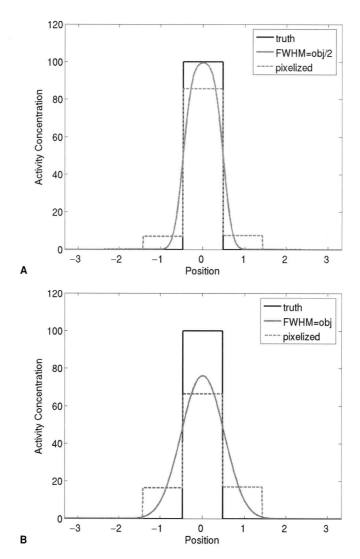

Figure 2-15. Partial volume effect. (**A**) The true activity distribution in the object is shown in black. If the resolution FWHM of the system is less than or equal to half of the object size, then the activity concentration is blurred (black), but the correct maximum may still be recovered. Another factor that must be considered though is the image voxel size. If the voxel size is too large, the activity will also be averaged over the voxel volume, and this can further reduce the apparent activity concentration (black dashed). (**B**) When the resolution of the system is greater than half of the object size, the activity is spread over a larger volume and the activity concentration is diminished.

ACKNOWLEDGMENT

The authors thank Tyler Dumouchel for his assistance with this chapter.

REFERENCES

1. Brownell GL, Sweet WH. Localization of brain tumors with positron emitters. *Nucleonics.* 1953;11:40.
2. Ter-Pogossian M, Spratt JS Jr, Rudman S, Spencer A. Radioactive oxygen 15 in study of kinetics of oxygen of respiration. *Am J Physiol.* 1971;201:582 [PMID: 13775945].
3. Rankowitz S, Robertson JS, Higinbotham WA, Rosenblum MJ. Positron scanner for locating brain tumors. *IRE Int Conv Record.* 1962;9:49.
4. Ter-Pogossian MM, Phelps ME, Hoffman EJ, et al. A positron-emission transaxial tomograph for nuclear imaging (PETT). *Radiology.* 1975;114:89. [PMID: 1208874].
5. Slart RH, Bax JJ, van Veldhuisen DJ, et al. Prediction of functional recovery after revascularization in patients with coronary artery disease and left ventricular dysfunction by gated FDG-PET. *J Nucl Cardiol.* 2006;13:180 [PMID: 16580957].
6. Dorbala S, Vangala D, Sampson U, Limaye A, Kwong R, Di Carli MF. Value of vasodilator left ventricular ejection fraction reserve in evaluating the magnitude of myocardium at risk and the extent of angiographic coronary artery disease: A 82Rb PET/CT study. *J Nucl Med.* 2007;48:349 [PMID: 17332611].
7. Sharir T, Germano G, Kavanagh PB, et al. Incremental prognostic value of post-stress left ventricular ejection fraction and volume by gated myocardial perfusion single photon emission computed tomography. *Circulation.* 1999;100:1035 [PMID: 10477527].
8. Bailey DL, Townsend DW, Valk PE, Maisey MN, eds. *Positron Emission Tomography – Basic Sciences.* Springer-Verlag London Limited; 2005.
9. Lecomte R. Technology challenges in small animal PET imaging. *Nucl Instrum Methods Phys Res A.* 2004; 527:157.
10. Panin V, Kehren F, Michel C, Casey M. Fully 3-D PET Reconstruction with System Matrix Derived From Point Source Measurements. *IEEE Trans Med Imag.* 2006; 25:907–921.
11. Machac J, Bacharach SL, Bateman TM, et al. Positron emission tomography myocardial perfusion and glucose metabolism imaging. *J Nucl Cardiol.* 2006;13:e121 [PMID: 17174789].
12. Melcher CL. Scintillation crystals for PET. *J Nucl Med.* 2000;41:1051. [PMID: 10855634].
13. Saint-Gobain Crystals. Physical properties of common inorganic scintillators. www.detectors.saint-gobain.com. Accessed 2007.
14. Cherry SR, Sorenson JA, Phelps ME. *Physics in Nuclear Medicine.* 3rd ed. Elsevier Science; 2003.

ADDITIONAL READING

Cherry SR, Sorenson JA, Phelps ME. *Physics in Nuclear Medicine.* 3rd ed. Philadelphia, PA: Elsevier Science; 2003.

Phelps ME. *PET—Molecular Imaging and Its Biological Applications.* Springer-Verlag New York; 2004.

Wernick MN, Aarsvold JN, eds. *Emission Tomography—The Fundamentals of PET and SPECT.* San Diego, CA: Elsevier Academic Press; 2004.

SECTION 2

RADIOPHARMACEUTICALS

CHAPTER 3

Basic Principles of Flow Tracers

Haris Athar

Gary V. Heller

INTRODUCTION

In recent years, important advances have taken place in stress myocardial perfusion imaging in patients with suspected or known coronary artery disease (CAD) for the detection of ischemia, assessment of prognosis, preoperative risk assessment, evaluation of myocardial viability, and determination of the efficacy of revascularization in patients undergoing coronary artery bypass surgery or percutaneous intervention. New ^{99m}Tc-labeled perfusion agents have emerged to enhance the diagnostic accuracy of SPECT and to provide additional information regarding regional and global left ventricular systolic function via ECG gating of images. The quality of images obtained with these new ^{99m}Tc-labeled radionuclides has been shown to be superior to that of images obtained with ^{201}Tl because of the more favorable physical characteristics of ^{99m}Tc imaging. However, all of the present perfusion tracers have limitations. This chapter outlines properties of contemporary myocardial perfusion imaging agents with regard to tracer kinetics, extraction, distribution, and retention characteristics of individual tracers as well as their strengths and weaknesses.

TRACER KINETICS

The major role of nuclear cardiology in clinical practice is the evaluation of regional myocardial blood flow and viability under rest or stress conditions. Current tracers used for perfusion imaging have provided valuable clinical information. Ongoing developments will further enhance the detection rate of coronary artery lesions and impact of medical therapy.

The ideal tracer should

- track myocardial blood flow across the entire physiological range;
- be taken up rapidly (high myocardial extraction rate);
- be extracted as completely as possible out of the bloodstream;

49

- exhibit a linear relationship between myocardial uptake and blood flow;
- be retained in myocardium for a sufficient period to be imaged;
- be taken up independent of changes in metabolic conditions;
- exhibit low extracardiac uptake;
- show myocardial redistribution;
- be easily labeled; and
- exhibit stability of the labeled compound.

CHARACTERISTICS OF FLOW TRACERS

Myocardial perfusion abnormalities detected during either exercise or pharmacologic stress are caused by differential blood flow between normal and stenotic arteries. Radiotracers reflect the changes in blood flow induced by the stressors because of their high myocardial extraction, which should be maintained throughout the range of blood flow. To accurately reflect myocardial blood flow the most important characteristics of each tracer is its extraction fraction and linearity with blood flow. In clinical imaging, the radiotracers are not completely extracted. The amount of tracer uptake by the myocardium after bolus injection is the product of extraction fraction and myocardial blood flow. Generally, tracers with higher first-pass extraction will track blood flow over a wider range compared to tracers of lower first-pass extraction.

Virtually all myocardial perfusion imaging agents show a linear relationship between myocardial blood flow and tracer uptake during resting conditions. With increasing blood flow during stress tracer uptake becomes nonlinear after a two- to fourfold increase from resting conditions (Figure 3-1). This plateau effect differs between tracers. Theoretically, the flow tracer closest to linearity with microspheres will most accurately reflect differences in ischemia between stress and rest conditions. Conversely, flow tracers with the least linearity might not exhibit

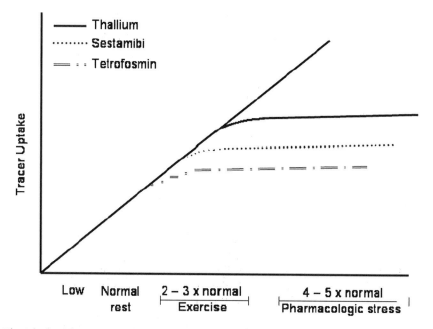

Figure 3-1. The ideal perfusion tracer would track myocardial blood flow across the entire range of physiological flows. The available perfusion tracers "roll off" at higher levels of flow. Each tracer tracers reaches a plateau at differing levels of myocardial blood flow.

Table 3-1

Comparison of Perfusion Agents Used in Clinical Practice

Characteristic	^{201}Tl	^{99m}Tc tetrofosmin	^{99m}Tc sestamibi	Rubidium-82
Cell uptake	Na/K ATPase	Passive mitochondrial	Passive mitochondrial	Active
Clearance	Moderate	Slow	Slow	Decay
Extraction fraction	0.85	0.54	0.55–0.65	Higher than 65%
Redistribute	Yes	Partial	Minimal	No
Measure of blood flow	Good	Adequate	Adequate	Good
Gated images	Poor–adequate	Excellent	Excellent	Excellent
Photon energy	70 keV	140 keV	140 keV	511 keV
Half-life	73 h	6 h	6 h	75 s
Clearance	Renal	Hepatic	Hepatic	Renal

differences between rest and stress conditions. For example, Tc-99m-labeled teboroxime has the highest percentage of extraction in the myocardium.

Five myocardial tracers are available for clinical use. These include Tl-201; three technetium-based agents: sestamibi, teboroxime, tetrofosmin; and the positron emission tomography (PET) tracer rubidium-82. Teboroxime and two other PET tracers (0-15-H$_2$O and N-13-NH) are rarely used clinically because of lack of availability (Table 3-1). The relationship between increasing blood flow and uptake of these radionuclides is illustrated in Figure 3-2.

Clearance of each agent is also varied. For example, thallium complete clearance is slow but begins within 10 minutes, whereas sestamibi and tetrofosmin are retained for several hours. On the other hand, teboroxime clearance is the most rapid, and imaging must commence immediately after injection. We present different characteristics of each tracer that are important for clinical applications.

Tc-99m Teboroxime

Tc-99m-labeled teboroxime, with the highest extraction fraction, exhibits the closest to linear

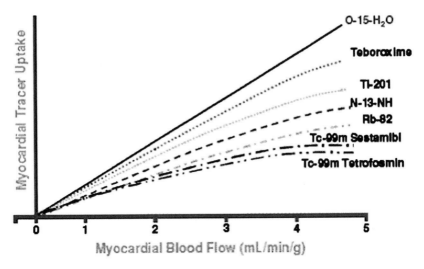

Figure 3-2. Relationship of increasing blood flow and tracer uptake. The ideal agent would reflect a linear relationship over wide clinical range of blood flow.

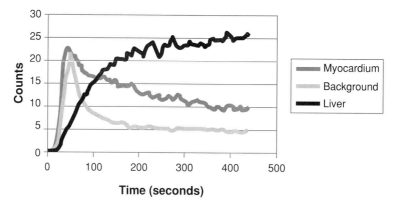

Figure 3-3.   Teboroxime uptake curves. A high initial myocardial uptake is followed by a rapid washout. Note the rapidly increasing hepatic activity.

correlation within the range of pharmacologic stress of all SPECT radionuclear tracers (Figure 3-3). Animal vasodilator models suggesting a linear correlation of myocardial teboroxime uptake maintained up to 5 mL/min/g flow rate led to initial enthusiasm, as this plateau was significantly higher than other SPECT agents. Myocardial extraction of Tc-99m teboroxime approaches 100%, the highest among all single-photon tracers. These properties would suggest teboroxime as an ideal tracer to reflect accurately blood flow throughout the entire spectrum of pharmacologic and exercise stress. However, the very high initial uptake of Tc-99m teboroxime is followed by a rapid myocardial washout and a rapidly increasing hepatic activity, significantly limiting clinical use. For standard SPECT imaging the choice is to start acquiring very soon after injection, leading to artifacts as a result of inconsistencies between projections, or to wait to acquire when the activity over the myocardium and liver are stable, leading to a very poor myocardium to liver ratio and imaging artifacts.

Tc-99m teboroxime remains—despite the technical limitations related to its use—an attractive myocardial blood flow single-photon tracer. Its unique pharmacodynamic characteristics offer an interesting niche for specific clinical applications. Although it is currently not used clinically, Tc-99m teboroxime may again become an op-

tion because of the availability of ultrafast SPECT technology. Owing to its neutral lipophilic properties, Tc-99m teboroxime comes close to being a freely diffusible radiotracer similar to xenon-133. After initial uptake, redistribution of Tc-99m teboroxime is similar to that of Tl-201. Therefore, viable regions demonstrate defect reversibility while nonviable regions remain nonreversible.

Thallium-201

Although Tl-201 is considered biologically similar to potassium, its myocardial uptake is greater than that of potassium. With 87% at normal flow rate, Tl-201 has the highest extraction fraction of the myocardial tracers currently in clinical use. As shown in animal models, Tl-201 activity corresponds to blood flow in a linear relationship to at least 3 mL/min/g. At this level a plateau effect occurs, resulting in stable thallium activity despite increases in blood flow. The plateau effect is at a higher blood flow than other current tracers of sestamibi and tetrofosmin (Figure 3-4).

Technetium-99m Sestamibi

The most common clinically used technetium-based tracer is sestamibi. The extraction fraction of sestamibi is less than thallium (55%–65% range) but greater than tetrofosmin. Experimental

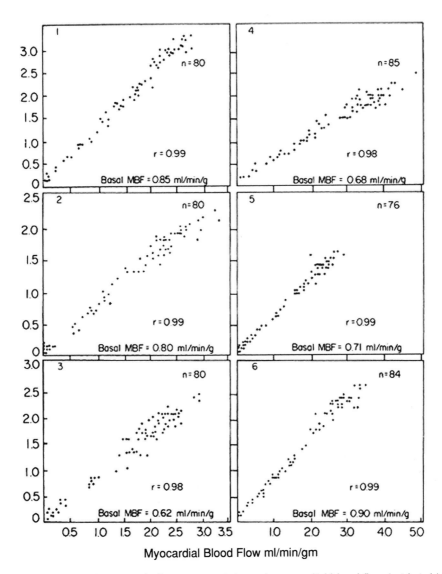

Figure 3-4.   The relationship between thallium-201 activity and myocardial blood flow (mL/min/g) in six dogs during exercise and ischemia. *n* = number of samples analyzed.

studies have demonstrated a linear relationship of uptake of sestamibi to level of 2 mL/min/g, above which a nonlinear relationship is noted to increasing flow. Although this plateau effect ensues at a lower blood flow than seen with Tl-201 and theoretically might decrease the sensitivity to detect flow differences, a clinical effect has not been shown to be relevant (Figure 3-5).

Tc-99m Tetrofosmin

Tc-99m tetrofosmin is a diphosphine complex of Tc-99m that shows similar myocardial uptake, retention, and blood clearance kinetics as Tc-99m sestamibi. The agents are different in some respects: compared with Tc-99m sestamibi, Tc-99m tetrofosmin's initial myocardial uptake is slightly

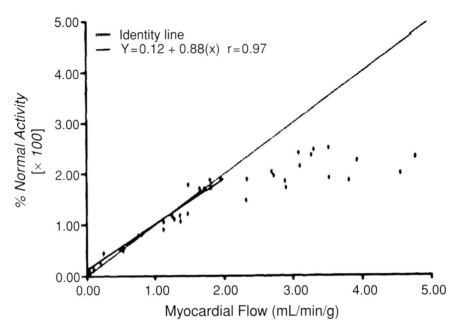

Figure 3-5.   Technetium-99m Sestamibi.

lower, its clearance from both the liver and the lung is faster, and its preparation does not require a heating period. In animal models, regional uptake of Tc-99m tetrofosmin relates to regional myocardial blood flow, but there is an underestimation of flow at rates exceeding 1.5 to 2.0 mL/min/g. However, this behavior is common among all single-photon myocardial perfusion tracers. The mechanism for myocardial uptake of Tc-99m tetrofosmin is believed to be similar to sestamibi— it is dependent on mitochondrial membrane activity. Human studies have shown a stable myocardial retention of Tc-99m tetrofosmin, at least up to 4 hours after intravenous injection. It should be pointed out, however, that in animal experiments, retention of this agent was different than in humans, highlighting the fact that animal experimental data may not readily be applied to humans. The slightly lower myocardial extraction of Tc-99m tetrofosmin has raised concerns about the ability of this agent to detect mild ischemia. Tetrofosmin also demonstrates a plateau during

stress, which may be lower than that of sestamibi[1] (Figure 3-5).

Rubidium-82

The diagnosis of CAD by PET is based on the evaluation of regional myocardial blood flow with myocardial perfusion tracers. Three PET tracers are currently available: O_{14}, N_{13} ammonium, and rubidium-82 (Rb-82). The most commonly used positron-emitting tracer is Rb-82, with a half-life of 75 seconds. It is generator produced and does not require on-site cyclotrons. Rb-82 is a cation, the intracellular uptake of which across the sarcolemmal membrane reflects active cation transport. The short half-life of this agent facilitates rapid sequential rest–stress examinations. However, exercise studies with short-lived PET perfusion tracers are difficult, and chest motion during exercise will impair both image quality and attenuation correction. Most PET studies have used pharmacologic vasodilator stress with

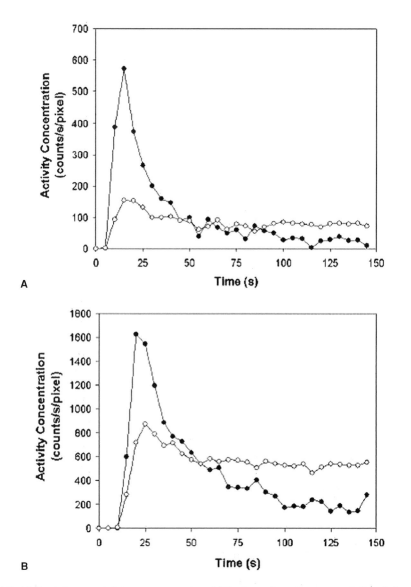

Figure 3-6. (**A**) Rubidium time–activity curves at rest and (**B**) after adenosine stress. Solid circles represent the activity concentration in the left atrium and the open circles represent the activity concentration in myocardial tissue.

intravenous dipyridamole or adenosine to assess relative regional myocardial blood flow and flow reserve. Experimental studies[2–4] demonstrated a first-pass myocardial extraction of 50% to 60%, which remained relatively linear up to 2.5 to 3 times resting baseline flow varying under a variety of physiological and pathophysiological conditions. However, net uptake of rubidium plateaus at the hyperemic flows often achieved with pharmacologic stress. Nonetheless, qualitative assessment of relative rubidium perfusion defects have correlated well with those obtained from microspheres.

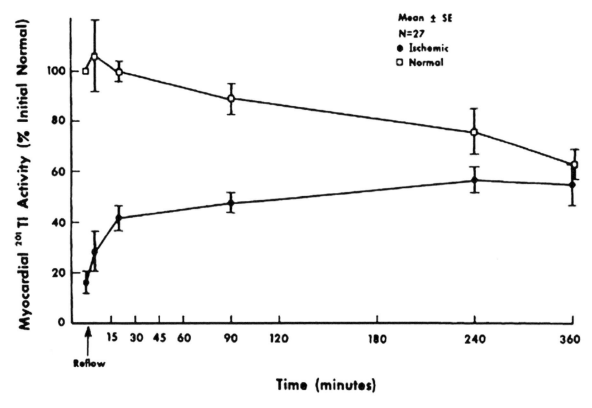

Figure 3-7. Serial determination of myocardial thallium-201 (Tl-201) activity, expressed a percent of initial (before reflow) normal Tl-201 activity in all five groups of dogs occluded for 20 minutes and reperfused for 5, 20, 90, 240, and 360 minutes. The initial value of Tl-201 activity in the ischemic region was obtained before reflow and represents the mean ± SEM for all 27 dogs. Near equalization of Tl-201 concentration in normal and ischemic myocardial regions appears by 4 hours. (From Beller et al.[5])

Clinically, rubidium PET has both high sensitivity and specificity for detecting CAD (Figure 3-6).

TRACER RETENSION

The radiotracer must be retained in the myocardium long enough to acquire an image of the tracer distribution. Tracers currently in clinical use differ greatly in mechanism and extent of retention. For example, Tl-201 as a potassium analog enters the myocardial cell through active channels and is retained in the viable cells in the potassium pool with an intact transmembrane potas-

sium gradient. In contrast, Tc-99m sestamibi and tetrofosmin are neutral compounds that diffuse freely through the cell membrane but sequester within mitochondria by large negative transmembrane potentials. This washout is dependent on myocardial flow.

TRACER DISTRIBUTION

After tracer injection, most of the tracer is distributed through all body compartments and only 3% to 5% of the tracer is delivered to the myocardium. After the initial extraction, the tracer washed out from the myocardium is not linear and depends on specific redistribution characteristics of the tracers and is not simply related to myocardial blood flow.

The initial activity of Tl-201 in blood decreases by 92% in 5 minutes. The remaining activity exhibits a half-life of 40 minutes. Myocardial uptake of Tl-201 is not static. This stress redistribution is one of the most clinically important characteristics of Tl-201 and clinically utilized to diagnose the presence of CAD. Generally, 3 to 5 hours after the injection at stress a perfusion defect will show normalization for the thallium uptake (Figure 3-7). In contrast, Tc-99m sestamibi binds irreversibly to myocardial cells because of the negatively charged mitochondrial membrane gradient and does not redistribute to a significant extent. This leads to a very slow myocardial clearance after its initial myocardial uptake (fractional clearance of 10%–15% in 4 hours).

TRACER CLEARANCE

The effective half-life of the current myocardial tracers vary significantly and depend on both biological half-life and radionuclide decay. The PET tracer rubidium-82 decays rapidly to strontium and is renally excreted. The primary elimination pathway for thallium is through excretion into the feces, but renal elimination may be substantial (approximately 35%). Technitium-99m sestamibi is not metabolized and has an elimination half-life of 6 hours, and 27% of it is renally excreted and more than 60% of a dose has been recovered in urine and bile during the first 24 hours after injection. The hepatobiliary system is the major pathway for clearance; activity from the gallbladder appears in the intestine within 1 hour of injection. The effective half-life of clearance is approximately

3 hours, which is considerably shorter than the half-life of thallium-201 (73 hours).

SUMMARY

In summary, the clinical implication of flow-dependent tracer extraction is that with higher extraction coefficient a better correlation with actual flow impairment is achieved.

A plateau effect in various degrees is noted with all myocardial tracers. Tracer retention needs to be long enough to allow adequate imaging. Redistribution is determined by membrane transport rather than blood flow. The clinical impact of each tracer's ability to reflect blood flow may be important but have not been shown to represent meaningful clinical difference in comparative studies.

REFERENCES

1. Soman P, Taillefer R, DePuey EG, et al. Enhanced detection of reversible perfusion defects by Tc-99m sestamibi compared to Tc-99m tetrofosmin during vasodilator stress SPECT imaging in mild-to-moderate coronary artery disease. *J Am Coll Cardiol.* 2001;37: 458–462.
2. Mullani NA, Goldstein RA, Gould KL, et al. Myocardial perfusion with rubidium-82. I. Measurement of extraction fraction and flow with external detectors. *J Nucl Med.* 1983;24:898–906.
3. Goldstein RA, Mullani NA, Marani SK, et al. Myocardial perfusion with rubidium-82. II. Effects of metabolic and pharmacologic interventions. *J Nucl Med.* 1983;24: 907–915.
4. Wilson RA, Shea M, Landsheere CD, et al. Rubidium-82 myocardial uptake and extraction after transient ischemia: PET characteristics. *J Comput Assist Tomogr.* 1987;11:60–66.
5. Beller GA, Watson DD, et al. Time course of thallium-201 redistribution after transient myocardial ischemia. *Circulation.* 1980;61(4):791–797.

CHAPTER 4

PET Radiopharmaceuticals

Gavin Noble

INTRODUCTION TO PET IMAGING

Nuclear cardiology has addressed many aspects of cardiovascular disease; however, its greatest strength has been in the diagnosis and risk stratification of coronary artery disease. Despite a plethora of studies documenting the benefits of SPECT imaging, limitations remain. Single-vessel disease is still not optimally detected, balanced ischemia presents a challenge, and attenuation artifact is prevalent and the correction of this is complex.[1,2] Positron emission tomography (PET) imaging offers another alternative with the ability to overcome many of these limitations. Higher resolution, higher-energy photons, shorter half-lives, and simpler attenuation correction (AC) can result in better images, lower radiation doses, higher accuracy, and shorter protocols.

PET has been available for many years; however, the recent proliferation of PET scanners for oncologic evaluations has opened new avenues for cardiac PET, both research and clinical applications. Most institutions began performing clinical PET for oncologic studies but do not fill the scanner all day. This opens the possibility of sharing the scanner with other specialties, and, indeed, this is a common way to begin doing cardiac PET. This overcomes one of the initial obstacles, the cost of the scanner, while simultaneously solving the problem of the underutilized resource of the existing, expensive camera.

There have been many PET radiopharmaceuticals studied for cardiac imaging. Many of these have presented challenges related to their short half-life and the consequent need for an on-site cyclotron. This has limited their application to research institutes with the resources necessary to sustain these operations. However, metabolic studies with fluorine-18-radiolabeled deoxyglucose (F-18 FDG) have become relatively common because of its long half-life ($T_{1/2}$ 110 minutes), which allows regional distribution from a central radiopharmacy. Recently, commercial

59

development of a rubidium-82 generator has facilitated the performance of PET myocardial perfusion studies in centers without on-site cyclotrons. Additionally, there are a number of other radiotracers that have yielded important information on blood flow, metabolism, and inflammation, despite the current limitations on their clinical implementation.

There are many important features of positron emitting isotopes that offer significant real and theoretical advantages over other available agents. Three common positron emitters, carbon-11, nitrogen-13 and oxygen-15, are also important elements in all biologic systems. These molecules can be incorporated into standard compounds to provide targeted imaging of biologically active systems. F-18 can replace a hydroxyl group in many molecules and, thus, also gain entry to metabolic pathways. Rubidium-82 is a potassium analog and, thus, has an obvious entry pathway into metabolically active cells via the K^+/Na^+ AT-Pase transporter. The 511-keV photon of PET has better intrinsic tissue penetration than the photon used in SPECT imaging (attenuation coefficient 0.09 cm^{-1} vs. 0.15 cm^{-1}).[3] Many positron emitters have short half-lives (75 seconds to 110 minutes), permitting higher doses and increased counts, while maintaining safe radiation exposure. Additionally, AC unrelated to the depth of origination of the photons is more straightforward and easily applied to PET than the depth-dependent AC used in SPECT imaging.

POSITRON EMISSION AND ANNIHILATION IMAGING

More people are familiar with SPECT imaging than with PET, so it is useful to compare the two modalities for similarities and differences as a way of explanation. Both PET and SPECT are nuclear techniques relying on the emission of photons to identify metabolic or physiologic activity. Both can use filtered backprojection or iterative reconstruction. Both can use multiple different tracers, although there is essentially no overlap, that is no

SPECT tracers are used for PET and no PET tracers are used for SPECT. Both modalities have AC available, although this is relatively simple, and always applied for PET, and more complex and less routinely used with SPECT imaging. All positron emission results in annihilation, resulting in two photons, each with 511 keV, whereas multiple different decay methods with a wide range of gamma and X-rays are possible with SPECT imaging.

All positron emitters share a common mechanism of decay, positron decay, also called beta-positive decay (Figure 4-1). Positron decay is the emission of a positron, a positively charged electron, from the nucleus, with the resultant conversion of a proton to a neutron, whereas beta-negative decay is the emission of a negatively charge electron from the nucleus with the conversion of a neutron to a proton. During positron decay the atomic number (Z, number of protons) decreases by one while the mass number (A, protons + neutrons) remains the same. Positron decay is

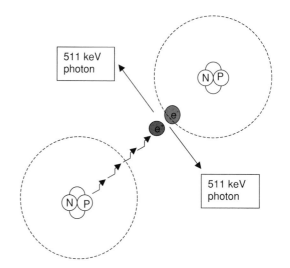

Figure 4-1. A proton (P) is converted to a neutron (N) in the nucleus with the subsequent ejection of a positron (e$^+$). The positron collides with an electron (e$^-$), either in the same atom or in a nearby atom, with resultant annihilation and conversion of the rest mass of both particles to photons with 511 keV, each traveling in opposite directions.

analogous to electron capture, which also converts a proton to a neutron, although in that case with the emission of characteristic X-rays. The positron that is emitted travels a short distance, typically 1 to 2 mm, and collides with a nearby electron. These two particles annihilate with one another, converting all of their mass into energy. The rest mass of an electron (0.9108×10^{-30} kg each) is equivalent to 511 keV as predicted by Einstein's theory of relativity ($E = mc^2$). Since there are two particles, each of which creates a photon with an energy of 511 keV, we have two photons simultaneously produced and traveling in nearly opposite directions. The photons travel at almost 180 degrees to one another in order to preserve momentum; any residual momentum is accounted for in the slight variation of angles (non-colinearity). Typically, non-colinearity will result in a loss of resolution of 1 to 2 mm. These photons arrive at the detectors nearly simultaneously, providing the basis for coincidence detection. The coincidence window is often on the order of 10 nanoseconds. If a photon is 30 cm closer to one detector than the other, the difference in arrival will be approximately 1 nanosecond. Detector systems that can distinguish these nanosecond differences in arrival are called time-of-flight detectors, and they are under development.

The positrons are emitted from the nucleus with a characteristic range of energies. The average energy is approximately one third of the maximum energy. The distance a positron travels before annihilating with an electron is directly related to the energy of that positron. Thus, low-energy positron emitters will have inherently better resolution capabilities than high-energy positron emitters.

Attenuation can affect PET imaging as well but is much simpler to deal with than in SPECT imaging. The challenge in SPECT imaging is that it is impossible to determine exactly how deep a measured electron began, and, thus, how much of the measured attenuation map needs to be applied to correct for the depth-dependent attenuation. In PET imaging, the amount of attenuation is related to the overall length of tissue that both photons go through. The overall distance the photons travel in tissue is greater in PET because even if the annihilation occurs near the surface on one side of the body, one of the photons is going to have to travel through nearly the whole body to escape to the other detector for coincidence imaging to occur. Therefore, while more attenuation occurs to the photons in PET, correction is depth independent in PET, since all photon pairs must be corrected for, based on the total amount of tissue and its characteristics on any line of acquisition (Figure 4-2).

PET RADIOTRACERS

As discussed above, there are five common radiotracers used in PET imaging.[4] Three of them require an on-site cyclotron, oxygen-15 (O-15), nitrogen-13 (N-13), and carbon-11 (C-11); one can be produced from a generator, rubidium-82 (Rb-82), and one is available through regional distributors as the radiopharmaceutical F-18 FDG. These can be used in the synthesis of many biologically active molecules (i.e., O-15 H_2O, N-15 ammonia, and C-11 acetate) or administered directly (Rb-82). Each of these tracers has positive and negative attributes relating to positron energy, inherent resolution, half-life, and methods of production and delivery, as will be discussed below.

FLUORINE-18

F-18 is essentially a pure positron emitter, with a negligible (3%) number of photons emitted following electron capture. It is frequently produced from O-18-enriched water in a cyclotron according to the reaction O-18(p,n)F-18, in which a proton replaces a neutron in the nucleus, and the atomic number (Z) increases by 1 while with mass number (A) remains the same. One hour of target irradiation can typically produce approximately 800 mCi of F-18. F-18 has a half-life of 110 minutes, facilitating its production at a central radiopharmacy and subsequent regional distribution.[5] F-18 decays via positron emission to O-18 as the proton converts back into a neutron, as

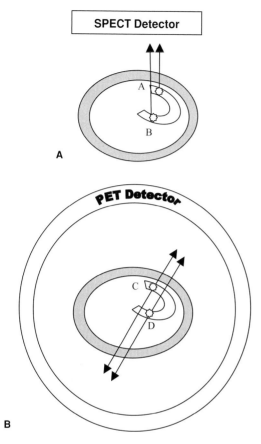

Figure 4-2.   Differences in attenuation between PET and SPECT. In panel **A**, One SPECT detector is shown with two possible photons that may be received. It is not possible to determine how deep the photon originated, and thus it is complicated to apply attenuation correction. Photon A originates nearer to the surface and has less tissue to traverse, whereas photon B has significantly more tissue to interact with and likely more attenuation, but the detector cannot distinguish this difference. In contrast, PET attenuation is demonstrated in panel **B**. In this situation, both photons must exit, and thus the line of colinearity traverses the whole body along the particular line that is being acquired. The attenuation that affects the photons originating at points C and D is essentially the same. The overall distance the photons travel in PET is greater, and thus, even though they have a lower attenuation coefficient, there is more total attenuation. This ease of correction more than makes up for this and has been routinely applied to PET imaging from the beginning of this technology.

demonstrated in Figure 4-3. F-18 is most frequently administered as the compound F-18-labeled 2-flouro-2-deoxy-D-glucose (FDG). F-18 FDG is taken up by cells through facilitated diffusion by cell membrane glucose transporters.

Fluorine has a relatively low-energy positron with a consequently shorter range in tissue than many other radioisotopes (Table 4-1). The tissue retention is high because of metabolic trapping, so that nearly all of the blood-pool activity has cleared by the time imaging is undertaken. These features and FDG's relatively long half-life combine to provide high-quality images with sharp contrast to background.

F-18 FDG, in most instances, is produced in a central facility, which is responsible for all quality control issues related to the radiopharmaceutical. The FDG is then delivered in unit doses, which have been ordered the day before. Unit doses are calibrated for a specific time of day for injection, thus limiting the flexibility of the imaging facility to some degree.

As in all situations utilizing medical radiation, it is critical to minimize the dose both to the patient and to the technologists and other staff working in the area. It is helpful to compare dose rates to technetium-99m. One hour after a patient receives a dose of 15 mCi of F-18 FDG, the dose rate at 1 m from the patient is 6.2 mrem/h, while the dose rate to technologists from 15 mCi of TC-99m is approximately 0.06 mrem/h.[3]

Newer tracers, such as F-18-labeled FTHA, are permitting investigation of fatty acid oxidation with potentially higher specificity than C-11-labeled isotopes mentioned later.[6]

GLUCOSE METABOLISM

F-18 is most commonly utilized as a component of F-18 FDG, and thus a brief review of myocardial glucose metabolism is warranted. Normally, myocardial cells preferentially utilize fatty acids for energy, but, while damaged or stressed, but still living, myocardial cells undergo a metabolic shift toward glucose metabolism. This physiologic shift is the principle underlying PET viability imaging.

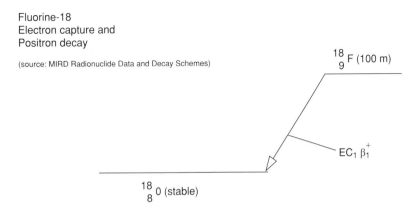

Fluorine-18
Electron capture and
Positron decay

(source: MIRD Radionuclide Data and Decay Schemes)

$^{18}_{9}F$ (100 m)

$EC_1 \beta_1^+$

$^{18}_{8}O$ (stable)

Figure 4-3.   Nuclear decay scheme for flourine-18.

Viability is an important issue, because there are more than 400,000 new cases of congestive heart failure in the United States each year. The identification of those likely to benefit from surgery, while avoiding unnecessary risk in those unlikely to benefit, is the goal of viability testing.

FDG is a glucose analog, which undergoes nearly identical uptake and phosphorylation compared to glucose, thus becoming trapped in the cell. However, the missing hydroxyl group prevents further conversion to fructose-6-phosphate, prohibiting further involvement in glucose metabolism. The steps in which FDG participates are the rate-limiting steps in glucose metabolism, and thus FDG uptake is proportional to glucose uptake, but not a direct measure of glucose metabolism. Metabolic states, which increase glucose uptake, also increase FDG uptake in the myocardium.

The most frequent cardiac application of FDG is for viability assessment. As mentioned before, damaged, but viable, myocardium has a preference for glucose utilization rather than free fatty acids (FFAs), which are preferred by healthy myocardial cells. This uptake can be further enhanced by glucose loading, and insulin or nicotinic acid derivative administration. Glucose loading stimulates the release of endogenous insulin, decreases the level of FFA, and stimulates the mobilization of glucose transporters to the cell membrane. This shifts the myocardium, particularly injured myocardium, toward glucose utilization. This can be done with either an oral glucose load or a hyperinsulinemic, euglycemic clamp. Many patients, particularly those with diabetes, require exogenous insulin to help drive myocardial glucose uptake. In many cases, an oral glucose protocol (similar to a glucose-tolerance test) provides diagnostic quality images, but in patients with diabetes, the more time-consuming clamp may be required.

However, FDG competes with glucose for uptake primarily via the GLUT 1 and 4 transporters, and thus FDG uptake will be inversely related to glucose level. If needed, insulin can be administered to obtain a blood glucose level below 200 mg/dL, ideally less than 140 mg/dL. Lowering the glucose level, thus, increases relative FDG uptake.

VIABILITY PROTOCOL

Metabolic viability testing with F-18 FDG has two components: resting perfusion and metabolism. Areas of myocardium with normal or near-normal perfusion are inherently viable. However, areas of significantly decreased or absent perfusion may be either viable or nonviable. In these areas, enhanced glucose uptake, as indicated by regional FDG uptake, indicates ongoing metabolism, and thus viability. Therefore, a study demonstrating

Table 4-1

Intrinsic Properties of Positron Emitters Used in Cardiology

Isotope	$T_{1/2}$	Avg. β^+ Energy (MeV)	Max β^+ Energy (MeV)	β^+ Range Average (mm)	β^+ Range Maximum (mm)	Production	Delivery
Fluorine-18	110 min	0.250 (100%)	0.64	0.64	2.3	Accelerator O-18(p,n)F-18	Offsite radiopharmacy, regional distribution of unit doses
Carbon-11	20.4 min	0.385 (99.8%)	0.96	1.03	3.9	Accelerator N-14 (p,α)C-11	On-site cyclotron, semiautomated chemistry laboratory
Nitrogen-13	9.97 min	0.492 (99.8%)	1.19	1.32	5.1	Accelerator O-16(p,α)N-13	On-site cyclotron, semiautomated chemistry laboratory
Oxygen-15	122 s	0.735 (99.9%)	1.72	2.01	8.0	Accelerator N-14(d,n)O-15	On-site cyclotron, direct infusion to imaging room
Rubidium-82	75 s	1.523 (83.3%) 1.157 (10.2%)	3.35	4.29	16.5	Generator Sr-82/Rb-82	Generator, direct infusion into patient

Average β^+ energies are given along with the percentage of decays in which they occur.
After Jadvar and Parker.[3]

mismatch, that is decreased perfusion with enhanced metabolism, is considered viable. Areas with perfusion and metabolism match, both are decreased, are nonviable.

Essentially any technique could be used to demonstrate resting perfusion: thallium-201 SPECT, Tc-99m-labeled agents, Rb-82, O-15 H_2O or N-13 NH3 PET, or potentially CT or MR. These images are then compared to the FDG images. The goal of viability testing is enhanced sensitivity for viable cells; thus, glucose metabolism is stimulated, typically with oral glucose loading (25–100 g), to stimulate insulin secretion and glucose uptake, with FDG injection (5–15 mCi) when blood glucose has normalized. FDG imaging should be initiated 45 to 60 minutes after injection. Patients with diabetes frequently require an IV hyperinsulinemic, euglycemic clamp to obtain diagnostic images. Image acquisition typically lasts 10 to 30 minutes, depending on the count rate and system being utilized. ECG gating is optional. A detailed explanation of the factors involved in designing a protocol is available in the recent guidelines of the American Society of Nuclear Cardiology.[5]

RUBIDIUM-82

Rubidium-82 (Rb-82) emits primarily positrons (decay 95% positron, 5% electron capture, 776-keV gamma 15% abundance, 1395-keV gamma 0.5% abundance), with the added benefit that it is generator produced and does not require an on-site cyclotron (Figure 4-4). Rb-82 is a potassium analog, similar to thallium-201, and relies on the same K^+/Na^+ ATPase transporter. Rb-82 has a half-life of 75 seconds and, thus, requires direct injection into the patient with immediate imaging.

The generator is similar in function to a Mo-99/Tc-99m generator. The parent strontium-82 (Sr-82) is adsorbed on a stannic oxide column, while the daughter, Rb-82, is soluble in normal saline. The two isotopes exist in secular equilibrium, the half-life of the parent (Sr-82, $T_{1/2}$ 25 days) being much greater than that of the daughter (Rb-82, $T_{1/2}$ 75 seconds). The relationship allows Rb-82 levels to build up to full equilibrium levels in 10–12 minutes. Full doses can be obtained every 10 minutes, facilitating rapid serial studies. Rb-82 decays to krypton-82, which is stable.

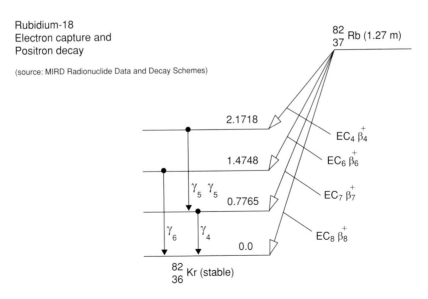

Figure 4-4. Nuclear decay scheme for rubidium-82.

The short $T_{1/2}$ of Rb-82 requires direct injection into the patient. Currently this requires a proprietary infusion cart, which is available through the manufacturer of the generator, Bracco (Princeton, NJ). This cart includes shielding for the generator, an infusion/elution pump to circulate saline, a pressure-sensitive switch to divert the elution to a waste container if high pressures are encountered, and a radiation detector to measure the dose that has been administered. These components are connected directly to the infusion line, so the patient receives nearly all of the eluted dose that had been requested. The available dose decreases over the course of the 1-month lifetime of the generator in proportion to the decrease in remaining Sr-82 activity. The generator is typically replaced every 28 days.

Quality control is the responsibility of the administering facility. The main factor that must be accounted for is Sr-82 and Sr-85 breakthrough. This is monitored by holding the first elution of the day for all Rb-82 to decay and then assaying the remaining activity. The allowable level of Sr-82 is 0.02 mCi per mCi of Rb-82 and for Sr-85 is 0.2 mCi per mCi of Rb-82.[7]

Rubidium is used clinically for myocardial perfusion imaging studies. Either a stand-alone PET scanner with line-source transmission capabilities or a PET/CT scanner can be used. Rubidium has been imaged with good results using all types of detectors in both 2D and 3D mode. ECG-gated images are readily acquired using current protocols, and software has been developed to display tomographic images in very similar formats to SPECT images that many are familiar with. Rubidium is a potassium analog and localizes to viable cells in a flow-dependent manner. It has somewhat decreased extraction at high flow rates, intermediate between sestamibi and thallium-201 (Figure 4-5). The short half-life of Rb-82 presents challenges to imaging. Optimal imaging must strike a balance between blood-pool clearance and radioactive decay. A typical protocol involves rest imaging, followed by the stress test, which is then followed by stress imaging (Figure 4-6). The rest and stress acquisitions typically use the same dose and imaging parameters. PET/CT scanners typically require a scout and transmission scan before each PET acquisition, while line source detectors can perform the transmission scan either before or

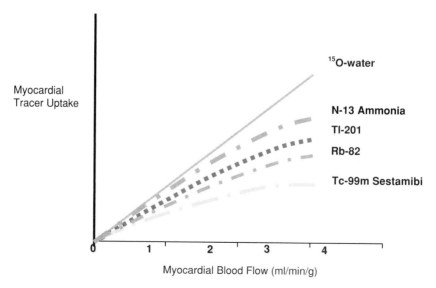

Figure 4-5. Relative myocardial uptake in relation to blood flow ("roll off") for commonly used medical isotopes.

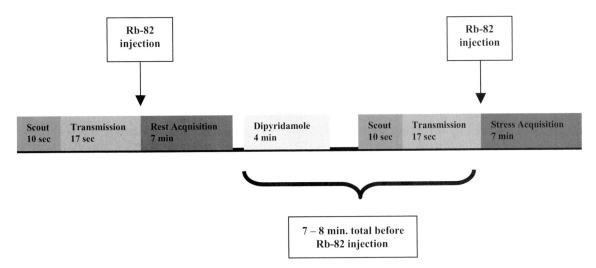

Figure 4-6. Rubidium myocardial perfusion imaging protocol. The scout film is used to position the table to acquire the entire cardiac silhouette in the field of view of the camera. Transmission CT scan is then performed. Without moving the patient on the table, the table then moves to the PET detector for Rb-82 acquisition. Rb-82 imaging incorporates the 1- to 2-minute delay for blood-pool clearance and 5-minute count acquisition. The table is then brought out of the camera for stress agent administration. After dipyridamole is finished, the scout, transmission, and table repositioning are repeated, which often takes 3 to 4 minutes at which time peak vasodilation has been reached and the stress dose of Rb-82 can be administered and then imaged.

after acquisition. Rb-82 injection is done using the cart described above and typically requires 20 to 30 seconds to complete. Following this, there is a delay of 1 to 2 minutes to allow for blood-pool clearance. As lower doses are being acquired at the end pf the generator life, shorter delays are used. In situations where one expects delayed blood-pool clearance, such as severe left ventricular dysfunction, longer delays are used. Acquisition is typically 5 minutes long, for a total scan time of 6 to 7 minutes. Longer delays will have poor counts, and shorter delays are complicated by poor target-to-background ratio. By the time rest image acquisition and the stress modality have been completed, the generator has returned to equilibrium and another full dose is ready for stress acquisition. The rest dose should have completely decayed in the patient and not interfere with stress counts.

Currently most protocols utilize dipyridamole, adenosine, and less commonly dobutamine for the stress agent. Exercise presents challenges as a stress

modality related to room design, breathing artifact, and patient positioning, but is currently being explored and may be a viable option in the future.

Positioning and limiting motion are critical to obtaining high-quality imaging. Misregistration artifacts can create artificial defects, which can mimic coronary artery disease. These artifacts can be the result of breathing, cardiac motion, patient motion during PET acquisition, or, most commonly, patient motion between the CT scan and Rb-82 acquisition. Software solutions are currently in development and should be readily available in the near future.

NITROGEN-13 AMMONIA

Nitrogen-13 (N-13) is a cyclotron-produced positron emitter, which requires an on-site cyclotron as a result of its short half-life ($T_{1/2} = 9.96$ minutes). Decay is primarily by positron emission.

Maximum and average positron energies are mid-range at 1.19 and 0.492 MeV, respectively (Table 4-1). This tracer requires synthesis of ammonia after production of the radioisotope, which is possible with semiautomated chemistry stations. N-13 is produced by the nuclear equation ^{16}O (p,α) ^{13}N and decays to carbon-13, which is stable.[8] Sub-batches are tested for chemical and radionuclidic purity before each batch is administered to the patient. Prior to the availability of Rb-82 generators, most PET myocardial perfusion was studied with N-13 ammonia, although this may be changing as Rb-82 expands to sites without cyclotrons.

Neutral ammonia (NH_3) easily diffuses across cell membranes. Rapid metabolism of ammonia to N-13 glutamine by glutamine synthase traps the N-13 in the tissue, where it is incorporated into the cellular amino acid pool. Ammonia is rapidly cleared, with 85% being removed from the circulation within 1 minute. Because of the relatively low-energy positron and relatively long half-life, high-quality images with good resolution can be obtained. There is essentially no blood-pool activity remaining at the time of imaging, so no subtraction of this activity is required as it is with O-15 H_2O. Myocardial uptake is nearly linear with

increasing myocardial flow until approximately 3 mL/mg/min, at which point it begins to plateau. This is favorable compared to other common radiotracers (Figure 4-5).

Clinically, N-13 ammonia is used for 1 day rest/stress myocardial perfusion protocols. The relatively long half-life requires a waiting period between rest and stress for decay of the N-13, which is on the order of 45 minutes to 1 hour. Often patients are staggered, with the second patient completing their rest scan before the first patient has their pharmacologic stress and stress acquisition. The protocol is demonstrated in Figure 4-7 (adapted from Ref. 9). ECG-gated or ECG-ungated images may be acquired, and a separate dynamic acquisition may be used to permit quantification.[10] Image quality is very high, but the duration of the overall protocol can easily extend past 2 hours.

Very-high-quality images can be obtained with N-13 ammonia in either the 2D or the 3D acquisition mode. One peculiar aspect of N-13 ammonia is a decrease in counts in the lateral wall, even in normal volunteers, which must be recognized. The mechanism of this heterogeneous uptake is not known.[11] As with all radiotracers, N-13 ammonia is susceptible to uptake in noncardiac

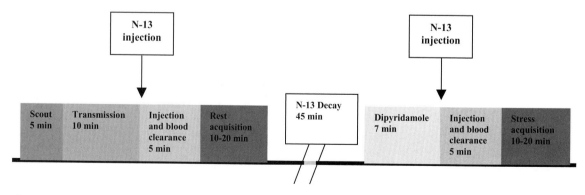

Figure 4-7. N-13 ammonia myocardial perfusion imaging protocol. Similar to Rb-82, a transmission map is acquired, often prior to any PET acquisition. This protocol demonstrates transmission with a scanning line source, although CT scan can be used as well. After N-13 ammonia injection a delay for blood clearance is necessary, and, because of the longer half-life than rubidium, adequate counts remain. Lower doses are administered compared to Rb-82, but the longer half-life allows a longer acquisition period and more than adequate counts are obtained.

structures obscuring the area of interest, particularly liver and lung uptake, although this does not frequently limit interpretation.[12]

CARBON-11

Carbon is an essential element in the human body and can be incorporated into many biological molecules. Semiautomated systems are available to assist in the synthesis of many of these molecules. Additionally, the half-life of carbon-11 (20.4 minutes) is such that there is time to make relatively complex radiotracers such as fatty acids and receptor agonists and antagonists and other molecules targeting many biologic pathways in the body. Carbon-11, like O-15 and N-13, requires an on-site cyclotron because while the half-life is long enough to permit synthesis, it is not long enough to permit regional distribution, as is the case with F-18.

The isotope is produced through the reaction $^{14}N(p,\alpha)^{11}C$. Carbon-11 decays by positron emission and electron capture to boron-11, which is stable.[8] The positron has low to intermediate energy (average ß+ energy 0.385 MeV) and, consequently, a short distance traveled prior to annihilation (average ß+ range 1.03 mm). Frequently, C-11 is synthesized into acetate or palmitate, which are incorporated into the Krebs cycle and can measure oxidative metabolism in the heart. Both C-11 acetate and C-11 palmitate may also provide an opportunity to evaluate myocardial perfusion and blood flow as well, but currently they are not used clinically for this purpose. Palmitate may have longer tissue retention and therefore simpler kinetics compared to acetate because acetate is more readily converted to CO_2 and released from the myocardium. These measures of beta-oxidation trace the metabolism of FFAs. Currently, these tracers are limited to research applications.

Under normal conditions, fatty acids are the preferred energy source in the myocardium; however, this requires significant amounts of oxygen. Under ischemic conditions, fatty acid metabolism is decreased and glucose metabolism is upregulated, as described in the section on viability. The clinical utility of fatty acid metabolism imaging is unclear but may have a role in ischemic memory imaging, as the normalization from glucose metabolism back to fatty acid utilization can be delayed 24 to 48 hours after ischemia has resolved. Furthermore, fatty acid metabolism may be altered in cardiomyopathies such as hypertrophic cardiomyopathy (HCM) out of proportion to blood flow disturbance.[13]

Carbon-11 can also be incorporated into other molecules such as hydroxyephedrine, epinephrine, phenylephrine, pindolol, prazosin, and acetylcholine receptor antagonists for investigation into sympathetic and parasympathetic nervous systems.

SUMMARY

PET imaging has many advantages related to the physics of positron emission and coincidence imaging. Additionally, the available radiotracers offer dramatic flexibility in targeting physiologic pathways and molecular processes because of the ability to incorporate positron-emitting isotopes of essential elements into common molecules. Positron emitters have a common end point, annihilation, but many differences, including positron energy, inherent resolution, half-life, and method of delivery. Current clinical cardiac PET imaging is dominated by metabolic imaging with F-18 FDG and perfusion imaging with N-13 ammonia and Rb-82, while many centers are actively involved in research utilizing O-15 H_2O and C-11 molecules. Research is under way to incorporate the optimal characteristics of F-18 into other molecules targeted toward myocardial perfusion or plaque imaging. Limiting factors for PET imaging include the need for an on-site cyclotron and synthetic radiopharmacy skills to take advantage of many of the molecules of interest. The spread of PET scanners initially dedicated to oncologic imaging has removed one of the financial barriers to cardiac PET imaging and ushered in an era of rapid advancement in clinical cardiac PET.

REFERENCES

1. Kong BA, Shaw LS, Miller DD, et al., Comparison of accuracy for detecting coronary artery disease and side-effect profile of dipyridamole thallium-201 myocardial perfusion imaging in women versus men. *Am J Cardiol*. 1992;70:168–173.
2. Case JA, Cullom, SJ, Bateman TM. Myocardial perfusion single-photon emission computed tomography attenuation correction. In: Iskandrian AE, Verani MS, eds. *Nuclear Cardiac Imaging Principles and Practice*. 3rd ed. New York: Oxford University Press; 2003:106–120.
3. Jadvar H, Parker JA. *Clinical PET and PET/CT*. London: Springer-Verlag; 2005:1–68.
4. Schwarz SW, Caehle GG, Welch MJ. Accelerators and positron emission tomography (PET) Radiopharmaceuticals. In: Sandler MP, Coleman RE, Patton JA, et al., eds. *Diagnostic Nuclear Medicine*. 4th ed. New York: Lippincott Williams and Wilkins; 2003:117–131.
5. Bacharach SL, et al. American Society of Nuclear Cardiology practice guidelines: PET myocardial glucose metabolism and perfusion imaging. *J Nucl Cardiol*. 2001;10(5):543–554.
6. Takala TO, Nuutila P, Pulkki K, et al. 14 (R,S)-[18F] fluoro-6-thiaheptadecanoic acid as a tracer of free fatty acid uptake and oxidation in myocardium and skeletal muscle. *Eur J Nucl Med*. 2002;29:1617–1622.
7. *CardioGen-82* [Package insert]. Princeton, NJ: Bracco Diagnostics; 2000.
8. Nuclear Decay in the MIRD Format. National Nuclear Data Center. 2006. http://www.nndc.bnl.gov/mird/.
9. Mahac J. Cardiac positron emission tomography imaging. *Semin Nucl Med*. 2005;35:17–36.
10. Sawada S, Muzik O, Beanlands RS, et al. Interobserver and interstudy variability of myocardial blood flow and flow-reserve measurements with nitrogen-13 ammonia-labeled positron emission tomography. *J Nucl Cardiol*. 1995;2:413–422.
11. Beanlands R, Muzik O, Hitchins G, et al. Heterogeneity of regional nitrogen 13-labeled ammonia tracer distribution in the normal heart: Comparison with rubidium-82 and copper-62-labeled PTSM. *J Nucl Cardiol*. 1994;35:1122–1124.
12. Tamaki N, Ruddy TD, Dekamp R, et al. Myocardial perfusion. In: Wahl RL, Buchanan JW, eds. *Principles and Practice of Positron Emission Tomography*. Philadelphia, PA: Lipincott, Williams & Wilkins; 2002:320–333.
13. Ohtsuki K, Sugihara H, Kuribayashi T, et al. Impairment of BMIPP accumulation at junction of ventricular septum and left and right ventricular free walls in hypertrophic cardiomyopathy. *J Nucl Med*. 1999;40:2007–2013.

CHAPTER 5

Fatty Acid Metabolic SPECT Imaging: Applications in Nuclear Cardiology

Christopher Pastore
Edouard Daher
John Babich
James E. Udelson

Free fatty acids are the major substrate for energy production in the heart under normal conditions of oxygen delivery. Approximately 60% to 80% of the heart energy demand is derived from fatty acids beta-oxidation, and the remaining demand is supplied from glucose metabolism. Under ischemic conditions, the heart shifts its metabolism from preferentially fatty acids to glucose, as this allows the myocardium to remain viable with low energy expenditure.[1] Thus, the study of fatty acid metabolism has been considered as a sensitive marker of myocardial ischemia.

Imaging of fatty acid metabolism has been accomplished using a variety of 123-labelled fatty acids to evaluate cardiac oxidative metabolism.[2]

FATTY ACID RADIOPHARMACEUTICALS

The ideal synthetic fatty acid analog for clinical metabolic imaging of the myocardium is one that avoids rapid catabolism, demonstrates high uptake, and is retained long enough in myocardial cells to allow acquisition via conventional gamma camera imaging by SPECT or by positron emission tomography (PET). The ideal fatty acid radiopharmaceutical should also be relatively stable and readily available when clinically needed. Each of these prerequisites is critical for the suitability and feasibility of fatty acid metabolic imaging of the myocardium in clinical settings, where an impact on clinical decision making is dependent on the production of reliable, high-quality images that can be generated with predictable pharmacokinetics of the administered radiotracer.

Initial noninvasive investigations of alterations in myocardial energy substrate utilization patterns used the positron-emitting radiotracer C-11 palmitate.[3,4] Widespread use of this method in human clinical studies is limited by the requirement of an on-site cyclotron and a PET camera. For this reason, gamma-emitting fatty acid radiopharmaceuticals that can be imaged with conventional

SPECT cameras have emerged as the focus of investigations examining the potential role for myocardial metabolic imaging in acute and chronic disease states.

Several radiopharmaceuticals have been developed for the purpose of evaluating myocardial energy substrate utilization patterns. Naturally occurring fatty acids such as palmitate are rapidly metabolized by ß-oxidation and cleared, thus limiting the feasibility of their utility in clinical noninvasive imaging. ^{123}I-iodophenylpentadecanoic acid (IPPA) is a straight-chain fatty acid that demonstrates myocardial uptake proportional to regional perfusion. Under nonischemic conditions IPPA is rapidly metabolized and released, resulting in rapid washout kinetics.[5] In the setting of ischemia, suppressed metabolism results in longer myocardial retention and a redistribution pattern on serial imaging.[6] In clinical trials, IPPA has been successfully used to diagnose coronary stenosis, detect myocardial ischemia,[7] determine myocardial viability,[8] and predict recovery of regional left ventricular dysfunction following revascularization.[9] Nevertheless, the rapid kinetics of IPPA metabolism and washout have limited the feasibility of its clinical utility.

ß-Methyl-*p*-(^{123}I)-iodophenylpentadecanoic acid (BMIPP) is a diagnostic radiopharmaceutical that has been designed to evaluate myocardial metabolic substrate utilization patterns. BMIPP is marketed in Japan as Cardiodine® and has been approved for use there since 1993 in the diagnosis of ischemic heart disease, cardiomyopathy, myocarditis, and valvular heart disease. BMIPP is an iodine-labeled branched-chain fatty acid that is retained predominantly in myocardial cells following intravenous administration and does not readily undergo ß-oxidation. The addition of the methyl group to the fatty acid substrate (Figure 5-1) results in intramyocardial trapping with limited catabolism, such that its metabolism is substantially slowed compared to natural fatty acids.[10,11] Prolonged intramyocardial retention of BMIPP, coupled with rapid clearance from the blood and limited extracardiac uptake, allows for high-quality planar and SPECT imaging to be

15-(p-Iodo-phenyl)-3-R,S-methylpentadecanoic acid (BMIPP)

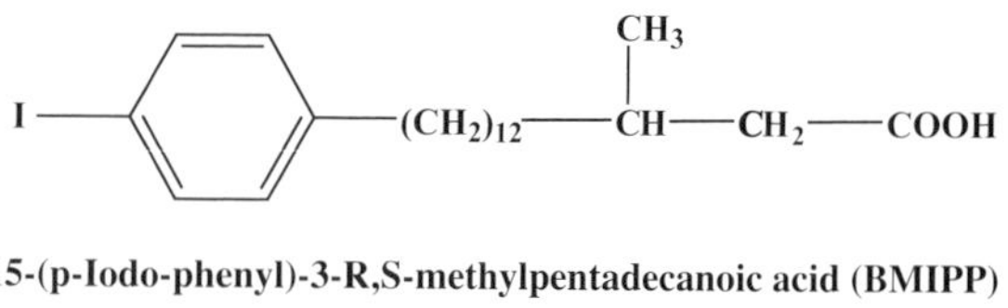

Figure 5-1. The structure of BMIPP.

obtained with high heart-to-background ratios as early as 15–30 minutes after tracer administration.[12]

The clinical utility of BMIPP imaging stems from the fact that alterations in fatty acid metabolism resulting from transient ischemia persist for prolonged periods, even after perfusion has returned to normal (ischemic memory).[13] In dysfunctional myocardium, a disproportionately greater decrease in BMIPP compared to a perfusion tracer uptake may represent a state of repetitive ischemia with recurrent stunning and has been shown to correlate with preserved inotropic reserve[14] and histological evidence of viability[15] and predict postrevascularization recovery of function.[16–18] On the other hand, a concordant, severe reduction in both BMIPP uptake and perfusion indicates predominantly infarcted tissue that is unlikely to recover function.

KINETICS OF BMIPP

Several studies have investigated tracer kinetics of myocardial metabolism with BMIPP. Animals and human experiments have shown BMIPP to be a potentially useful radiotracer of cardiac fatty acid metabolism, as a result of the high first extraction of the tracer by the myocardium (60%–80%), high retention (60%) by residing in the triglyceride (TG) pool, slow clearance from the myocardium (25% in 2 hours), and minimal back diffusion (~8%).[19] In addition, the target to background ratio is favorable for cardiac imaging, with high myocardial-to-lung and myocardial-to-blood ratios at the time of imaging. BMIPP uptake in the myocardium is believed to reflect accumulation of fatty acids in the TG pool and is, therefore, affected by TG synthesis, and has been shown to be closely related to the level of ATP in the myocardium, which is critical to the acetylation into BMIPP-CoA, which then is stored into the TG storage pool. Experimental studies have been performed to evaluate the effect of different substrates levels on the uptake and storage of BMIPP in the TG pool. Nohara et al.[19] found that infusion of lipid substrate significantly decreased the uptake and extraction of BMIPP and increased the washout through back-diffusion. Similarly, increase lactate levels had the same effects. In contrast, infusion of glucose substrate had minimal impact on BMIPP uptake and washout. This should be taken into consideration when interpreting BMIPP images, since this may underestimate the amount of ischemia or viable myocardium based on fatty acid level in the blood.

IMAGING BMIPP

Patient Preparation

Patients have traditionally been asked to fast overnight to make sure that a steady metabolic state is maintained. For the purpose of evaluation of myocardial viability and cardiomyopathy, a 20-minute resting SPECT BMIPP imaging has generally been performed approximately 20 to 30 minutes after tracer administration. Image analysis may be performed in conjunction with a SPECT perfusion tracer such as Tl-201 or more recently with Tc-99m radioactive tracers, with perfusion data acquired at a separate sitting. BMIPP imaging has been compared to Tl-201 and Tc-99m SPECT imaging by numerous investigators,[20] and it is believed that the initial distribution of BMIPP 2 to 5 minutes after injection reflects myocardial perfusion, while 20 to 30 minutes later it reflects more metabolism and myocardial viability. More recent data have challenged this concept. Finally, approximately 0.2% to 1% of the patients will have absent uptake of BMIPP in the myocardium, which is believed to be caused by either a deficiency of the membrane transporter involved in fatty acids

uptake in the myocardium or a shift in cardiac metabolism to glucose, which is more likely to happen in cases of severe ischemia, or anaerobic metabolism because of lactate accumulation.

ACQUISITION PROTOCOLS

SPECT imaging can be performed after the injection of 3 to 4 mCi of BMIPP using a double- or triple-headed gamma camera equipped with either a low-energy all-purpose (LEAP) or a low-energy high-resolution (LEHR) collimator, the latter resulting in significant improvement in signal-to-noise ratio. Ideally, medium-energy collimators could be used although are not as widely available. For BMIPP SPECT acquisition, a symmetrical window of 10% to 20% is set around the 159-keV photopeak of BMIPP. SPECT images are then obtained approximately 10 minutes after injection for "early" images, and 20 to 30 minutes later for approximately 20 minutes for the "late" images. Both are acquired in a step and shoot mode. Images can be acquired over either 180- or 360-degree circumference and stored on a 64×64 digital matrix.

Recent investigations have attempted to optimize the acquisition of I-123-based tracers, as the standard SPECT collimators (such as LEHR collimators) are not ideal. Abundant high-energy photons can penetrate the septa of LEHR collimators, degrading imaging quality, and a proportion the peak 159-keV photons are blocked. These issues are minimized with the use of medium-energy all-purpose (MEAP) collimators, but these are not widely available. Chen and colleagues[21] have recently demonstrated that by incorporating a technique known as deconvolution of septal penetration (DSP) into the processing algorithm, I-123 images acquired with LEHR collimators can be optimized, with the resulting tracer distribution accurate enough to allow the creation of quantitative databases. This approach will be very important in the current development of BMIPP and other I-123-based tracers, as clinicians in recent years have become more comfortable and accepting of quantitative programs.

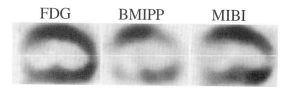

FDG   BMIPP   MIBI

Figure 5-2. Energy substrate utilization patterns in ischemia and infarction as detected by FDG, BMIPP, and ^{99m}Tc-sestamibi SPECT imaging. Vertical long-axis SPECT images of a 66-year-old man with anterior myocardial infarction and old inferior myocardial infarction. A mismatch pattern with reduced BMIPP uptake with relatively preserved sestamibi uptake is seen in the anterior wall, correlating with viability by FDG imaging in that wall. (Adapted from Sato et al.[32])

Image Analysis and Interpretation

The myocardium can be divided into a 17- or 20-segment model, and segments can be quantified according to recommended guidelines on a 5-point scoring system. Summed scores can then be calculated for either stress and rest perfusion or perfusion–metabolic mismatch (Figure 5-2). A >10% of the left ventricle mismatch is considered clinically significant and correlates with improvement in function after revascularization.[20] Three main patterns of perfusion (Tl-201 or Tc-99m radioactive tracers) and metabolism (BMIPP tracer) have been recognized in the literature and correlated with distinct clinical scenarios. In patients with regional myocardial dysfunction, matched defects between perfusion and BMIPP are suggestive of predominant scar and will not improve postrevascularization, while a mismatch pattern with lower uptake of BMIPP compared to a perfusion tracer has been correlated with viable myocardium and is predictive of improvement in regional function after revascularization. In patients with hypertrophic cardiomyopathy a heterogeneous uptake of BMIPP in the myocardium or with lower BMIPP uptake in the septum and apical areas has been reported. This pattern has been shown to preclude any glucose abnormality by FDG imaging, or perfusion abnormality with Tl-201.[22] Recently, gated BMIPP SPECT imaging has been

introduced by Inubushi et al.[23] and found to be able to accurately and simultaneously assess myocardial free fatty acid utilization and left ventricular function as calculated by a quantitative gated SPECT software.

POTENTIAL CLINICAL APPLICATIONS

Fatty Acid Imaging in the Assessment of Acute Chest Pain

The appropriate triage of patients with chest pain presenting to the emergency department remains a challenge to the health-care system in the United States. This challenge is defined by the number (more than 6 million) of ED presentations for chest pain each year, 40% of which result in hospitalization for further evaluation of suspected acute coronary syndrome (ACS).[24] Of these patients admitted for the "rule out of myocardial infarction," many are later found to be either disease free or suffering from lower acuity conditions. The associated cost of care for these patients may exceed $3 billion annually.[25] This cost is absorbed by our health-care system, given the overriding concern for the need to achieve rapid reperfusion and myocardial salvage in the approximate 1 million chest pain presentations determined to represent acute myocardial infarction, and for the appropriate treatment of the additional 1 million chest pain presentations consistent with unstable angina. Furthermore, it is estimated that 2% to 3% of all acute myocardial infarctions are missed in emergency departments each year.

However, patients presenting with clear ECG changes of ST elevation or depression do not constitute a large majority of those ultimately diagnosed with an ACS. The rapidity of achieving an accurate diagnosis in cases of suspected, but not obvious, ACS is hindered by atypical descriptions of symptoms, the delayed time course of serum cardiac biomarkers, and equivocal ECG findings. The need for a more rapid and accurate diagnostic test for chest pain is underscored by the persistent inability of many acute care centers to consistently avoid delay in diagnosis and to achieve adequate door to balloon times in cases of acute ST elevation myocardial infarction.[26] The primary objectives of the development of myocardial metabolic imaging for the assessment of patients with acute chest pain are, therefore, to minimize unnecessary hospitalizations and inappropriate discharges, while facilitating and expediting definitive medical or revascularization therapy in the setting of ACS.

Rest SPECT Perfusion Imaging: Strengths and Limitations A resting myocardial perfusion scan is an important diagnostic tool for the assessment of acute chest pain of unclear etiology, based on the concept that SPECT imaging of the myocardium following the injection of a perfusion tracer reflects myocardial blood flow at the time of injection. Rest perfusion imaging is a powerful predictor of myocardial infarction when performed early after presentation to the emergency department with chest pain.[27] Patients with active chest pain are risk stratified with a single injection of perfusion tracer, followed by rest acquisition of SPECT myocardial images. Substantial observational data as well as data from randomized, controlled trials have resulted in high-level class IA recommendation for resting SPECT perfusion imaging in this clinical setting.[28]

However, most data suggest that resting SPECT perfusion is of optimal diagnostic value during symptoms, or relatively early after symptom resolution, and may be of more limited diagnostic utility greater than 2 to 3 hours after the resolution of chest pain. The injection of perfusion tracer at rest beyond 2 hours after the cessation of symptoms is, therefore, likely to result in a suboptimally diagnostic study.[27] Thus, in the absence of active chest pain, a reliable diagnostic evaluation of chest pain (to make a diagnosis of ACS and/or underlying CAD) requires provocative exercise or pharmacologic stress testing in order to induce a reversible perfusion defect (once very recent infarction has been ruled out with sufficient probability). It is important to note that normal resting SPECT perfusion imaging studies have been shown to identify a patient with low-risk ED chest

pain even when injected out to 6 hours after symptom resolution.[29]

Ischemic Memory

Fatty acid imaging of the myocardium with BMIPP SPECT offers potential advantages over the conventional resting perfusion scan because it theoretically extends the window of opportunity for imaging to approximately 30 hours after the cessation of chest pain symptoms. Following an ischemic event, myocardial blood flow normalizes long before metabolism returns to steady state. While myocardial blood flow, as detected by SPECT imaging, returns to baseline within 2 to 3 hours following an ischemic event, the ischemia-induced shift from fatty acid to glucose metabolism persists for a prolonged period that allows for fatty acid imaging of a metabolic imprint called "ischemic memory." This reversible process of prolonged metabolic alteration has also been referred to as "metabolic stunning."

The utility of BMIPP SPECT for the assessment of acute chest pain in patients with ED was reported by Kawai and associates in 2001.[30] In a prospective study, 111 patients with acute chest pain and without obvious myocardial infarction underwent resting tetrofosmin SPECT within 24 hours of the last episode of chest pain, followed by BMIPP SPECT and coronary angiography on the next day (Figure 5-3). Coronary angiography revealed a significant stenosis (luminal narrowing >75%) or coronary spasm in 87 patients. In this group, resting perfusion abnormalities corresponding to the territory of the diseased vessel were found in 33 patients (sensitivity 38%), whereas reduced uptake of BMIPP in corresponding segments on resting SPECT images were found in 64 patients (sensitivity 74%; $p < 0.001$). Of 24 patients with no angiographic evidence of coronary disease, 23 patients had normal resting perfusion and 22 patients had normal BMIPP uptake (specificity 96% and 92%, respectively; $p =$ NS).

An open-label Phase 2A clinical trial investigating the utility of BMIPP SPECT to detect

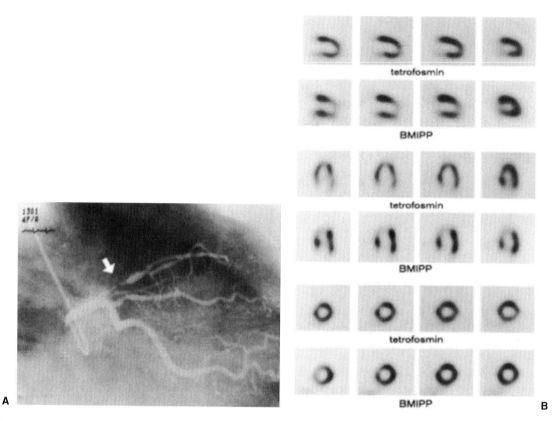

Figure 5-3. BMIPP and tetrofosmin SPECT imaging in the evaluation of acute chest pain. (**A**) Coronary arteriogram of a 65-year-old woman with effort angina. Severe stenosis is seen in the left anterior descending coronary artery (arrow). (**B**) Sequential tetrofosmin images. No significant abnormal perfusion is observed on the tetrofosmin images obtained at the time of hospital admission. However, the BMIPP images obtained on the next day show severely reduced uptake in the apex and anteroseptal regions. (Adapted from Kawai et al.[30])

myocardial ischemic memory up to 30 hours, following exercise-induced demand ischemia, was conducted and reported by Dilsizian et al. in 2005 (13). In this study, 32 patients who were found to have exercise-induced ischemia on a clinically indicated thallium SPECT imaging study underwent rest SPECT imaging 10 minutes (early) and again 30 minutes (delayed) after BMIPP injection. The ability of BMIPP to detect an ischemic abnormality was evidenced by agreement between BMIPP and thallium data with both early (91% agreement, 95% CI, 75%–98%) and delayed imaging (94% agreement, 95% CI, 79%–99%) (Figure 5-4). Agreement between BMIPP and thallium

data for the presence of an abnormality was similar, whether performed on the same day (mean of 6 hours after ischemia) or on the following day (mean of 25 hours after ischemia) (95% vs. 91%, respectively, $p = $ NS). A significant correlation was found between the magnitude of the resting BMIPP metabolic defect and the magnitude of the exercise-induced thallium perfusion defect ($r = 0.6$, $p = 0.001$, for early BMIPP; $r = 0.5$, $p = 0.005$, for delayed BMIPP).

In summary, initial small clinical trials investigating the diagnostic utility of BMIPP in the assessment of acute chest pain have demonstrated the ability of fatty acid imaging with BMIPP

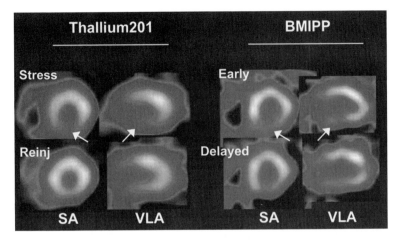

Figure 5-4.   BMIPP detection of ischemic memory after demand ischemia. (**Left**) Thallium-201 stress and reinjection (Reinj) images after treadmill exercise in the short axis (SA) and vertical long axis (VLA) SPECT tomograms (left). Thallium images demonstrate a severe reversible inferior defect (arrows), consistent with exercise stress-induced ischemia. (**Right**) A similar defect is seen on the early BMIPP images in the same tomographic cuts (arrows), with BMIPP injected 22 hours after the stress-induced ischemia. The defect on the delayed BMIPP image is less prominent than on the early image. These image data suggest that BMIPP detects prolonged postischemic suppression of fatty acid metabolism for up to 22 hours after stress-induced ischemia. (Adapted from Dilsizian et al.[13]) (See color insert.)

SPECT to identify an ischemic imprint up to 30 hours following the onset of both "supply-type" ischemia because of ACS and "demand-type" ischemia induced by exercise. Future clinical trials of larger size are needed to further investigate larger patients groups and to assess the anatomical correlation of fatty acid imaging with the site and severity of coronary disease found at cardiac catheterization, to further define the time window of suppression of fatty acid metabolism after ischemia and to compare both the clinical effectiveness and the cost effectiveness of this approach to other emerging diagnostic imaging techniques.

Fatty Acid Imaging for Prediction of Left Ventricular Functional Recovery After Acute Myocardial Infarction

The extent of myocardial salvage is often unclear at the time of mechanical or thrombolytic revascularization for acute myocardial infarction. Despite restoration of culprit epicardial coronary vessel pa-

tency, some patients are found to have varying degrees of left ventricular dysfunction early after acute myocardial infarction. Left ventricular dysfunction at this early time point can be because of reversible causes such as myocardial stunning or persistent ischemia, or because of irreversible infarct. An early predictive test of left ventricular functional recovery would be of significant value in terms of determining prognosis, risk stratification for future adverse events, and identification of candidates for further revascularization and/or adjunctive therapy.

An analysis of the metabolic state of the myocardium following acute myocardial infarction may provide important predictive information. As previously described, the myocardium undergoes a protective metabolic shift in energy substrate utilization from fatty acids to glucose in response to acute ischemic injury. Increasing experimental evidence supports the concept that the impairment of recovery of normal energy substrate metabolism may be the mechanism responsible for stunning or reperfusion injury and that the predominance of glucose metabolism is required to support optimal functional recovery.[31] In the isolated perfused rat heart model of ischemia and reperfusion, an increase in carbohydrate metabolism is accompanied by a significant improvement of contractile function during reperfusion of ischemic hearts.[2] Furthermore, the concentration-dependent inhibition of glucose oxidation by fatty acids may adversely affect the recovery of function.[31] A postischemic recovery mode characterized by a prolonged predominance of glucose metabolism corresponds to viable myocardium with the potential for functional recovery. Recovery of the myocardium from ischemia is facilitated by the predominant oxidation of glucose, since this is the most efficient metabolic substrate for high-energy ATP production.

Reduced uptake of BMIPP on SPECT images corresponds to the metabolic shift from fatty acid to glucose utilization that is characteristic of metabolic recovery following acute myocardial infarction. A postinfarct dual isotope SPECT imaging study that demonstrates uptake of a technetium-99m perfusion tracer, but decreased uptake of BMIPP, suggests the presence of viable myocardium that is in a state of metabolic recovery. A perfusion/metabolism "mismatch" may be semiquantified by the subtraction of the BMIPP uptake score from the uptake score of the perfusion tracer, using a 17-segment model for instance.

The extent of functional recovery following coronary revascularization was predicted by the assessment of perfusion/metabolism mismatch in a study reported by Sato et al.[32] In this study, 30 consecutive patients with ischemic myocardial dysfunction underwent resting myocardial SPECT imaging with ^{99m}Tc-sestamibi (MIBI), fluorodeoxyglucose (FDG), and BMIPP prior to coronary revascularization. Myocardial segments demonstrating high metabolic mismatch (FDG/BMIPP and MIBI/BMIPP) had the lowest regional wall motion score at baseline, representing the most severely impaired ischemic myocardium, and had the greatest improvement in regional wall motion score after revascularization.

The presence and magnitude of perfusion/metabolism uptake mismatch on dual ^{99m}Tc/BMIPP SPECT imaging also positively correlates with functional recovery when the imaging study is performed after coronary revascularization for acute myocardial infarction.[33] In the post-MI setting, robust metabolic recovery mode is detected by extensive perfusion/metabolism mismatching on ^{99m}Tc/BMIPP SPECT imaging. Conversely, the resumption of steady-state metabolism, as detected by predominant fatty acid utilization and corresponding lack of perfusion/metabolism mismatch, may mark the cessation of functional recovery. A series of small clinical studies (see Table 5-1) has demonstrated the ability of defect mismatch on dual SPECT imaging with BMIPP and a perfusion tracer to predict functional recovery following myocardial infarction.

Risk Stratification for Sudden Cardiac Death

Fatty acid imaging is potentially useful in the determination of the risk spectrum for sudden cardiac death and, thus, theoretically for more efficient patient selection for an implantable cardioverter defibrillator (ICD), particularly in the controversial early period after acute MI. Fatty acid imaging early after myocardial infarction may provide supplementary risk stratification by predicting left ventricular functional recovery and residual left ventricular ejection fraction. Left ventricular ejection fraction, an independent risk factor for sudden death, has become the basis for determining a patient's eligibility for an ICD following myocardial infarction. Current American College of Cardiology—American Heart Association guidelines for the management of acute myocardial infarction recommend the implantation of an ICD 1 month or more after myocardial infarction in patients with a left ventricular ejection fraction of 30% or less and in those with a left ventricular ejection fraction of 40% or less and additional evidence of electrical instability.[34] It is important to note that current Medicare regulations do not

Table 5-1

Studies of BMIPP—Prediction of Left Ventricular Functional Recovery After Myocardial Infarction

Study, Publication Year	N	Imaging Study	Index of LV Function	Follow-up Period	Comment
Hashimoto, 1995	29	BMIPP/^{201}Tl SPECT	Radionuclide ventriculography	60 days	Difference between thallium and BMIPP scores during acute phase correlated with improvement in LVEF at follow-up in the PTCA group ($r = 0.65$, $p < 0.005$)
Hashimoto, 1996	56	BMIPP/^{201}Tl SPECT	Left ventriculogram	3 months	BMIPP/thallium mismatch correlated with improvement in wall motion at follow-up ($r = 0.65$, $p < 0.005$)
Franken, 1996	18	BMIPP/^{99m}Tc-sestamibi SPECT	Echocardiographic wall motion score	6 months	BMIPP/sestamibi mismatch predictive of functional recovery with 85% accuracy, 94% positive predictive value, and 94% negative predictive value. Improved wall motion in 82% of mismatched segments; unchanged wall motion in 90% of matched segments
Ito, 1996	37	BMIPP/^{201}Tl SPECT	Left ventriculogram	1 month	BMIPP/thallium mismatch strongly correlated with improvement in WMS ($r = 0.86$, $p < 0.0001$) and EF at follow-up ($r = 0.85$, $p < 0.0001$)
Nishimura, 1998	167	BMIPP/^{201}Tl SPECT	Left ventriculogram	90 days	LVEF at discharge and follow-up more closely correlated to extent of ^{201}Tl defect than extent of BMIPP defect ($r = -0.60$ vs. $r = -0.47$ and $r = -0.53$ vs. $r = -0.43$, respectively)
Fujiwara, 1998	23	BMIPP/^{99m}Tc-sestamibi SPECT	Left ventriculogram	1 month	Improved regional wall motion and LVEF in patients with discordant tracer retention
Hambye, 2000	18	BMIPP/^{99m}Tc-sestamibi SPECT	Gated SPECT	3 months	Functional recovery correlated with extent of BMIPP/^{99m}Tc-sestamibi mismatch ($r = 0.68$, $p = 0.001$)
Akimoto, 2000	18	BMIPP/^{99m}Tc-tetrofosmin SPECT	Left ventriculogram	Acute to chronic phase	Improvement in LV function correlated to BMIPP/^{99m}Tc-tetrofosmin discordance score ($r = 0.691$, $p = 0.037$)
Yasugi, 2002	35	BMIPP and ^{201}Tl SPECT	Echocardiographic wall motion score	6 months	Positive predictive value and negative predictive value of dual SPECT imaging = 76% and 67%, respectively, for functional recovery
Akutsu, 2004	32	BMIPP/^{201}Tl SPECT	Echocardiographic wall motion score	1 month	Magnitude of functional recovery and contractile reserve correlated with extent of BMIPP/^{201}Tl SPECT mismatch
Tani, 2004	30	BMIPP and ^{201}Tl SPECT	Echocardiographic wall motion score	5 months	Low-dose dobutamine echocardiography superior to BMIPP in sensitivity and specificity in predicting functional improvement in hypokinetic segments

WMS, wall motion score; LVEF, left ventricular ejection fraction; PTCA, percutaneous transluminal coronary angioplasty.

allow reimbursement for ICD therapy less than 40 days following myocardial infarction.[35] Nevertheless, the VALIANT trial demonstrated that the risk of sudden death is highest in the first 30 days after myocardial infarction among patients with left ventricular dysfunction and/or heart failure.[36] Thus, the ability of fatty acid imaging to predict left ventricular recovery early after myocardial infarction may play a role in the early implementation of strategies to prevent sudden death in patients at high risk.

The fact that the DINAMIT findings did not support the use of early ICD therapy in a high-risk population after myocardial infarction[37] may, in part, reflect an overreliance on the left ventricular ejection fraction as a risk stratification tool. Metabolic assessment through fatty acid imaging may add incremental value to risk stratification over measurement of the left ventricular ejection fraction alone, given that, in the acute phase of myocardial infarction, the metabolic consequences of severe ischemia may trigger ventricular fibrillation, even though ventricular function was often normal before the event.[38] Recently reported population-based data confirm prior observations that only a minority of sudden deaths occur in patients previously identified as having significant left ventricular dysfunction.[39] Evidenced by recent reimbursement support from the Centers for Medicare & Medicaid Services (CMS) for supplementary risk stratification tests such as microvolt T wave alternans testing, increasing budgetary pressure, exists to develop an accurate, predictive test for the purpose of better determining ICD candidacy through the identification of patients most likely to benefit from this therapy.

Future Directions in Fatty Acid Imaging

Although the current research direction for fatty acid imaging focuses on patients with acute chest pain in the emergency department, one can envision numerous potential clinical scenarios in which information regarding the metabolic status of the myocardium may be clinically useful, possible areas for future research.

Clarifying Positive Biomarkers in Clinical Syndromes Other Than ACS Fatty acid imaging may play an important role in the risk stratification of patients in whom the significance of elevations of cardiac biomarkers is unclear. Elevated levels of cardiac troponin are found in acute myocardial infarction but are also observed in the absence of ACS. Numerous disease states, including pulmonary embolism, heart failure, tachycardia, sepsis, renal failure, and myocarditis, can be associated with elevated troponin level.[40] This laboratory finding represents a frequent reason for cardiology consultation. As in cases of acute chest pain, however, very early provocative testing is contraindicated because the extent of underlying coronary disease, and the certainty of the presence of an ACS, is unclear. For this reason, a resting perfusion/metabolism study using fatty acid imaging may be a potentially useful diagnostic tool in the differentiation of cardiac enzyme elevations secondary to ACSs from other etiologies.

Simultaneous Dual-Isotope Perfusion Metabolic Testing to Assess Stress-Induced Ischemia and Viability Given the preliminary data on "ischemic memory" imaging,[13] an imaging protocol can be envisioned, whereby a patient with suspected CAD exercises on a treadmill becomes ischemic or not, has no immediate isotope injection during peak stress but, rather, is injected with *both* a perfusion tracer such as thallium and a fatty acid imaging agent such as BMIPP together at some point *after* exercise. If the tracers could then be simultaneously imaged successfully, the BMIPP image should reflect the metabolic imprint of ischemia that had been recently induced on the treadmill, while the perfusion image represents resting perfusion. If indeed simultaneous imaging could be accomplished technically, then the full spectrum of information usually obtained from separate stress and rest perfusion acquisitions—the extent of stress-induced ischemia, rest perfusion, and viability—could be obtained with only one "spin" of the SPECT camera, boosting throughput and increasing laboratory efficiency. At the moment this approach remains conceptual; nonetheless, it is an attractive route for development, and recent advances suggest that simultaneous dual-isotope imaging may be a reality in the near term.[41,42]

Beyond the Myocardium In the future, continued development of the field of fatty acid imaging may extend beyond the myocardium. Metabolic evaluation of the lower extremity may aid in the assessment of the potential benefit of revascularization therapy in peripheral arterial disease. The elucidation of the mechanisms of metabolic recovery from tissue level hypoxia may also enhance our understanding of the potential for functional recovery in other organ systems. Fatty acid imaging may also be of future interest in nonpathologic assessment of exercise physiology and optimal metabolic performance.

The development of emerging imaging modalities such as fatty acid imaging will be balanced by the societal need for health-care cost containment. The Medicare Payment Advisory Committee's report to Congress in March 2005 expressed concern about the recent apparent increase in the use of imaging services within the Medicare program and suggested several steps for reform. In response, the AHA Science Advisory and Co-ordinating Committee recently published several principles regarding the use of emerging imaging modalities.[43] These recommendations appear to mandate a simultaneous coupling of cost analysis with rigorous scientific evidence as the standard for the development of new imaging techniques. In summary, the successful development of fatty acid imaging will depend on continued assessments of its cost effectiveness.

The application of fatty acid imaging in the assessment of acute chest pain and heart failure may prove to have an important impact on both clinical practice and health-care economics. As the field of metabolic imaging progresses, it may soon become apparent that neglect of metabolism, the "lost child" of cardiology,[44] may signal a new and clinically useful approach for a more sophisticated understanding of certain clinical syndromes.

REFERENCES

1. Taegtmeyer H, King LM, Jones BE. Energy substrate metabolism, myocardial ischemia, and targets for pharmacotherapy. *Am J Cardiol.* 1998;82:54K–60K.
2. Lopaschuk G. Regulation of carbohydrate metabolism in ischemia and reperfusion. *Am Heart J.* 2000;139: S115–S119.
3. Goldstein RA, Klein MS, Welch MJ, Sobel BE. External assessment of myocardial metabolism with C-11 palmitate in vivo. *J Nucl Med.* 1980;21:342.
4. Schon HR, Schelbert HR, Robinson G, et al. C-11 labeled palmitic acid for the noninvasive evaluation of regional myocardial fatty acid metabolism with positron-computed tomography. I. Kinetics of C-11 palmitic acid in normal myocardium. *Am Heart J.* 1982;103:532.
5. Reske SN, Biersack HJ, Lackner K, et al. Assessment of regional myocardial uptake and metabolism of omega-(p-123I-phenyl) pentadecanoic acid with serial single-photon emission tomography. *Nuklearmedizin.* 1982;21:249.
6. Yang JY, Ruiz M, Calnon DA, et al. Assessment of myocardial viability using 123I-labeled iodophenylpentadecanoic acid at sustained low flow or after acute infarction and reperfusion. *J Nucl Med.* 1999;40:821.
7. Caldwell JH, Martin GV, Link JM, et al. Iodophenylpentadecanoic acid-myocardial blood flow relationship during maximal exercise with coronary occlusion. *J Nucl Med.* 1990;31:99.
8. Murray G, Schad N, Ladd W, et al. Metabolic cardiac imaging in severe coronary disease: Assessment of viability with iodine-123-iodophenylpentadecanoic acid and multicrystal gamma camera, and correlation with biopsy. *J Nucl Med.* 1992;33:1269.
9. Verani MS, Taillefer R, Iskandrian AE, et al. 123I-IPPA SPECT for the prediction of enhanced left ventricular function after coronary bypass graft surgery. Multicenter IPPA Viability Trial Investigators. 123I-iodophenylpentadecanoic acid. *J Nucl Med.* 2000;41:1299.
10. Goodman MM, Kirsch G, Knapp FF. Synthesis and evaluation of radioiodinated terminal p-iodophenyl-substituted α- and ß-methyl branched fatty acids. *J Med Chem.* 1984;27:390–397.
11. Knapp FF, Kropp J. Iodine 123-labelled fatty acids for myocardial single-photon tomography: Current status and future perspectives. *Eur J Nucl Med.* 1995;22: 361–381.

12. Tamaki N, Kawamoto M, Yonekura Y, et al. Regional metabolic abnormality in relation to perfusion and wall motion in patients with myocardial infarction: Assessment with emission tomography using an iodinated branched fatty acid analog. *J Nucl Med.* 1992;33:659.

13. Dilsizian V, Bateman TM, Bergmann SR, et al. Metabolic imaging with ß-methyl-*p*-[123I]-iodophenyl-pentadecanoic acid identifies ischemic memory after demand ischemia. *Circulation.* 2005;112:2169–2174.

14. Hambye AS, Vaerenberg MM, Dobbeleir AA, et al. Abnormal BMIPP uptake in chronically dysfunctional myocardial segments: Correlation with contractile response to low-dose dobutamine. *J Nucl Med.* 1998; 39:1845.

15. Kudoh T, Tadamura E, Tamaki N, et al. Iodinated free fatty acid and 201Tl uptake in chronically hypoperfused myocardium: Histologic correlation study. *J Nucl Med.* 2000;41:293.

16. Franken PR, Dendale P, De Geeter F, et al. Prediction of functional outcome after myocardial infarction using BMIPP and sestamibi scintigraphy. *J Nucl Med.* 1996; 37:718.

17. Ito T, Tanouchi J, Kato J, et al. Recovery of impaired left ventricular function in patients with acute myocardial infarction is predicted by the discordance in defect size on 123I-BMIPP and 201Tl SPECT images. *Eur J Nucl Med.* 1996;23:917.

18. Hashimoto A, Nakata T, Tsuchihashi K, et al. Postischemic functional recovery and BMIPP uptake after primary percutaneous transluminal coronary angioplasty in acute myocardial infarction. *Am J Cardiol.* 1996;77:25.

19. Nohara R, Hosokawa R, Hirai T, et al. Basic kinetics of 15-(p-iodophenyl)-3-R,S-methylpentadecanoic acid (BMIPP) in a canine myocardium. *Int J Cardiac Imaging.* 1999;15:11–20.

20. Tamaki N, Morita K, Kuge Y, et al. The role of fatty acids in cardiac imaging. *J Nucl Med.* 2000;41:1525–1534.

21. Chen J, Garcia EV, Galt JR, Folks RD, Carrio I. Optimized acquisition and processing protocols for I-123 cardiac SPECT imaging. *J Nucl Cardiol.* 2006; 13:251–260.

22. Nishimura T. *β*-Methyl-*p*-(123-I)-iodophenyl pentadecanoic acid single-photon emission computed tomography in cardiomyopathy. *Int J Cardiac Imaging.* 1999;15:41–48.

23. Inubushi M, Tadamura E, Kudoh T, et al. Simultaneous assessment of myocardial free fatty acid utilization and left ventricular function using 123-I-BMIPP-gated SPECT. *J Nucl Med.* 1999;40:1840–1847.

24. Ryan TJ, Anderson JL, Antman EM, et al. ACC/AHA guidelines for the management of patients with acute myocardial infarction. A report of the American College of Cardiology/American Heart Association Task Force on Practice Guidelines (Committee on Management of Acute Myocardial Infarction). *J Am Coll Cardiol.* 1996;28:1328–1428.

25. Burt CW. Summary Statistics for acute cardiac ischemia and chest pain visits to United States EDs, 1995–1996. *Am J Emerg Med.* 1999;17:552–559.

26. Brodie BR, Hansen C, Stuckey TD, et al. Door-to-balloon time with primary percutaneous coronary intervention for acute myocardial infarction impacts late cardiac mortality in high-risk patients and patients presenting early after the onset of symptoms. *J Am Coll Cardiol.* 2006;47(2):289–295.

27. Udelson JE, Beshansky JR, Ballin DS, et al. Myocardial perfusion imaging for evaluation and triage of patients with suspected acute cardiac ischemia; a randomized controlled trial. *JAMA.* 2002;288: 2693–2700.

28. Klocke FJ, Baird MG, Lorell BH, et al. ACC/AHA/ ASNC guidelines for the clinical use of cardiac radionuclide imaging—executive summary: A report of the American College of Cardiology/American Heart Association Task Force on practice guidelines (ACC/ AHA/ASNC Committee to revise the 1995 guidelines for the clinical use of cardiac radionuclide imaging). *Circulation.* 2003;108:1404–1418.

29. Tatum JL, Jesse RL, Kontos MC, et al. Comprehensive strategy for the evaluation and triage of the chest pain patient. *Ann Emerg Med.* 1997;29:116–125.

30. Kawai Y, Tsukamoto E, Nozaki Y, et al. Significance of reduced uptake of iodinated fatty acid analogue for the evaluation of patients with acute chest pain. *J Am Coll Cardiol* 2001;38(7):1888–1894.

31. Taegtmeyer H, Goodwin GW, Doenst T, Frazier OH. Substrate metabolism as a determinant for postischemic functional recovery of the heart. *Am J Cardiol.* 1997;80:3A–10A.

32. Sato H, Iwasaki T, Toyama T, et al. Prediction of functional recovery after revascularization in coronary artery disease using (18)F-FDG and (123)I-BMIPP SPECT. *Chest* 2000;117(1):65–72.

33. Seki H, Toyama T, Higuchi K, et al. Prediction of functional improvement of ischemic myocardium with 123I-BMIPP SPECT and 99mTc-tetrofosmin SPECT imaging: A study of patients with large acute myocardial infarction and receiving revascularization therapy. *Circulation J.* 2005;69(3):311–319.

34. Antman EM, Anbe DT, Armstrong PW, et al. ACC/AHA guidelines for the management of patients with ST-elevation myocardial infarction: A report of the American College of Cardiology/American Heart Association Task Force on practice guidelines (Committee to revise the 1999 guidelines for the management of patients with acute myocardial infarction). *Circulation.* 2004;110:e82–e292.

35. Al-Khatib SM, Sanders GD, Mark DB, et al. Implantable cardioverter-defibrillators and cardiac resynchronization therapy in patients with left ventricular dysfunction: Randomized trial evidence through 2004. *Am Heart J.* 2005;149(6):1020–1034.

36. Solomon SD, Zelenkofske S, McMurray JJV, et al., for the Valsartan in Acute Myocardial Infarction Trial (VALIANT) Investigators. *N Engl J Med.* 2004;325:2581–2588.

37. Hohnloser SH, Kuck KH, Dorian P, et al. Prophylactic use of an implantable cardioverter-defibrillator after acute myocardial infarction. *N Engl J Med.* 2004;351:2481–2488.

38. Buxton AE. Sudden death after myocardial infarction-who needs prophylaxis, and when? *N Engl J Med.* 2004;325:2638–2640.

39. Stecker EC, Vickers C, Waltz J, et al. Population-based analysis of sudden cardiac death with and without left ventricular systolic dysfunction: Two year findings from the Oregon sudden unexpected death study. *J Am Coll Cardiol.* 2006;47:1161–1166.

40. Jeremias A, Gibson CM. Narrative review: Alternative causes for elevated cardiac troponin levels when acute coronary syndromes are excluded. *Ann Int Med.* 2005;142(9):786–791.

41. El Fakhri G, Sitek A, Zimmerman RE, Ouyang J. Generalized five-dimensional dynamic and spectral factor analysis. *Med Phys.* 2006;33(4):10016–10024.

42. El Fakhri G, Habert MO, Maksud P, et al. Quantitative simultaneous 99mTc-ECD/123I-FP-CIT SPECT in Parkinson's disease and multiple system atrophy. *Eur J Nucl Med Mol Imaging.* 2006;33(1):87–92.

43. Gibbons RJ, Eckel RH, Jacobs AK, et al., for the Science Advisory and Coordinating Committee. The utilization of cardiac imaging. *Circulation.* 2006;113:1715–1716.

44. Taegtmeyer H. Metabolism—the lost child of cardiology. *J Am Coll Cardiol.* 2000;36:1386–1388.

CHAPTER 6

Cardiac Neuronal Imaging with ^{123}I-mIBG

Mark I. Travin

INTRODUCTION

The heart is densely innervated with autonomic fibers, sympathetic and parasympathetic. This autonomic innervation, along with circulating autonomic mediators such as norepinephrine, plays a crucial role in regulating cardiac function. There is a complex balance between sympathetic and parasympathetic effects that maintain heart rate and blood pressure within a narrow range, with the system being able to respond to cardiac workload demands by affecting appropriate changes in chronotropic and inotropic cardiac function.

The presence of cardiac pathology from coronary artery disease and/or other disease entities can disrupt proper autonomic function and upset the appropriate balance between sympathetic and parasympathetic cardiac control. Cardiac autonomic dysfunction impairs the ability of the heart to respond to workload demands, often leading to patient symptoms and activity limitations. At the same time, such autonomic abnormalities

have been shown to increase a patient's susceptibility to adverse cardiac events, particularly life-threatening arrhythmias and cardiac death. Thus, the ability to image the functional status of cardiac autonomic innervation can provide important information in patients with cardiac disease, enhancing risk stratification and potentially guiding therapy.

IMAGING OF SYMPATHETIC NERVE TERMINALS

Numerous radiotracer compounds that can visualize cardiac innervation have been developed, although all are limited to investigational status in the United States at this time. Such imaging has focused predominantly on the synaptic junction of the sympathetic system that is the predominant autonomic innervation of the ventricles (parasympathetic fibers are mainly present in the atria).

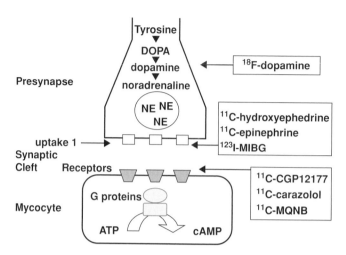

Figure 6-1.   Synaptic neuronal synapse. Schematic representation with commonly used tracers for assessment of neuronal function. ATP, adenosine triphosphate; DOPA, dihydroxyphenylalanine; MIBG, metaiodoben-zylguanidine; NE, norepinephrine. (From Carrió[1] with permission.)

As in Figure 6-1, some tracers have been designed to image presynaptic anatomy and function, while others visualize postsynaptic function via receptor binding.[1] Most published clinical work has described imaging of presynaptic sympathetic anatomy and function, the focus of the following discussion.

Imaging of presynaptic innervation uses analogs of the naturally occurring mediator of sympathetic function, norepinephrine. As in Figure 6-1, norepinephrine (noradrenaline) is produced in the presynaptic sympathetic nerve terminal by a series of steps originating with tyrosine, and this molecule is stored at high concentration in vesicles. In response to an appropriate stimulus, the norepinephrine-filled vesicles fuse with the neuronal membrane, releasing norepinephrine into the synaptic space to bind with postsynaptic receptors, resulting in various physiologic responses. In order to closely regulate sympathetic stimulation, there is a transporter protein-mediated, sodium- and energy-dependent reuptake of norepinephrine, i.e., "uptake-1" into the presynaptic terminal for storage or catabolic disposal, in effect terminating the sympathetic

response. Some norepinephrine is also taken up by non-neuronal cells, probably by sodium-independent passive diffusion, i.e., the "uptake-2" system.[2]

Guanethidine is a false neurotransmitter analog of norepinephrine that can enter the uptake-1 pathway. Chemical modification of guanethidine produces a molecule that can be labeled with radioactive iodine—metaiodobenzylguanidine (*m*IBG)—and therefore imaged (Figure 6-2). When first developed in the late 1970s, *m*IBG was labeled with ^{131}I and was used for detection of neural crest tumors, neuroblastomas, and pheochromocytomas. [131]I-*m*IBG imaging of such tumors is currently the only FDA-approved use of radiolabeled *m*IBG in the United States. As ^{131}I gives off relatively high-energy γ emissions of 365 keV, emits β^- particles, and has a relatively long half-life of approximately 8.02 days, ^{123}I labeling has been developed and thus [123]I-*m*IBG is the preferred tracer. [123]I emits predominantly γ photons with energy of 159 keV and has a half-life of 13.2 hours, therefore easily imaged and well tolerated by patients. (Note: [123]I also emits multiple but low-abundance higher-energy photons, to

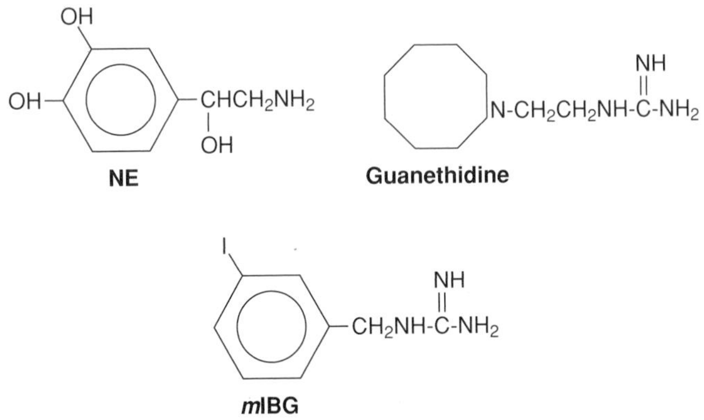

Figure 6-2. Molecular structures of norepinephrine (NE), guanethidine, and ^{123}I-mIBG (metaiodobenzylguanidine).

be discussed subsequently). ^{123}I-mIBG has been used extensively in Europe and Japan for cardiac imaging but is currently not FDA approved in the United States for cardiac imaging (although it can be obtained from various institutions and commercial centers that have appropriate approvals and can be used at physicians' discretion as an off-label use). Use of ^{123}I-mIBG for cardiac imaging is considered to be investigational in the United States.

As an analog of norepinephrine and guanethidine, intravenously administered ^{123}I-mIBG accumulates in the presynaptic nerve terminal via the uptake-1 pathway. However, unlike norepinephrine, ^{123}I-mIBG is not catabolized by monoamine oxidase (MAO) or catechol-o-methyltransferase, allowing it to localize in myocardial sympathetic nerve endings in a higher cytoplasmic concentration than NE.[2–4] There is also the potential for the non-neuronal uptake-2 process to occur, but this appears minimal at the relatively low concentrations used for cardiac imaging.[5]

Cardiac neuronal uptake of ^{123}I-mIBG is illustrated in Figure 6-3. Myocardial imaging allows assessment of both global and regional tracer uptake, providing information on both the anatomic integrity of cardiac sympathetic innervation and the physiologic function.

PROCEDURE FOR ^{123}I-mIBG ADMINISTRATION

^{123}I-mIBG is performed at rest and needs only minimal preparation. Current recommendations are to keep the patients' NPO (except for water) after midnight for morning testing, but patients who are having afternoon imaging may have a light breakfast. Medications that can interfere with catecholamine uptake, such as various antidepressants, antipsychotics, and some calcium channel blockers, should be held for 24 hours prior to tracer injection and imaging. Patients should be questioned regarding allergies to iodine, which may preclude ^{123}I-mIBG imaging.

There is disagreement with regard to the need for administration of thyroid-blocking agents such as potassium iodide, potassium perchlorate, or Lugol's solution, prior to MIBG administration. Historically, such blockade has been undertaken to shield the thyroid from exposure to unbound radionuclide impurities such as ^{124}I and ^{125}I. With modern production methods the amount of such unbound impurities, as well as unbound ^{123}I, is minimal, and thus many investigators feel that such pretreatment is unnecessary. Such pretreatment should therefore be based on local and institutional regulations and may be clarified further when or if ^{123}I-mIBG

Sympathetic Nerve Terminal

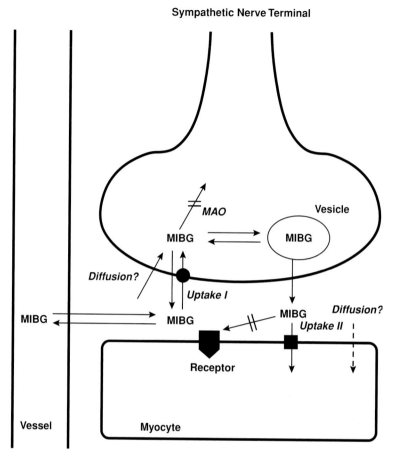

Figure 6-3. MIBG uptake at neuronal synapse. Neuronal uptake is mostly via the energy-dependent uptake-1 pathway. Non-neuronal uptake-2 also occurs, but usually at higher concentrations of MIBG. MAO, monoamine oxidase; MIBG, metaiodobenzylguanidine. (From Hattori and Schwaiger[6] with permission.)

obtains FDA approval for cardiac and oncologic imaging.

The amount of tracer to administer has not been formally established. In several published investigations, a dose of 3–5 mCi (111–185 MBq) of ^{123}I-mIBG administered over a 1-minute period has been used, and this is generally satisfactory for planar image analysis.[7,8] However, because it is often difficult to obtain satisfactory SPECT images using these tracer doses in patients with severe cardiac dysfunction and heart failure, a dose of up to

10 mCi (370 MBq) may be appropriate and is under investigation.[5]

It is recommended that patients lie quietly in a supine position for at least 5 minutes before tracer administration. As the initial images are obtained a few minutes later, the tracer is best administered while the patient is lying under the camera or at least in close proximity.

Reported adverse reactions to ^{123}I-mIBG have been very uncommon. Among the side effects that have been reported from Japan and Europe when the tracer is administered too quickly are palpitations, shortness of breath, heat sensations, transient hypertension, and abdominal cramps. There is also the rare possibility of an anaphylactic reaction.

PROCEDURE FOR ^{123}I-*m*IBG IMAGING

Much published work with ^{123}I-*m*IBG has dealt with planar imaging and the parameters that can be measured from it. However, SPECT imaging should also be done, as more recent studies show that important information is derived from it as well.[7,9] As indicated above, higher administered tracer activity may be required to obtain acceptable SPECT images in patients with depressed left ventricular function.

The parameters for planar and SPECT acquisition of ^{123}I-*m*IBG are not formally established, but current methods are described in various published reviews.[1,10] Planar images are obtained in the anterior view for 10 minutes using an energy window of 159 keV ± 20%. The patient should be positioned to include the entire heart and as much of the thorax as possible. One should avoid positioning the heart too close to the edge of the field or too close to the center; use of a radioactive marker may be helpful for consistent positioning between early and late images.

SPECT images are obtained using the 159 keV ± 20% energy window via a 180-degree circular acquisition from 45-degree RAO to 45-degree LPO, using a total of 60 stops (30 stops per head if done with a dual-headed camera) at 30 seconds per stop. While a circular orbit is preferred to avoid apical artifacts on reconstructed images, noncircular orbits can be used with long-bore collimators or if there is sufficient gap during passage of the camera around the apex.

SPECT image reconstruction and reorientation are the same as for standard perfusion images, with adjustment of filters as needed to obtain quality images, particularly if counts are low. Pro-

cessing is currently done most often with filtered back projection, but iterative reconstruction is being investigated and may give truer results. The use of attenuation correction is also being investigated.

While low-energy collimators have been routinely used for ^{123}I-*m*IBG acquisition, multiple, low-abundance higher-energy photons (including one of 529 keV) that are emitted by ^{123}I more freely penetrate the septa and degrade image quality. Work is under way using a measured point spread function to perform 3D deconvolution of the septal penetration, in order to compensate for this effect and improve image accuracy.[11,12]

Planar and SPECT images are routinely obtained at approximately 15 minutes following ^{123}I-*m*IBG administration (early), and again 4 hours later (delayed). While many feel that only the 4-hour image should be used for interpretation and analysis because it represents actual neuronal uptake (as opposed to interstitial uptake in the early images), studies from Japan have shown that tracer washout between early and delayed images can provide important additional information (see discussion below).

IMAGE ANALYSIS AND INTERPRETATION

Planar Imaging

Much published work on ^{123}I-*m*IBG imaging has investigated the clinical implications of global tracer uptake, as measured by the heart mediastinal (H/M) count ratio on the anterior planar image (Figure 6-4). While the H/M ratio is a gross measurement, providing no regional innervation information, much of the prognostic literature is based on this parameter.

At least three analytic methods have been used to derive the H/M ratio. In one, squares or rectangular regions of interest (ROIs) are drawn in the center of the heart and the upper mediastinum, with a count per pixel ratio calculated.[14] In another, the ROI is drawn around the epicardial

ANALYSIS OF MIBG PLANAR IMAGES

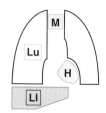

H/M Ratio

ROI's drawn around heart and mediastinum, counts per pixel determined for each, and ratio calculated

Myocardial Washout

[(Early-late counts corrected for I-123 decay) × 100]/early counts

Figure 6-4. Analysis of MIBG planar images to determine heart mediastinal ratio (H/M ratio) and tracer washout. H, heart; Li, liver; Lu, lung; M, mediastinum; MIBG, metaiodobenzylguanidine. (From Morozumi et al.,[13] with permission.)

border of the heart, including the valve plane.[15] Finally, some have drawn the cardiac ROI encompassing the myocardium alone, tracing the epicardial and endocardial borders, excluding the valve plane.[8] Interestingly, all methods appear to give similar results in any given patient study. Normal values for H/M ratio range from 1.9 to 2.8, with a mean of approximately 2.2.[6] A particularly poor prognosis has been noted for patients with H/M ratio less than 1.2.[16] The H/M ratio has been shown to improve after treatment for heart failure, and such improvement may indicate improved prognosis.[8] Examples of patients with normal and abnormal H/M ratios are shown in Figure 6-5. An international, multicenter study is currently being initiated to comprehensively investigate the prognostic utility of H/M ratio in patients with Class II–III congestive heart failure and a left ventricular ejection fraction ≤35% (MBG311 and MBG312, by GE Healthcare Ltd).

Among the problems that may affect the ability to determine an accurate H/M ratio are low myocardial counts and overlying tracer activity (such as from the lung and liver). In addition, a normal H/M ratio does not preclude severe disease, as patients may potentially have profound regional abnormalities but a normal H/M ratio.

Another frequently measured quantity from planar images is ^{123}I-mIBG washout, derived as

follows[17]:

$$\text{Cardiac I-123 MIBG washout}$$
$$= [(CD_{\text{heart-early}} - CD_{\text{heart-late}})/$$
$$(CD_{\text{heart-late}})] \times 100\%$$

where CD = count densities in heart after subtraction of mediastinal background and after decay correction.

Ogita et al. determined the normal washout value in control subjects to be 9.6% ± 8.5%. In their study, patients with heart failure who had MIBG washout more than 27% (>2 SD from normal mean) had a dramatically increased mortality compared with patients who had lower values.[18]

SPECT Imaging

Analysis of ^{123}I-mIBG SPECT images is less well established but increasingly used. SPECT imaging allows assessment of regional sympathetic innervation. It has been suggested that regional denervation, while not only a sign of significant cardiac disease, may also create an area of electrical supersensitivity, predisposing to potentially lethal cardiac arrhythmias.[19]

In order to properly evaluate SPECT ^{123}I-mIBG, one must establish that any defect seen is the result of denervation rather than hypoperfusion. Thus, a SPECT perfusion image study at rest should also be performed, preferably with a ^{99m}Tc-based agent. Areas of mismatch (^{123}I-mIBG defect with preserved perfusion) indicate regional denervation (Figure 6-5). Sympathetic nerves are more sensitive to ischemic insults than the myocardium, and thus such mismatches are frequently seen following both ST and non-ST segment elevation myocardial infarctions, and after ischemic episodes.[5]

While there is no officially established method of scoring SPECT ^{123}I-mIBG images, analysis can be performed similar to that used for conventional SPECT perfusion imaging. The SPECT images can be divided into 17 segments (four for the apical short-axis slice, six each for the mid and basal short-axis slices, and one, the apex, for the

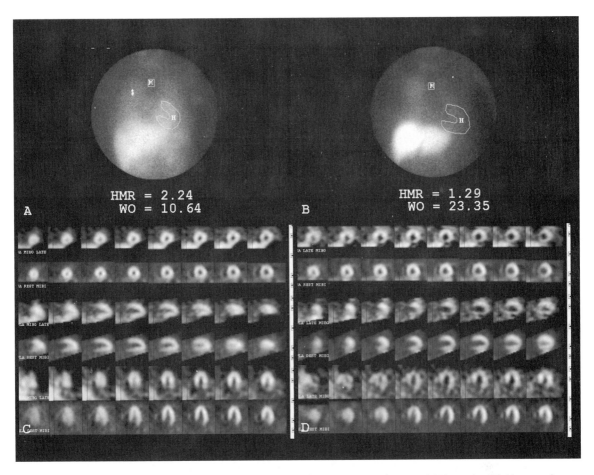

Figure 6-5.   Examples of ^{123}I-mIBG images. (**A**) Normal planar image with normal H/M ratio. (**B**) Abnormal planar image with abnormally reduced H/M ratio. (**C**) SPECT images (^{123}I-mIBG [*top rows of pairs*] and ^{99m}Tc-sestamibi [*bottom rows of pairs*], in short axis (SA), vertical long axis (VLA), and horizontal long axis (HLA) orientations). These images show normal ^{123}I-mIBG and normal ^{99m}Tc-sestamibi tracer uptake. (**D**) Abnormal SPECT images, with a mismatching ^{123}I-mIBG defect of the inferior and apical wall (in relation to ^{99m}Tc-sestamibi images). HMR, heart mediastinal ratio; MIBI, ^{99m}Tc-sestamibi; WO, washout.

mid-vertical long-axis slice). Segments can be scored on a scale of 0 (normal tracer activity) to 4 (no tracer activity). One should also derive a standard summed perfusion image score for the rest perfusion images and subtract it from the ^{123}I-mIBG summed score to yield a mismatch score. Polar plots can also be created, and regional tracer distribution can be compared with normal controls.

The utility of SPECT image scores remains to be determined. A pilot study showed a correlation with the potential for implantable defibrillator shocks,[7] and it would be expected that summed score would correlate with prognosis in patients with heart failure and left ventricular dysfunction. ^{123}I-mIBG imaging could potentially help identify patients who would benefit from an implantable defibrillator. Regional analysis may also help elucidate the mechanisms of primary arrhythmic abnormalities such as Brugada syndrome.[9]

EXTRANEOUS CONDITIONS THAT AFFECT *m*IBG IMAGING

Autonomic innervation may be affected by factors other than cardiac disease, and these must be considered when interpreting ^{123}I-*m*IBG images. Global and regional tracer uptake and washout appear to change as patients age, even in the absence of known heart disease. Inferior wall defects are common and appear more prominent in men compared with women. On the other hand, lateral wall defects appear more often in older women. For younger patients, washout appears lower in women.

Differences in autonomic tone, as measured, for example, by heart rate variability, may alter global uptake and washout in otherwise normal patients. Prolonged exercise has been shown to decrease global ^{123}I-*m*IBG uptake.

Diabetes can alter cardiac sympathetic tracer uptake in the absence of otherwise detectable cardiac disease. However, such abnormalities, both global and regional, may be indicative of subclinical disease that may increase a patient's risk of a cardiac event. Abnormalities in diabetic patients, including those without clinical evidence of neuropathy, should not be considered artifacts, and such patients should not be used as "normal controls" for studies.

Medications that affect autonomic function can affect cardiac ^{123}I-*m*IBG imaging. A variety of antidepressant, neuropsychiatric, sympathomimetic antiarrhythmic, and antihypertensive agents (e.g., calcium blockers) may potentially interfere with tracer uptake.

Other cardiac medications that improve cardiac conditions, such as β-blockers, angiotensin-converting enzyme inhibitors, and angiotensin receptor blockers, have been shown to alter ^{123}I-*m*IBG image results in association with other parameters (e.g., LVEF, NYHA class, etc.), reflecting improvement in the cardiac condition. Mechani-

cal devices, such as pacemakers and implantable defibrillators, can affect ^{123}I-*m*IBG tracer uptake by damaging the myocardium and sympathetic innervation at sites of the device's electrical output.

Cardiac transplant, by severing the autonomic innervation of the ventricles, will affect ^{123}I-*m*IBG images. Renervation that can be measured with ^{123}I-*m*IBG imaging may help track the improvement of patients who have had a heart transplant.

NEURONAL TRACERS FOR PET

In general positron emission tomographic (PET) radiotracers produce better images than single photon compounds. In addition, PET isotopes can be incorporated into a wider variety of biologic molecules. For neuronal imaging, PET tracers are closer to norepinephrine in composition and thus have distinct advantages. The most commonly used neuronal PET tracer is ^{11}C-*meta*-hydroxyephedrine (HED). Among the advantages of HED compared with MIBG is higher uptake-1 selectivity (i.e., lower nonspecific non-neuronal uptake), resulting in better differentiation between innervated and denervated myocardium, recently found to be of particular advantage in evaluating neuronal heterogeneity in hibernating myocardium.[20] HED also appears to have more homogeneous uptake than MIBG (less heterogeneity in the inferior wall).

Other less well-studied ^{11}C neuronal tracers include ^{11}C-epinephrine and ^{11}C-phenylephrine. The latter is rapidly metabolized by MAO and as a result could potentially play a role in assessment of vesicular storage function. Various ^{18}F tracers, such as ^{18}F 6-fluorodopamine are also being studied. ^{18}F is more conveniently obtained than ^{11}C, and its longer half-life may allow assessment of tracer clearance for a longer period of time.[21]

CONCLUSION

Cardiac autonomic innervation plays a crucial role in cardiac function. Abnormalities of innervation contribute much to disease processes and appear to greatly increase the incidence of adverse cardiac events, particularly sudden arrhythmic death. Investigational studies of cardiac autonomic imaging with ^{123}I-mIBG have shown much promise in risk-stratifying patients and better understanding the mechanisms of various arrhythmic conditions. Nevertheless, the lack of routine clinical use in the United States has impaired exploration of the full potential of ^{123}I-mIBG and related PET tracers. Large-scale trials are under way to help further understand the potential of cardiac neuronal imaging and help it become established in the United States.

REFERENCES

1. Carrió I. Cardiac neurotransmission imaging. *J Nucl Med*. 2001;42:1062–476 [PMID: 11438630].
2. Sisson JC, Wieland DM. Radiolabelled meta-iodobenzylguanidine pharmacology: Pharmacology and clinical studies. *Am J Physiol Imaging*. 1986;1:96–103 [PMID: 3330445].
3. Kline RC, Swanson DP, Wieland DM, et al. Myocardial imaging in man with I-123 Meta-iodobenzylguanidine. *J Nucl Med*. 1981;22:129–132 [PMID: 7463156].
4. Wieland DM, Brown LE, Rogers WL, et al. Myocardial imaging with a radioiodinated norepinephrine storage analog. *J Nucl Med*. 1981;22:22–31 [PMID: 7452352].
5. Flotats A, Carrio I. Cardiac neurotransmission SPECT imaging. *J Nucl Cardiol*. 2004;11:587–602 [PMID: 15472644].
6. Hattori N, Schwaiger M. Metaiodobenzylguanidine scintigraphy of the heart. What have we learned clinically? *Eur J Nucl Med*. 2000;27:1–6 [PMID: 10654140].
7. Arora R, Ferrick KJ, Nakata T, et al. I-123 MIBG imaging and heart rate variability analysis to predict the needs for an implantable cardioverter defibrillator. *J Nucl Cardiol*. 2003;10:121–131 [PMID: 12673176].
8. Gerson MC, Craft LL, McGuire N, Suresh DP, Abraham WT, Wagoner LE. Carvedilol improves left ventricular function in heart failure with idiopathic dilated cardiomyopathy and a wide range of sympathetic nervous system function as measured by iodine 123 metaiodobenzylguanidine. *J Nucl Cardiol*. 2002;9:608–615 [PMID: 12466785].
9. Wichter T, Matheja P, Eckardt L, et al. Cardiac autonomic dysfunction in Brugada syndrome. *Circulation*. 2002;105:702–706 [PMID: 11839625].
10. Patel AD, Iskandrian AE. MIBG Imaging. *J Nucl Cardiol*. 2002;9:75–94 [PMID: 11845133].
11. Chen J, Galt JR, Folks RD, Garcia EV. SPECT acquisition and processing protocols to optimize quantification of I-123 cardiac studies: Preliminary results. *J Nucl Med*. 2005;46:259P (abstract).
12. Chen J, Galt JR, Folks RD, Garcia EV. Optimization of acquisition and processing protocols for I-123 cardiac SPECT imaging with low-energy high-resolution collimators. *J Nucl Cardiol*. 2005;12:S124 (abstract).
13. Morozumi T, Kusuoka H, Fukuchi K, et al. Myocardial iodine-123-metaiodobenzylguanidine images and autonomic nerve activity in normal subjects. *J Nucl Med*. 1997;38:49–52 [PMID: 8998149].
14. Agostini D, Belin A, Amar MH, et al. Improvement of cardiac neuronal function after carvedilol treatment in dilated cardiomyopathy: A ^{123}I-MIBG scintigraphic study. *J Nucl Med*. 2000;41:845–851 [PMID: 10809201].
15. Yamada T, Shimonagata T, Fukunami M, et al. Comparison of the prognostic value of cardiac iodine-123 metaiodobenzylguanidine imaging and heart rate variability in patients with chronic heart failure. *J Am Coll Cardiol*. 2003;41:231–238 [PMID: 12535815].
16. Merlet P, Valette H, Dubois-Randé JL, et al. Prognostic value of cardiac metaiodobenzylguanidine imaging in patients with heart failure. *J Nucl Med*. 1992;33:471–477 [PMID: 1552326].
17. Somsen GA, Verberne HJ, Fleury E, Righetti A. Normal values and within-subject variability of cardiac I-123 MIBG scintigraphy in healthy individuals: Implications for clinical studies. *J Nucl Cardiol*. 2004;11:126–133 [PMID: 15052243].
18. Ogita H, Shimonagata T, Fukunami M, et al. Prognostic significance of cardiac ^{123}I metaiodobenzylguanidine imaging for mortality and morbidity in patients with chronic heart failure: A prospective study. *Heart*. 2001;86:656–660 [PMID: 11711461].
19. Verrier RL, Antzelevich C. Autonomic aspects if arrhythmogenesis: The enduring and the new. *Curr Opin Cardiol*. 2004;19:2–11 [PMID: 14688627].
20. Luisi AJ, Suzuki G, deKemp R, et al. Regional ^{11}C-hydroxyephedrine retention in hibernating myocardium: Chronic inhomogeneity of sympathetic innervation in the absence of infarction. *J Nucl Med*. 2005;46:1368–1374 [PMID: 16085596].
21. Bengel FM, Schwaiger M. Assessment of cardiac sympathetic neuronal function using PET imaging. *J Nucl Cardiol*. 2004;11:603–616 [PMID: 15472645].

PRINCIPLES AND TECHNIQUE
CONSIDERATIONS FOR STRESS TESTING

CHAPTER 7

Exercise Testing

Brian G. Abbott

INTRODUCTION

Exercise stress testing has been widely employed in the assessment of patients with known or suspected coronary artery disease (CAD). Stress testing serves as one of the mainstays in the evaluation of ischemic heart disease. Given the ease with which the test can be performed, including in an office-based setting, exercise electrocardiography (ECG) has been in widespread clinical use since its inception more than 50 years ago. The test is highly useful for diagnosis and risk assessment of patients with suspected CAD and can be performed alone in or conjunction with an imaging modality such as myocardial perfusion imaging or echocardiography. Stress testing is used in a wide variety of patient populations, ranging from screening in selected asymptomatic patients,[1,2] to emergency department patients with chest pain,[3] and patients with known CAD after an acute coronary syndrome (ACS),[4,5] or revascularization procedure.[6,7] This chapter focuses on how to safely perform and effectively interpret an exercise stress electrocardiogram.

INDICATIONS

Exercise ECG is typically performed to diagnose obstructive CAD in patients with symptoms suggestive of ischemia, such as chest pain or exertional dyspnea. It is also useful in patients with known CAD for risk assessment and to evaluate response to medical therapy, and after an ACS or revascularization procedure. Other indications include the evaluation of functional capacity in patients with congestive heart failure, valvular disease, and certain arrhythmias.

Detection of CAD

As with any diagnostic test, the exercise ECG has its greatest utility when performed in patients with an intermediate pretest probability of the condition or disease being present. This can be codified using a table such as that derived by Diamond and Forrester, which incorporates age, gender, and type of chest pain to determine the likelihood of CAD based on these clinical variables alone.[8] This evaluation is helpful to confirm that the probability of CAD is such that the results of the test will impact the posttest probability of CAD and thus improve diagnostic certainty. Patients with low pretest probability of CAD will still have a low posttest probability even if the test is abnormal or "positive." In this manner, many of the abnormal tests in this population will be "false positives." As such, the exercise ECG is most valuable in patients with an intermediate pretest probability, adding significant incremental information to the pretest probability to aid diagnostic certainty (e.g., a posttest probability of <20% or >75%).[9,10]

The diagnostic accuracy of the exercise stress test has been studied extensively in a variety of patient populations, including patients with clinical characteristics that may confound interpretation of the stress ECG, such as baseline abnormalities secondary to digoxin or left ventricular hypertrophy,[11,12] as well as in women,[13] and have demonstrated that, overall, the sensitivity to detect CAD ranges from 23% to 100% and the specificity from 17% to 100%.[14] The substantial splay in the diagnostic accuracy can be attributed to variations in the pretest likelihood of disease in the groups studied, the bias toward further testing (i.e., coronary angiography) in patients with abnormal stress ECG results, and the criteria used for both a "positive" test (definition of an abnormal ECG response) and the definition of angiographic CAD (50% or 70% stenosis) used in the analysis. More selective studies have demonstrated that the mean sensitivity is 67% with a specificity of 72%.[14]

Risk Stratification in Patients with Known CAD

Exercise ECG is also a useful tool to evaluate patients with known CAD. Treadmill exercise is indicated in assessing a patient's response to antianginal medications, and to document exercise capacity prior to enrollment on a cardiac rehabilitation program after a cardiac event, such as an ACS or a coronary revascularization.[7,15,16] The use of exercise testing after an ACS is typically limited to patients who clinically are at low risk at the time of hospital discharge. A submaximal exercise test, performed 4 to 7 days post-ACS, or a symptom-limited test, 14 to 21 days afterward, can be helpful to document exercise capacity and evaluate residual ischemia. Given the clinical characteristics of this group, it is expected that some will need to undergo exercise testing with MPI because of the abnormal baseline ECG abnormalities, which preclude interpretation of ST-segment changes. If the results of the submaximal or symptom-limited exercise ECG are abnormal (e.g., low workload achieved, angina, or ischemic ECG changes), further evaluation with myocardial perfusion imaging to quantify the extent and severity of the ischemic burden and infarct size may be necessary.[14]

After revascularization procedures, particularly percutaneous coronary interventions, exercise testing is often helpful in evaluating patients with symptoms suggesting restenosis or incomplete revascularization. Although isolated cases of adverse events have been reported,[17,18] stress testing is generally considered safe in these patients.[19]

EXERCISE PHYSIOLOGY

While the focus of an exercise test is usually the exercise ECG, important diagnostic and prognostic information is also obtained from the hemodynamic data collected during exercise. As such, an understanding of the normal response to exercise is essential to performing and interpreting a stress test. The normal cardiac response to exercise is an increase in cardiac output caused by increases in heart rate, and cardiac contractility. Aerobic exercise exerts primarily a volume load on the heart, as systolic blood pressure rises while diastolic blood pressure stays the same or decreases slightly. Peripheral artery vasodilation and recruitment of capillary beds that are closed at rest serve to lower the peripheral vascular resistance. Despite this vasodilation, there is an increase in systemic arterial blood pressure because the cardiac output is increasing at a faster rate. Increased body temperature with exercise and increase in carbon dioxide from actively metabolizing tissues also serve to increase the dissociation of oxygen from hemoglobin to facilitate delivery to the muscles.

All of these physiologic changes represent important adaptations that the body undergoes during exercise. In the normal state, these changes serve to augment oxygen delivery to metabolically active tissues and muscles, in particular the myocardium. In the presence of a flow-limiting coronary stenosis, nutrient myocardial blood flow may be diminished. As myocardial oxygen demand increases, the resistance vessels eventually become maximally vasodilated, and ischemia develops when demand exceeds supply. The ischemic cascade that occurs begins with myocardial perfusion deficits, diastolic and then systolic dysfunction, followed by ischemic electrocardiographic changes (ST-segment depression), and finally angina (see Figure 7-1).

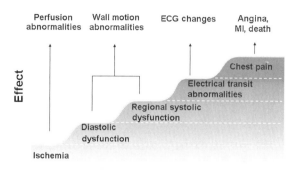

Figure 7-1. Ischemic cascade. The development of abnormalities associated with CAD generally follows a specific sequence of events, starting with decreases in flow that produce myocardial ischemia leading to detectable perfusion abnormalities. Progression of CAD leads to diastolic dysfunction followed by regional systolic dysfunction manifested as wall motion abnormalities. As the condition progresses, electrical transit abnormalities occur and are evident on the ECG. Symptoms of chest pain occur late in the ischemic sequence and may culminate in unstable angina, MI, or death. (CAD = coronary artery disease, ECG = electrocardiogram, MI = myocardial infarction).

PERFORMING THE EXERCISE STRESS TEST

Equipment

The majority of stress tests in the United States are performed using a motorized treadmill that can increase speed and incline, while exercise testing in Europe is typically performed using a bicycle ergometer. It is useful to note that arm ergometry can be performed in patients unable to exercise adequately because of lower extremity impairments. While automated blood pressure monitoring equipment is available, assessment of blood pressure using a manual sphygmomanometer is typically more accurate and reliable. Other necessary equipment includes continuous 12-lead ECG; an emergency kit or "code cart" containing all the necessary equipment for advanced cardiac life support, including intravenous cardiac medications; and an external defibrillator.

Patient Evaluation and Preparation

Prior to the performance of the exercise stress test, the procedure should be explained in detail to the patient, with an opportunity to have questions and concerns addressed. Written informed consent should then be obtained. Patients are typically instructed to fast for a few hours before the test. Pretest instructions should also advise the patient to wear clothes suitable for exercising. The referring physician should provide instructions with respect to continuing medication use, particularly drugs that may limit the heart rate response such as beta-blockers, calcium channel antagonists, and digoxin. This is of particular importance if the reason for the stress test is to diagnose CAD, since achievement of target heart rate is essential to achieve optimal sensitivity. For most diagnostic evaluations, all antianginal medications should be withheld for at least three medication half-lives. Medications may be continued in patients with known CAD who undergo testing for risk stratification, or even to assess the response to an anti-ischemic regimen.

Prior to the test, it is important to evaluate the patient with a brief history and physical examination focused on the cardiovascular system. Important historical elements include the patient's overall activity level, symptoms, prior medical and cardiac history including events and procedures, and a list of current medications. A directed physical examination to evaluate for signs of cardiac insufficiency should include auscultation of the lungs and heart. Abnormal signs or symptoms noted on initial evaluation may prompt modification to the exercise protocol used, or even cancellation of the examination.

Exercise testing is generally safe; however, myocardial infarction or death occurs at a rate of 1 to 4 per 10 000 tests performed, depending on the population studied.[2,20,21] For this reason, it is imperative to evaluate patients for high-risk features that may be exacerbated by the exercise test. As outlined in Table 7-1, absolute contraindications to stress testing include the presence of cardiac instability that would ordinarily require specific therapy and that stress testing is likely to worsen the condition such as an ACS, severe congestive heart failure, uncontrolled tachyarrhythmias, symptomatic bradycardia or heart block, severe aortic stenosis, and uncontrolled hypertension (systolic >200 mm Hg and/or diastolic >110 mm Hg). It should be noted that stress testing can be employed safely in patients with moderate aortic stenosis, in order to assess exercise capacity; however, these patients should be monitored very closely with frequent assessment of exercise blood pressures.[22] Relative contraindications include medications, and electrolyte or endocrine disorders, which may interfere with the heart rate response or stress ECG interpretation.

After the test has been thoroughly explained to the patient and informed consent to proceed is obtained, the ECG electrodes should be applied to the chest. The precordial leads (V1–V6) are affixed similar to a routine resting ECG; however,

Table 7-1

Contraindications to Exercise Stress Testing

Absolute
- Recent acute myocardial infarction (within 2 d)
- High-risk unstable angina
- Symptomatic or hemodynamically unstable cardiac arrhythmias
- Symptomatic severe aortic stenosis
- Uncontrolled symptomatic heart failure
- Acute pulmonary embolus or pulmonary infarction
- Acute myocarditis or pericarditis
- Acute aortic dissection

Relative
- Left main coronary stenosis
- Moderate stenotic valvular heart disease
- Electrolyte abnormalities
- Severe arterial hypertension (>200 mm Hg and/or diastolic blood pressure >110 mm Hg)
- Tachyarrhythmias or bradyarrhythmias
- Hypertrophic cardiomyopathy and other forms of outflow tract obstruction
- High-degree atrioventricular block

Adapted from Ref.[14]

most exercise laboratories modify the position of the limb leads, placing the arm leads over the pectoralis minor just below the clavicle and the leg leads on the trunk just below the costophrenic angle in the midclavicular line. The leads are commonly connected to a module that can be attached to a belt that the patient wears while exercising. Shaving any chest hair under where the electrodes will be placed, wiping the skin with alcohol to remove skin oils, and lightly scratching the skin with fine sandpaper to remove the superficial layer of skin may be helpful to improve electrode adherence to the skin and avoid electrodes falling off as a result of sweat production during exercise. The resting heart rate and blood pressure are recorded, and a standard 12-lead ECG should be recorded at rest in the supine and standing positions as the ECG can appear slightly different. During exercise, the 12-lead ECG should be recorded every minute, with the heart rate and blood pressure being assessed at least once per stage. Once the test is terminated, monitoring should continue for at least 5 minutes into recovery, and, until heart rate and blood pressure return to baseline, as important hemodynamic information, such as heart rate recovery,[23–25] and ischemic electrocardiographic changes[26] are often observed solely in recovery.

Exercise Protocols

A variety of protocols have been used to perform stress testing in patients with known or suspected CAD. The goal is to customize the protocol so that the patient completes at least 9 minutes of exercise. Bicycle ergometry can be performed using a ramp protocol, with the subject pedaling at 60 cycles per minute, and increasing the resistance from 50 W (or starting at 25 W for a modified protocol) until the target heart rate is achieved. The Bruce protocol, developed by Robert Bruce in Seattle, Washington, USA, is the protocol used most widely today for treadmill testing in most subjects[14] and is outlined in Table 7-2.[27] A modified Bruce protocol is also employed, which involves two "warm-up stages," 3 minutes each, with a speed of 1.7 miles per hour and a flat then 5% grade; these preliminary stages are usually referred to as "Stage 0" and "Stage 1/2." Other protocols include the Naughton protocol, which is less intense but of longer duration.[29]

Test End Points

The goal of the exercise test should be to have the patient exercise maximally in order to assess for the development of symptoms, ECG changes, or hemodynamic evidence of cardiac insufficiency. The test end point depends on the indication for the test. Accordingly, the development of angina and/or ischemic ECG changes during a test performed to diagnose or exclude CAD can be considered "positive" and terminated prior to the patient's maximum effort is achieved. In general, most tests should be performed with the goal that the patients exercise to their fullest. As such, the subject performs a "symptom-limited" test, stopping exercise because of inability to continue, fatigue, or desire to stop. Other end points that should prompt termination of the test include conduction abnormalities such as arrhythmias or heart block, the development of ST-segment depression >3 mm, ST-segment elevation >2 mm in leads without Q waves, and a hypotensive (decrease >10 mm Hg from baseline) or hypertensive (>250/115) blood pressure response. A test should also be stopped for any equipment malfunction, particularly any that prevents adequate monitoring of the blood pressure or ECG. If the test is being performed in conjunction with myocardial perfusion imaging, patients may need to notify the exercise test staff when they are approaching maximum effort in order to facilitate ejection of the radiotracer at peak stress and continue exercise for 1 to 2 minutes afterward, even if at a reduced workload, in order to permit adequate myocardial uptake. If the heart rate achieved is not close to the maximum predicted heart rate, usually at least 85% of this target, consideration

Table 7-2
BRUCE Protocol[27]

Stage	Time (min)	Speed (MPH)	Grade (%)	METS	Equivalent Activity Workload
1	3:00	1.7	10	4.6	Activities of daily living
2	6:00	2.5	12	7.0	Escalating one to two flights of stairs
3	9:00	3.4	14	10.0	Swimming and doubles' tennis
4	12:00	4.2	16	12.9	Singles' tennis and skiing
5	15:00	5.0	18	15.0 ⎫	Competitive athletes
6	18:00	5.5	20	18.0 ⎭	

Adapted from American Heart Association Exercise Standards[27] and the Duke Activity Status Index.[28]

should be given to defer injection of the radio-pharmaceutical and then converting the patient to a pharmacologic stress test.

INTERPRETATION OF THE STRESS TEST

A substantial amount of data is collected during a routine exercise stress test, which can be interpreted and applied to formulate a diagnosis and considered in determining prognosis. These data are outlined in Table 7-3.

Clinical Variables

The development of the symptoms during exercise that prompted the evaluation is, perhaps, the most useful piece of information obtained during an exercise test and may be sufficient to consider the test abnormal despite a normal ECG response. The overall workload achieved is important in that the greater the workload achieved, especially without chest pain or ECG changes, is known to be an independent predictor of cardiac events and even all-cause mortality.[2,30] In fact, a study of 6213 consecutive men referred for treadmill exercise testing found that men with a lower maximal heart rate, blood pressure, and overall exercise capacity achieved had a significantly worse survival during a mean follow-up of 6 years. After adjustment for age, the peak exercise capacity measured in metabolic equivalents (METS) was the strongest predictor of the risk of death among both normal subjects and those with cardiovascular disease, so much that each 1-MET increase in exercise capacity was associated with a 12% improvement in survival.[31] Similar findings have been described recently by Gulati and colleagues in a large cohort of women referred for stress testing, with the risk of death among asymptomatic women, whose exercise capacity was <85% of that predicted for age (based on a derived formula of MET = 14.7 − (0.13 × age)), being twice that among women whose exercise capacity exceeded 85%.[32]

Table 7-3

Data Collection During an Exercise Electrocardiogram

Clinical
  Symptoms (angina typical, dyspnea, and fatigue)
  Functional capacity
    Exercise duration
    Workload achieved
    Metabolic equivalents achieved
Hemodynamics
  Heart rate (peak, recovery)
    % age-predicted maximum HR (target HR) achieved
  Blood pressure (peak, hypertensive hypotensive)
  Rate pressure product (peak HR × peak systolic BP)
Electrocardiography
  ST-segment changes (severity (mm), onset, and duration into recovery)
    Morphology (upsloping, downsloping, and horizontal)
    Number and location of leads with changes
  ST-segment elevation
  Arrythmias

Hemodynamic Variables

The hemodynamic data acquired during a stress test can also be important. Exercise-induced hypotension, defined as a drop in systolic pressure >10 mm Hg from baseline, is associated with more advanced CAD and worse prognosis.[33–35] While much attention focuses on the achievement of "peak heart rate" (typically defined as >85% of the age-predicted maximum heart rate and calculated as 220 patients' age in years) for diagnostic purposes, the heart rate response to exercise has also been demonstrated to have prognostic significance. Many studies have confirmed that the lack of a heart rate reduction by at least 12 to 18 beats per minute in the first minute was associated with more significant CAD, left ventricular dysfunction, and decreased survival.[24,25,36,37]

Electrocardiographic Variables

The exercise ECG identifies CAD by detecting subtle alterations in electrical transit in the myocardium during repolarization in the presence of ischemia. It is generally accepted that the ST segment is compared to the isoelectric line or T-P segment on the baseline or rest ECG. The degree of ST-segment depression below this line is measured at the isoelectric point 60 to 80 milliseconds after the J point. J points in three consecutive beats is abnormal and consistent with ischemia. Upsloping ST-segment depression is a less specific finding,[38] although many consider ≥1.5 mm measured 80 milliseconds after the J point as an abnormal response. ST-segment depression at baseline is known to suggest CAD and may preclude a diagnostic test. However, additional change of ≥2 mm of horizontal or downsloping changes over baseline is a specific abnormal finding. Most, if not all, ECG changes noted on the stress ECG will occur in lead V5 and/or lead II. Accordingly, unlike ischemic changes on the rest ECG during symptoms, ischemic changes with stress do not localize to the vascular distribution (i.e., inferior or anterior).[39]

ST-segment elevation in leads without Q waves in 0.1% of patients who undergo exercise treadmill testing. With the exception of lead aVR and V1, the finding of ≥1 mm ST elevation in leads without Q waves should be considered evidence of impending myocardial injury, and the test terminated immediately. In contrast to ST-segment depressions, stress-induced ST elevations do localize to the coronary artery distribution involved. Representative ECG findings are displayed in Figure 7-2.

Right-sided and posterior leads have also been used in conjunction with stress testing and in several studies have demonstrated improved sensitivity[40]; however, the routine use of these additional leads is controversial and not universally accepted.

Duke Treadmill Score

Since reduced exercise capacity, the development of symptoms, particularly angina, and an ischemic ECG response are all associated with an increase in the likelihood of significant CAD and a worse

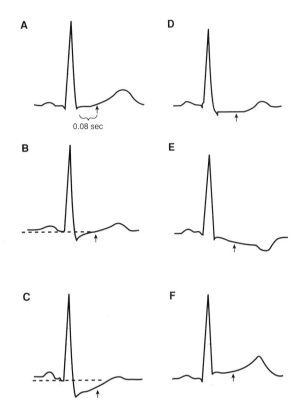

Figure 7-2.   Representative ECG changes during exercise. Schematic representation of various ST-segment patterns potentially produced by exercise. A: normal; B: junctional depression that returns to baseline (level of PR segment) within 0.08 s (arrow); C: junctional depression that remains below baseline at 0.08 s; D: horizontal ST depression; E: downsloping ST depression; F: ST elevation. (Reprinted with permission from Tavel.[42])

prognosis, the interplay of all these variables is likely to be useful as well. Registry data from 4083 participants in the Coronary Artery Surgery Study who did not undergo surgical revascularization showed that, as expected, mortality was inversely associated with exercise time and increased with a more ischemic ECG response. Those patients unable to achieve more than 5 METS of exercise and with >1 mm ST depression had an annual mortality of 5%, compared to <1% in those able to achieve at least 10 METS without ischemic changes. Based

Table 7-4

Duke Treadmill Score

Treadmill Score	Annual Mortality (%)
≤−11	5.25
+4 to −10	1.25
≥+5	0.25

The Duke Treadmill Score is calculated as follows: Exercise time (min) − 5 × (ST-segment depression in mm) − 4 × (angina score).

The exercise time is from a standard BRUCE protocol as outlined in Table 7-2, and the angina score is 0 if no angina occurred, 1 if angina developed, and 2 if exercise was limited by angina.

Adapted from Ref.[41]

on these findings, Mark and colleagues from Duke University analyzed an extensive database to determine the combined influence of these parameters in combination. As a way of combining the data elements above, a formula was derived, which incorporated the weighted impact of these findings on prognosis. The Duke Treadmill score[41] is outlined in Table 7-4.

Reporting of Exercise ECG Results

In addition to ensuring that the exercise test is performed safely in appropriate patients and analyzed correctly, similar attention should be provided to the reporting of the test results. Whether the exercise test is being interpreted alone or as part of a noninvasive imaging study, attention to detail in the reporting of the findings and conclusion is imperative. As many of these tests may be referrals from physicians who do not routinely perform stress testing, it is important to communicate the results and impression in a manner that will serve to guide the further management of the patient. A complete report should list the salient findings including the indication for the test, exercise time, protocol used, rest and stress hemodynamic data, and any symptoms that developed including the reason the test was terminated. An interpretation of the rest ECG should be included, and any ECG changes that occurred should describe the time of onset, lead location, peak deviation, and duration in recovery. The impression listed under the findings should begin with whether the test is normal, abnormal, or equivocal/nondiagnostic. A more descriptive impression is generally more helpful in distilling the results into a clinically relevant and meaningful conclusion. Alternatively, the entire report can be summarized in a paragraph such as outlined in Figure 7-3. Finally, when the study is markedly abnormal or very high risk, direct communication with the referring physician, such as by telephone, should be undertaken.

Indication_____

Findings:

The patient exercised for _____ minutes and _____ seconds of the _____ protocol achieving ___ METS of exercise, with (symptoms) beginning in stage ___ lasting___ into recovery. The test was terminated for (symptom(s)). Heart rate increased from ___ to____beats per minute, representing _____% of the age-predicted maximum heart rate, and blood pressure increased/decreased from ___/___ to ___/___ at peak exercise, for a calculated rate pressure product of _____. The rest electrocardiogram demonstrated _____. Beginning at Stage____, there were ST segment_____ in the _(leads), becoming _____mm at peak exercise, and lasting ____minutes into recovery.

Impression:

Normal/Abnormal/Equivocal/Nondiagnostic exercise stress electrocardiogram.

Figure 7-3.   Template for an exercise ECG report.

REFERENCES

1. Michaelides AP, Fourlas CA, Pitsavos C, et al. Exercise testing in asymptomatic patients with heterozygous familial hypercholesterolaemia. *Coron Artery Dis.* 2004; 15:461–465.

2. Balady GJ, Larson MG, Vasan RS, et al. Usefulness of exercise testing in the prediction of coronary disease risk among asymptomatic persons as a function of the Framingham risk score. *Circulation.* 2004;110:1920–1925.

3. Amsterdam EA, Kirk JD, Diercks DB, et al. Immediate exercise testing to evaluate low-risk patients presenting to the emergency department with chest pain. *J Am Coll Cardiol.* 2002;40:251–256.

4. Jensen-Urstad K, Samad BA, Bouvier F, et al. Prognostic value of symptom limited versus low level exercise stress test before discharge in patients with myocardial infarction treated with thrombolytics. *Heart (Br Cardiac Soc).* 1999;82:199–203.

5. Hamm LF, Crow RS, Stull GA, et al. Safety and characteristics of exercise testing early after acute myocardial infarction. *Am J Cardiol.* 1989;63:1193–1197.

6. Coplan NL, Curkovic V, Allen KM, et al. Early exercise testing to stratify risk for development of restenosis after percutaneous transluminal coronary angioplasty. *Am Heart J.* 1996;132:1222–1225.

7. Goto Y, Sumida H, Ueshima K, et al. Safety and implementation of exercise testing and training after coronary stenting in patients with acute myocardial infarction. *Circ J.* 2002;66:930–936.

8. Diamond GA, Forrester JS. Analysis of probability as an aid in the clinical diagnosis of coronary-artery disease. *N Engl J Med.* 1979;300:1350–1358.

9. Detrano R. Optimal use of literature knowledge to improve the Bayesian diagnosis of coronary artery disease. *J Clin Epidemiol.* 1989;42:1041–1047.

10. Detrano R, Yiannikas J, Salcedo EE, et al. Bayesian probability analysis: A prospective demonstration of its clinical utility in diagnosing coronary disease. *Circulation.* 1984;69:541–547.

11. Gianrossi R, Detrano R, Mulvihill D, et al. Exercise-induced ST depression in the diagnosis of coronary artery disease. A meta-analysis. *Circulation.* 1989;80:87–98.

12. Detrano R, Gianrossi R, Froelicher V. The diagnostic accuracy of the exercise electrocardiogram: A meta-analysis of 22 years of research. *Prog Cardiovasc Dis.* 1989;32:173–206.

13. Mieres JH, Udelson JE. Meta-analysis of exercise testing to detect coronary artery disease in women [comment]. *Am J Cardiol.* 1999;84:1454–1456.

14. Gibbons RJ, Balady GJ, Bricker JT, et al. ACC/AHA 2002 guideline update for exercise testing: Summary article. A report of the American College of Cardiology/American Heart Association Task Force on Practice Guidelines (Committee to Update the 1997 Exercise Testing Guidelines). *J Am Coll Cardiol.* 2002; 40:1531–1540.

15. Williams MA. Exercise testing in cardiac rehabilitation. Exercise prescription and beyond. *Cardiol Clin* 2001;19:415–431.

16. Abboud L, Hir J, Eisen I, et al. Long-term value of exercise testing after acute myocardial infarction: influence of thrombolytic therapy. *Chest.* 2000;117:556–561.

17. Parodi G, Antoniucci D. Late coronary stent thrombosis associated with exercise testing. *Catheter Cardiovasc Interv.* 2004;61:515–517.

18. Maraj R, Fraifeld M, Owen AN, et al. Coronary dissection and thrombosis associated with exercise testing three months after successful coronary stenting. *Clin Cardiol.* 1999;22:426–428.

19. Pierce GL, Seferlis C, Kirshenbaum J, et al. Lack of association of exercise testing with coronary stent closure. *Am J Cardiol.* 2000;86:1259–1261.

20. Gibbons L, Blair SN, Kohl HW, et al. The safety of maximal exercise testing. *Circulation.* 1989;80:846–852.

21. Myers J, Voodi L, Umann T, et al. A survey of exercise testing: methods, utilization, interpretation, and safety in the VAHCS. *J Cardiopulm Rehabil.* 2000;20:251–258.

22. Chung EH, Gaasch WH. Exercise testing in aortic stenosis. *Curr Cardiol Rep.* 2005;7:105–107.

23. Morshedi-Meibodi A, Larson MG, Levy D, et al. Heart rate recovery after treadmill exercise testing and risk of cardiovascular disease events (The Framingham Heart Study). *Am J Cardiol.* 2002;90:848–852.

24. Watanabe J, Thamilarasan M, Blackstone EH, et al. Heart rate recovery immediately after treadmill exercise and left ventricular systolic dysfunction as predictors of mortality: The case of stress echocardiography. *Circulation.* 2001;104:1911–1916.

25. Nishime EO, Cole CR, Blackstone EH, et al. Heart rate recovery and treadmill exercise score as predictors of mortality in patients referred for exercise ECG. *JAMA.* 2000;284:1392–1398.

26. Soto JR, Watson DD, Beller GA. Incidence and significance of ischemic ST-segment depression occurring solely during recovery after exercise testing. *Am J Cardiol.* 2001;88:670–672.

27. Fletcher GF, Balady G, Froelicher VF, et al. Exercise standards. A statement for healthcare professionals from the American Heart Association. Writing Group. *Circulation.* 1995;91:580–615.

28. Hlatky MA, Boineau RE, Higginbotham MB, et al. A brief self-administered questionnaire to determine functional capacity (the Duke Activity Status Index). *Am J Cardiol.* 1989;64:651–654.

29. Handler CE, Sowton E. A comparison of the Naughton and modified Bruce treadmill exercise protocols in their ability to detect ischaemic abnormalities six weeks after myocardial infarction. *Eur Heart J.* 1984;5:752–755.

30. Roger VL, Jacobsen SJ, Pellikka PA, et al. Prognostic value of treadmill exercise testing: A population-based study in Olmsted County, Minnesota. *Circulation.* 1998;98:2836–2841.

31. Myers J, Prakash M, Froelicher V, et al. Exercise capacity and mortality among men referred for exercise testing. *N Engl J Med.* 2002;346:793–801.

32. Gulati. The prognostic value of a nomogram for exercise capacity in women. *N Engl J Med.* 2005;353:468–475.

33. Iskandrian AS, Kegel JG, Lemlek J, et al. Mechanism of exercise-induced hypotension in coronary artery disease. *Am J Cardiol.* 1992;69:1517–1520.

34. Watson G, Mechling E, Ewy GA. Clinical significance of early vs. late hypotensive blood pressure response to treadmill exercise. *Arch Intern Med.* 1992;152:1005–1008.

35. Hammermeister KE, DeRouen TA, Dodge HT, et al. Prognostic and predictive value of exertional hypotension in suspected coronary heart disease. *Am J Cardiol.* 1983;51:1261–1266.

36. Georgoulias P, Orfanakis A, Demakopoulos N, et al. Abnormal heart rate recovery immediately after treadmill testing: Correlation with clinical, exercise testing, and myocardial perfusion parameters. *J Nucl Cardiol.* 2003;10:498–505.

37. Cheng YJ, Lauer MS, Earnest CP, et al. Heart rate recovery following maximal exercise testing as a predictor of cardiovascular disease and all-cause mortality in men with diabetes. *Diabetes Care.* 2003;26:2052–2057.

38. Desai MY, Crugnale S, Mondeau J, et al. Slow upsloping ST-segment depression during exercise: Does it really signify a positive stress test? *Am Heart J.* 2002;143:482–487.

39. Miranda CP, Lehmann KG, Froelicher VF. Correlation between resting ST segment depression, exercise testing, coronary angiography, and long-term prognosis. *Am Heart J.* 1991;122:1617–1628.

40. Shry EA, Eckart RE, Furgerson JL, et al. Addition of right-sided and posterior precordial leads during stress testing. *Am Heart J.* 2003;164:1090–1094.

41. Mark DB, Hlatky MA, Harrell FE Jr, et al. Exercise treadmill score for predicting prognosis in coronary artery disease. *Ann Intern Med.* 1987;106:793–800.

42. Tavel, ME, Stress testing in cardiac evaluation: Current concepts with emphasis on the ECG. *Chest.* 2001;119:907–925.

CHAPTER 8

Pharmacologic Stress Testing in Myocardial Perfusion Imaging: Technical Application

Rami Doukky

INTRODUCTION

An increasing proportion of patients are unable to perform maximum exercise or for whom exercise is contraindicated (Table 8-1). Fortunately, pharmacologic stress testing provides an excellent alternative to exercise testing and is widely used with single photon emission computed tomography (SPECT) myocardial perfusion imaging (MPI) and other imaging modalities. In fact, the vast growth of nuclear cardiology applications in recent years is credited, in large part, to effective pharmacologic stress testing, as it is estimated that pharmacologic stress testing accounts for approximately 45% to 50% of all MPI studies performed in the United States.[1,2] The diagnostic and prognostic value of pharmacologic-stress MPI has been well demonstrated in numerous clinical trials in the past two decades. Recent advances in pharmacologic stress testing have further enhanced its role on MPI. Simultaneous low-level exercise with adenosine infusion has improved image quality and substantially reduced adenosine-associated side effects.[3] Finally, new promising selective adenosine (A2A) receptor agonists are likely to further perfect the use of pharmacologic stress in MPI.[4]

Generally, pharmacologic stress agents can be divided into two broad categories: coronary vasodilatory agents—adenosine and dipyridamole, and catecholamines, such as dobutamine. Vasodilators increase coronary blood flow, creating disparity of flow augmentation between normal and stenotic coronary arteries, resulting in heterogeneity of radioisotope uptake between myocardium supplied by normal coronary artery and that supplied by diseased artery. For the most part, adenosine and dipyridamole are the preferred pharmacologic stress agents, comprising the majority of clinical data. Catecholamines act primarily via increasing heart rate, rate–pressure product, and myocardial contractility leading to increased myocardial oxygen demand and potentially inducing myocardial ischemia.

Table 8-1

Indications for Pharmacologic Stress Myocardial Perfusion Imaging

Inability to exercise
- Musculoskeletal limitations: amputations, arthritis, etc.
- Neurologic limitations: CVA, ataxia, vertigo, etc.
- Cardiopulmonary: chronic lung disease, and CHF

Contraindication to exercise
- Aortic dissection or large aortic aneurysm
- Uncontrolled hypertension

Indications specific to vasodilator-stress MPI
- LBBB
- Ventricular pacemaker

CVA, cerebrovascular accident; CHF, congestive heart failure; MPI, myocardial perfusion imaging; LBBB, left bundle branch block.

DOBUTAMINE SRESS

Dobutamine stress is an alternative stress agent in patients who cannot exercise and have a contraindication to adenosine or dipyridamole use (Table 8-2). Dobutamine is a β1- and β2-adrenergic receptor agonist. Its action in pharmacologic stress is primarily related to β1-receptor stimulation, leading to positive inotropic and

Table 8-2

Contraindications to Adenosine and Dipyridamole Stress

- Asthmatic patients with ongoing wheezing
- Greater than first-degree AV block or sick sinus syndrome without pacemaker
- Systolic blood pressure less than 90 mm Hg
- Use of aminophylline or caffeinated foods or beverages
- Acute phase of myocardial infarction or acute coronary syndrome
- Hypersensitivity to adenosine or dipyridamole
- Relative contraindication, profound sinus bradycardia (heart rate <40/min)
- Use of dipyridamole-containing medications is a contraindication to adenosine use but not dipyridamole

chronotropic response. It also increases coronary blood flow in normal coronaries by approximately two to three times the baseline level, which creates flow disparities between normal and abnormal coronary arteries, leading to heterogeneity in radioisotope uptake by corresponding myocardium. Although dobutamine increases coronary blood flow, some concern has been raised that it may interfere with Tc-99m sestamibi uptake, which can interfere with its ability to detect CAD.[5,6] This is possibly related to dobutamine-induced calcium influx, which blunts the mitochondrial membrane driving potential, diminishing sestamibi uptake.

Procedure

Dobutamine is given as a continuous intravenous infusion using a programmable pump, since it has a short half-life of 2 minutes. Starting infusion rate is 5 or 10 μg/kg/min. Infusion rate is up-titrated in 3-minute intervals by 10 μg/kg/min increments. The maximum infusion rate is 40 or 50 μg/kg/min. Atropine (0.5–1 mg) may be administered intravenously to further enhance chronotropic response in patients who do not achieve adequate heart rate response, which is usually 85% of the patient's predicted maximum heart rate (220 − age). Radioisotope is administered intravenously as soon as patient achieves target heart rate. Dobutamine infusion is continued for 2 to 3 minutes following radioisotope administration, to maintain high heart rate while radioisotope is being extracted by the myocardium. Some laboratories administer one or multiple doses of intravenous β-blocking agents, such as metoprolol or esmolol, to expedite heart rate recovery and enhance laboratory turnover. Continuous electrocardiogram (ECG) recording during dobutamine/atropine infusion and recovery period is crucial. Patients are monitored for arrhythmias (ventricular and supraventricular) and myocardial ischemia.

Contraindications to dobutamine/atropine stress testing include acute phase of acute coronary syndromes, uncontrolled hypertension, hypotension, uncontrolled ventricular or supraventricular

Table 8-3

Contraindications to Dobutamine Stress

- Recent acute myocardial infarction
- Unstable angina
- Significant left ventricular outflow obstruction
- Severe aortic stenosis
- Supraventricular tachycardia with rapid ventricular response
- History of ventricular tachycardia
- Uncontrolled hypertension
- Aortic dissection or large aortic aneurysm

arrhythmias, and hemodynamic instability (Table 8-3).

Common adverse effects to dobutamine include chest pain (39%), hypotension (3.4%), and arrhythmias. Other side effects include dyspnea, palpitations, headache, and flushing[7] (Table 8-4). Although chest pain is common during dobutamine infusion, it does not always represent myocardial ischemia. Hypotension is a more common side effect in the elderly.[8] Aggressive volume replacement with normal saline would help prevent and manage this problem, and intravenous atropine administration is often helpful. Supraventricular tachyarrhythmias commonly encountered are atrial fibrillation, atrial flutter, and atrioventricular (AV) nodal reentry tachycardia.

These are often transient, and patients return to sinus rhythm when dobutamine effect dissipates with infusion discontinuation. Serious ventricular arrhythmias are less common (4%).[7] Patients with structural heart disease, especially prior myocardial infarction (MI), and electrolytes disturbances are at increased risk of such events.[7] Intravenous β-blocking agents (esmolol or metoprolol) can be administered to acutely reduce heart rate and potentially terminate adverse events and side effect. Overall, dobutamine/atropine MPI has demonstrated excellent safety profile when done with trained personnel.[7–9]

Clinical Value of Dobutamine Testing

Based on data pool from 20 studies, Geleijnse et al.[10] reported that sensitivity, specificity, and accuracy of dobutamine-stress MPI for the detection of CAD were 88%, 74%, and 84%, respectively. Ischemic ECG changes with or without chest pain during dobutamine infusions are common. Nevertheless, diagnostic accuracy of such findings is limited.[11–14] Nondiagnostic test results (absence of reversible perfusion defects with submaximal stress) do occur in approximately 10% of patients.[10]

In addition to its excellent diagnostic value, dobutamine–atropine stress SPECT MPI provides

Table 8-4

Incidence of Common Side Effects with Pharmacologic Stress Agents

	Adenosine (%) (n = 9256) [35]	Dipyridamole (%) (n = 3911) [29]	Dobutamine (%) (n = 1076) [7]
Chest pain	35	20	39
Flushing	37	3	<1
Dyspnea	35	3	6
Dizziness	9	3	4
Gastrointestinal discomfort	15	1	1
Headache	14	12	7
Arrhythmia	3	5	45
AV block	8	0	0
ST-segment changes	6	8	20–31
Any adverse effect	81	50	50–75

excellent prognostic information similar to other stress modalities used in MPI. Geleijnse et al.[15] demonstrated that patients with normal dobutamine-stress MPI had low annual major cardiac event rate (cardiac death, nonfatal MI) of 0.8%. In a high-risk group, Calnon et al.[16] reported higher annual event rate of 2.3% in patients with normal dobutamine-stress MPI. However, the same study demonstrated much higher event rate of 10% in patients with abnormal study. In the largest study published to date (721 patients followed for 37 months), Schinkel et al. reported 1% annual cardiac death rate in patients with normal scan vs. 5.1% annual rate in patients with abnormal one.[17] In most laboratories, patients who undergo dobutamine-stress MPI are typically higher-risk group of patients with multiple comorbidities. Nevertheless, studies confirm the ability of dobutamine-stress MPI to separate patients with low risk from those with high risk.

β-Blocking agents, as a competitive antagonist to dobutamine at $\beta 1$ receptor's level, can interfere with pharmacologic action of dobutamine and ability to achieve target heart rate. However, with atropine use diagnostic test is often accomplished. Huang et al.[18] demonstrated that β-blocker use does not affect sensitivity or specificity of dobutamine stress myocardial perfusion as long as target heart rate is achieved. They also demonstrated that patients receiving these agents are more likely to require the administration of intravenous atropine to achieve targeted heart rate (51%) as compared to subjects not receiving β-blocking agents (13%).

Atropine alone has been used as a pharmacologic stress agent with MPI, usually in conjunction with exercise testing.[19] As a result of its potent anticholinergic effect, it induces tachycardia and increased myocardial oxygen demand, resulting in myocardial ischemia in patients with flow limiting coronary stenoses, which, in turn, leads to inhomogeneity in myocardial radioisotope uptake detected by MPI. Anticholinergic side effects are common (dry mouth, blurred vision, etc.). Although firm diagnostic performance and risk prediction data are lacking, the use of atropine with exercise appears safe and potentially useful in patients who are unable to achieve an adequate heart rate response.

VASODILATOR (ADENOSINE AND DIPYRIDAMOLE) STRESS MPI

Adenosine and dipyridamole produce coronary vasodilatation through common mechanism of action. Adenosine is produced endogenously in vascular smooth muscle and endothelial cells and produces coronary vasodilatation by activating adenyl cyclase, which results in the opening of the potassium channels (Figure 8-1). Exogenous (intravenous injection) dipyridamole inhibits the cellular reuptake of adenosine, thereby increasing the amount of adenosine available for receptor binding and thus indirectly promoting vascular smooth muscle relaxation.[2,20,21] Both adenosine and dipyridamole can increase coronary blood flow by three to five times above baseline level in normal coronary arteries. With severe coronary stenoses present, no increase in coronary blood flow is created by these vasodilators, and this disparity in coronary flow reserve results in inhomogeneity in radiopharmaceutical uptake in the corresponding myocardium.[22,23] In some cases, vasodilator agents can cause an absolute decrease of coronary blood flow in poststenotic segments secondary to coronary "steal" phenomenon caused by shunting of blood away from diseased coronary arteries via collateral vessels.[24] Caffeine and methylxanthines (theophilline and aminophylline) act as adenosine receptor blockers (antagonists)[25,26] and may prevent vasodilatation. Therefore, they should be avoided before vasodilator (adenosine and dipyridamole) MPI, for perhaps up to 24 hours, although recent data on the need for caffeine restriction suggest that this may be unnecessary.

Among patients who are unable to exercise maximally, adenosine and dipyridamole stresses are the preferred modes of testing for MPI, except in the setting of specific contraindications. The presence of severe reactive airways disease, overt wheezing, high-degree AV block,

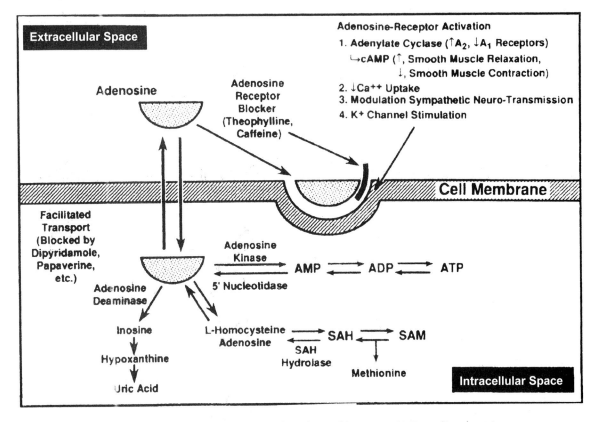

Figure 8-1. Mechanism of action of adenosine-mediated vasodilatation. cAMP, cyclic adenosine monophosphate; AMP, adenosine monophosphate; ADP, adenosine diphosphate; ATP, adenosine triphosphate; SAH, *S*-adenosyl homocysteine; SAM, *S*-adenosyl methionine. (Reprinted with permission from Verani.[20])

hypotension, and the recent ingestion of methylxanthines, such as caffeine, should be considered contraindications to performing vasodilator stress (Table 8-2).

Protocols

Dipyridamole Patients arrive for the test preferably fasting, so as to minimize abdominal discomfort and nausea. Caffeine-containing foods and aminophylline (given for reactive airway disease) should be withheld for 24 to 48 hours prior to the test. Dipyridamole is administered intravenously using a programmed infusion pump at 142 μg/kg/min for a 4-minute period. Dipyri-

damole produces maximum coronary vasodilatation within 5 minutes, which persists for 10 to 30 minutes after completion of infusion. Radiopharmaceutical agent is injected during period of maximum vasodilatation, usually 3 to 5 minutes after the dipyridamole infusion.

ECG and blood pressure monitoring is done during, and few minutes after, infusion. Typically, at peak vasodilatation, dipyridamole induces a mean of 15-beat/min increase in heart rate and a 15 mm Hg decrease in systolic blood pressure.[27] Poststress SPECT imaging should be started within 15 minutes following Tl-201 administration, to prevent redistribution of the tracer. When Tc-99m agents are used (tetrofosmin or sestamibi), imaging is typically done 45 to 60 minutes following radiopharmaceutical administration.[28] Dipyridamole effect can be quickly reversed by administration of aminophylline intravenously (75–150 mg).

Serious adverse events of dipyridamole (death, MI, and severe bronchospasm) are rare.[27] However, minor side effects (chest pain, headache, flushing, dyspnea, and dizziness) are very common.[29] The same study reported 8% incidence of ST-segment changes on ECG (Table 8-4). Brown et al.[30] demonstrated that dipyridamole pharmacologic stress is even safe as early as 2 days following uncomplicated acute MI. Dipyridamole infusion is contraindicated in patients with moderate-to-severe reactive airway disease, hypotension, acute phase of acute coronary syndrome, and hemodynamic instability.

Adenosine Similar to dipyridamole protocol, patients are instructed to be fasting and withholding caffeine-containing foods and aminophylline prescription medications (Table 8-2). Additionally, as dipyridamole will block the reuptake and prolong the effect of exogenously administered adenosine, dipyridamole-containing medications should not be given for at least 24 hours beforehand. Adenosine has a very short half-life, approximately 2 to 10 seconds, with the onset of action occurring in 5 seconds and maximum coronary dilatation occurring within 2 minutes. In MPI, adenosine is usually administered intravenously as continuous infusion, using a programmable electric pump at a rate of 140 μg/kg/min for a total of 6 minutes. Radioisotope is administered when maximum vasodilatation is achieved; this is typically done 2 to 3 minutes into the protocol (mid-point of infusion protocol). ECG is monitored continuously during and for few minutes following infusion for signs of myocardial ischemia and AV block.

Treuth et al.,[31] in a randomized 6- vs. 3-minute adenosine infusion MPI study, demonstrated that subjects experienced less adverse events during the 3-minute infusion protocol while maintaining 88% sensitivity for the detection of CAD. Nevertheless, perfusion defect size was slightly larger in patients with abnormal scans who received 6-minute infusion protocol. Other investigators[32,33] reported similar results when they addressed the same hypothesis. The results of these trials may not be applicable to other radiopharmaceutical agents (sestamibi, and especially tetrofosmin), since these agents have lower extraction fraction and inferior myocardial uptake in comparison with Tl-201. Still, newer data suggest that a 4-minute infusion may allow for a maximal hyperemic response and permit an adequate amount of time for radiotracer extraction. Therefore, a protocol with a 4-minute adenosine infusion is now generally considered acceptable,[34] although this deviates from the manufacture's recommendation.[28]

The hemodynamic effect of adenosine is slightly more profound than dipyridamole and causes higher increase in heart rate and higher incidence of side effects. In a study including 9256 patients, Cerqueira et al.[35] reported 80% incidence of side effects. Common side effects include chest pain (35%), flushing (37%), dyspnea (35%), dizziness (9%), gastrointestinal discomfort (15%), and headache (14%). Additionally, 8% of patients developed some degree of AV block, but less than 1% of patients had third-degree AV block. Ischemic ST-segment changes on ECG were reported in 6% of patients in the same study (Table 8-4). Nevertheless, given adenosine's very short half-life, these adverse effects reverse almost instantaneously as soon as adenosine infusion is terminated. Aminophylline rarely, if ever, needed to reverse its effect. As with dipyridamole, adenosine infusion is contraindicated in patients with moderate-to-severe reactive airway disease, hypotension, acute phase of acute coronary syndrome, and hemodynamic instability (Table 8-2). Adenosine may be used carefully in patients with mild controlled reactive airway disease as any adverse effect can be terminated quickly. Adenosine is contraindicated in patients with high-grade AV conduction abnormality.

Ischemic ECG changes during adenosine infusion suggest the presence of significant CAD and correlates with the finding of reversible perfusion defect on MPI.[36] In the past few years, growing body of evidence suggests that ischemic ECG changes during adenosine infusion caries significant negative prognostic implications irrespective of MPI findings. Abbott et al.[37] demonstrated in a study of patients with normal MPI that ischemic ECG changes during adenosine infusion were associated with significantly more adverse cardiac events than those without such changes (nonfatal MI, 7.6% vs. 0.5%; subsequent revisualization, 13.6% vs. 2.5%, respectively). Such findings have been replicated in several other studies.[38-40] Hence, ischemic ECG changes during adenosine MPI should warrant further evaluation, even when perfusion images are reassuring, which is different from the prognostic significance of ischemic ECG changes during dipyridamole infusion.[40,41]

False-positive finding of reversible septal defect on MPI is well documented in patients with baseline ECG abnormalities of left bundle branch block (LBBB), ventricular pre-excitation, and permanent ventricular pacing. False-positive imaging results are much less frequent with adenosine and dipyridamole[42-44] (10%) as compared to stress imaging with exercise (46%). Therefore, vasodilators (adenosine and dipyridamole) are stress agents of choice in this special group of patients. As with exercise, the use of dobutamine in patients with LBBB undergoing MPI is not recommended.[28]

β-Blockers are commonly prescribed to patients referred for stress testing. The effect of these agents on results of vasodilator-stress MPI is somewhat controversial. Taillefer et al.[45] clearly demonstrated that administration of intravenous metoprolol prior to dipyridamole-stress MPI reduces the sensitivity of the test for the detection of myocardial ischemia (71%), compared to control group (86%). Furthermore, summed stress score (SSS) and summed difference score (SDS) were significantly lower in the group of patients who received intravenous metoprolol, indicating that severity and extent of ischemia are also underestimated with β-blocker use. Sharir et al.[46] demonstrated similar effect to antianginal agents in general. Based on these data, withholding antianginals in general and β-blocking agents in particular is prudent prior to pharmacologic-stress MPI, especially when the purpose of the study is to establish the diagnosis of ischemic heart disease.

COMBINED VASODILATOR AND EXERCISE STRESS TESTING

Vasodilator pharmacologic stress agents (adenosine and dipyridamole) have a safety and diagnostic profile that is similar to exercise stress. The incidence of their adverse effects has been high. Since their effect is not limited to the coronary arteries, systemic vasodilatation leads to increased radioisotope uptake outside the heart, which degrades target to background ratio and leads to inferior image quality compared to that of exercise protocols. Combining low-level exercise with pharmacologic stress produces vasoconstriction in the splanchnic vessels and produces adrenergic response, which results in decreased adverse effects and reduced radioisotope uptake in nontarget organs.

Several studies have shown that dipyridamole, when combined with low-level exercise, is safe and improves patient tolerance, increases target-to-background ratios, and enhances image quality.[47-49] Stern et al.[50] evaluated various levels of exercise in combination with dipyridamole infusion and concluded that the addition of low-level treadmill exercise is superior to isometric handgrip and to dipyridamole infusion alone.

As with dipyridamole, several studies have established the role of simultaneous low-level exercise with adenosine infusion. Pennel et al.[51] were the first to investigate the combination of low-level bicycle exercise with adenosine and reported fewer side effects, improved target-to-background ratios, and more defect reversibility in patients undergoing the combined protocol. Several other European investigators reported similar findings using combined bicycle exercise with adenosine infusion.[49,52]

North American studies used treadmill exercise modality instead. Jamil et al.[53] provided the first report on the use of low-level treadmill exercise protocol with adenosine infusion. These

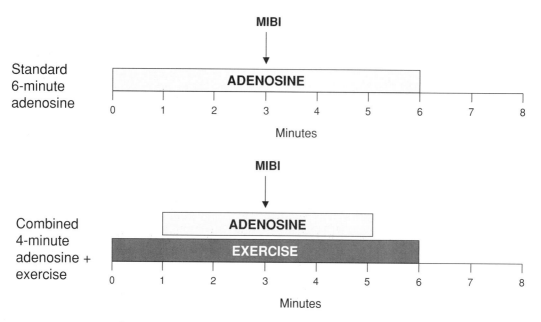

Figure 8-2. Schematic depicting standard 6-minute adenosine stress protocol and combined adenosine with low-level exercise protocol. MIBI, Tc-99m sestamibi. (Adapted with permission from Elliott et al.[57])

investigators used 4-minute adenosine infusion (140 μg/kg/min) with 6-minute treadmill exercise protocol (1.7 mph at 0% incline for 3 minutes, then 5% incline for the remaining 3 minutes). The exercise started 1 minute before and continued for 1 minute after adenosine infusion (Figure 8-2). Other studies have also shown the feasibility of combined adenosine and exercise protocols, using a variety of treadmill speeds and grades.[54] In all studies, adenosine infused at standard rate of 140 μg/kg/min and the radioisotope was injected at mid-point of adenosine infusion. In all cases, image quality and patient tolerability were improved with the use of adjunctive exercise.

Holly et al.,[55] in the BEAST trial, tested a very different hypothesis, adding pharmacologic stress to maximum symptom-limited treadmill exercise (Bruce protocol). Study subjects underwent both exercise MPI and exercise MPI with a 4-minute adenosine infusion on a separate day (Figure 8-3). This combined adenosine/maximal exercise protocol allows for full assessment of patient's functional capacity (Bruce protocol), in addition to

obtaining diagnostic pharmacologic-stress MPI regardless of patient's ability to achieve target heart rate, and hence maximizing the likelihood for obtaining a diagnostic MPI study. Detection of myocardial ischemia was enhanced using this novel protocol (Figure 8-4).

Most studies in print demonstrate that addition of exercise to adenosine infusion, in comparison to adenosine infusion alone, reduces most side effects including second- and third-degree AV block, sinus bradycardia, and hypotension.[51,54,56,57] Some studies suggested nonstatistically significant trend toward increased incidence of anginal chest pain.[49,54,58] Elliot et al.,[57] using crossover trial design, demonstrated marked reduction of patient-reported symptom-severity score with combined adenosine–exercise in comparison to adenosine-only protocol (Figure 8-5). Additionally, improvements in heart-to-background and heart-to-liver ratios were noted. Thomas et al.[56] also reported significant improvements in image quality. These authors clearly demonstrated the ability to obtain stress images

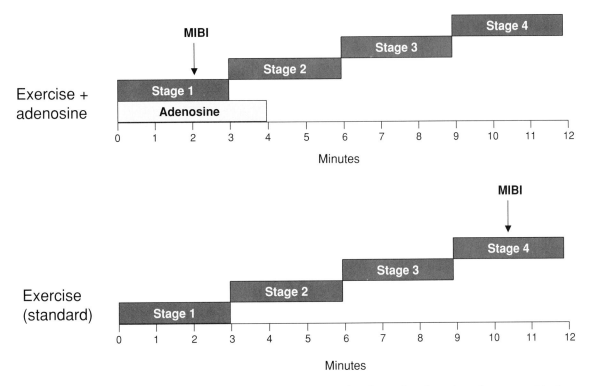

Figure 8-3.   Schematic depicting standard exercise stress protocol and exercise-plus-adenosine protocol in the BEAST study. In both protocols, patient underwent maximum symptom-limited exercise according to the Bruce Protocol. Tc-99m sestamibi (MIBI) was injected approximately 1 minute prior to termination of exercise in the standard protocol and 2 minutes into adenosine infusion in the exercise-plus-adenosine protocol. (Adapted with permission from Holly et al.[55])

earlier, following the combined stress protocol, which would shorten total test time. Several other trials have also reported improved image quality when exercise was added to vasodilator stress testing.[58]

Diagnostic accuracy may also be affected by adjunctive exercise. Exercise added to dipyridamole studies has demonstrated improved sensitivity.[47,48,50,59–61] In most adenosine-exercise studies, mild increase of sensitivity and defect reversibility has been observed.[51,52,54,55,57,58,62] Holly et al.[55] observed higher SSS and SDS in combined adenosine–exercise protocol compared with adenosine alone (Figure 8-4). Pennel et al.[51] reported similar findings. The mechanism of enhanced sensitivity for the detection of myocardial

ischemia is unclear but, may be because of combination of enhanced myocardial hyperemia,[63] α-adrenergic receptor-mediated exercise-induced spasm in astherosclerotic-diseased coronary arteries,[64,65] and/or improved diagnostic accuracy caused by improved image quality.

Combined adenosine–exercise stress testing also improves the value of MPI for predicting risk for cardiovascular events. In the Nuclear Utility in the Community (NUC) trial, Thomas et al.[66] investigated the prognostic value of combined adenosine–exercise stress modality and compared it with that of adenosine stress alone and exercise stress in 1612 outpatients. This study demonstrated, like with other stress modalities, the ability of the combined adenosine–exercise MPI to

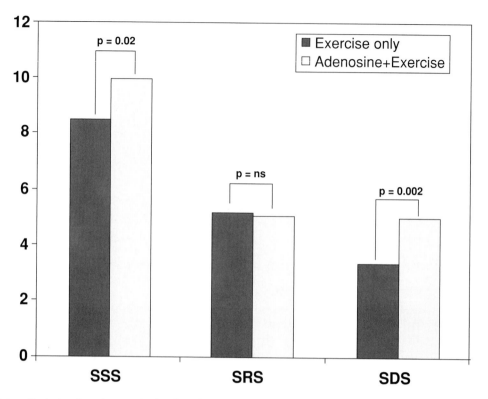

Figure 8-4.   Perfusion imaging results for the adenosine-only and adenosine-plus-exercise in the BEAST study. Compared with the exercise-only group, the summed stress scores (*SSS*) and summed difference scores (*SDS*) were significantly greater in the adenosine-plus-exercise group. There were no significant differences in the summed rest scores (*SRS*) between the two groups. (Adapted with permission from Elliott et al.[57])

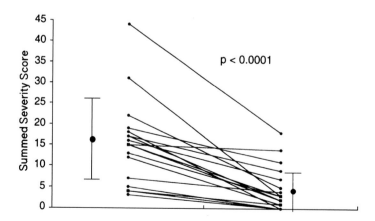

Figure 8-5.   Symptom severity scores for each patient during both adenosine protocols. Compared with a 6-minute adenosine protocol, an abbreviated adenosine infusion with low-level exercise resulted in a significant reduction in symptom severity scores ($P < 0.0001$). (Reprinted with permission from Elliott et al.[57])

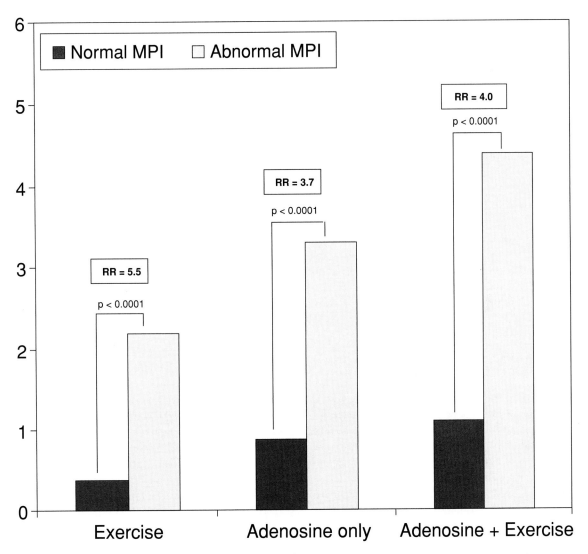

Figure 8-6. Incidence of adverse events in patients undergoing exercise, adenosine, and adenosine plus low-level exercise stress based on myocardial perfusion imaging results being normal or abnormal. As with adenosine and exercise protocols, combined adenosine plus low-level exercise stress protocol should separate patients into distinct risk strata based on the MPI findings. (Adapted from Thomas et al.[66])

predict very low risk of cardiac events in patients with normal MPI and separate those from patients with high risk, with abnormal MPI (Figure 8-6). Furthermore, the ability of the combined protocol to separate patient with high risk from those with low risk was better than adenosine alone (relative risk of abnormal to normal study was 3.9 for combined protocol vs. 3.2 for adenosine alone). Additionally, transient ischemic dilatation (TID) with the combined adenosine–exercise protocol was a better predictor of poor outcome that in patients with adenosine alone.

Left bundle branch block has been known to cause false-positive finding of septal ischemia in patients undergoing exercise MPI.[42,43] Similar problem is encountered in patients with right ventricular pacing.[67] Consequently, most trials investigating combined adenosine–exercise protocols have excluded patients with LBBB and paced ventricular rhythm.[55–57] Unless future data validate its use, the combined adenosine–exercise protocol should be avoided in these settings.

After exclusion of patients with LBBB and right ventricular pacing and those who are unable to perform any exercise, the majority of patients referred for pharmacologic-stress MPI are able to, and should, perform combined low-level exercise along with vasodilator stress testing. This practice results in improved image quality, superior patient tolerability, and possibly enhanced detection of myocardial ischemia.

SELECTIVE ADENOSINE A2A RECEPTOR AGONISTS

Despite their excellent diagnostic utility, dipyridamole and adenosine remain less-than-ideal pharmacologic stress agents. Although serious adverse events with these agents are exceedingly rare, their side effects are frequent and unpleasant and they are contraindicated in patients with bronchospastic disease and high-grade AV conduction abnormalities. Additionally, they require continuous intravenous infusion. These adverse events are primarily because of nonselective stimulation to adenosine receptors.

Four types of adenosine receptors have been identified: A1, A2A, A2B, and A3. AV conduction abnormalities and chest pain are thought to be mediated through A1 receptors.[68] A2A receptors are thought to mediate coronary vasodilatation,[69,70] whereas A2B receptors mediate peripheral vasodilatation and bronchoconstriction.[71] A3 receptor activation seems to elicit preconditioning against ischemic injury and stimulate mast cell degranulation.[72] Therefore, developing a selective A2A receptor agonist would be ideal for pharmacologic MPI, so as to induce coronary vasodilatation and myocardial hyperemia and avoid other adverse effects resulting from the stimulation of other adenosine receptors. Several selective A2A receptor agonists have been developed, which appear suitable for MPI. Two of these agents, regadenoson (also known as CVT-3146) and binodenoson (also known as MRE-0470 and WRC-0470), have now completed phase III clinical trials, with a third agent, apadenoson, demonstrating promise in a phase II study.

Regadenoson

Regadenoson (CVT-3146) is a selective, potent (10 times more potent than adenosine), low-affinity A2A receptor agonist. Its relative low-affinity property allows for rapid onset and termination of action.[73,74] Lieu et al.[75] demonstrated in human subjects that regadenoson produces dose-dependent increase in duration of coronary blood flow augmentation. They identified 400 μg to produce $\geq$2.5-fold increase in coronary blood flow, which was sustained for $\geq$2.5 minutes. In a pilot, phase II, crossover, open-label clinical trial Hendel et al.[76] evaluated regadenoson (400 and 500 μg doses) for tolerability and effectiveness as a pharmacological stress agent in MPI, in comparison with standard 6-minute adenosine infusion. Patients received regadenoson as rapid intravenous injection, followed by the radiopharmaceutical delivered within 1 minute. SPECT images were interpreted by three observers in blinded fashion. Overall agreement for ischemia extent and severity between the two agents were 86% and 83%, respectively. Overall, regadenoson was well tolerated; side effects (e.g., chest discomfort, flushing, and dyspnea) were generally mild in severity and self-limited. High-grade AV block and bronchospasm were not observed. A phase III clinical trial from 54 sites with 784 patients was recently published.[77] The bolus administration of a fixed dose of 400 μg demonstrated noninferior results when compared with adenosine. Flushing, chest pain, and dyspnea were less with regadenoson, but there was an increased incidence of headache. This agent will soon be considered for FDA approval for general clinical practice.

Binodenoson

Binodenoson (also known as MRE-0470 and WRC-0470) is a highly selective, high-affinity A2A receptor agonist, which is 200 times more potent than adenosine. It is more selective to A2A receptor than regadenoson. In comparison with regadenoson, binodenoson is slower in onset (3.3–5.5 minutes) and it has more prolonged duration of action (3.0–9.4 minutes).[78] In contrast to the rapid bolus injection of regadenoson, binodenoson is delivered by weight-based slow bolus for more than 30 seconds.

In multicenter, randomized, single-blinded, crossover trial, Udelson et al.[79] evaluated the safety, tolerability, and diagnostic accuracy of binodenoson (one of four dosing regimens) against standard 6-minute adenosine infusion in patients undergoing SPECT MPI. Agreement for the extent and severity of reversible perfusion defects ranged from 79% to 87%, indicating very-good-to-excellent agreement between binodenoson and adenosine. The risk of any side effects was significantly lower with any dose of binodenoson than with adenosine ($p \leq 0.01$). There was a reduction in the severity of chest pain, dyspnea, and flushing in all binodenoson doses compared with adenosine ($p < 0.01$), and the magnitude of severity reduction was dose related. There were no reports of high-grade AV block or bronchospasm.

Apadenoson

Apadenosone (BMS068645, ALT-146e) is a highly selective A2A with moderate receptor affinity, which has been shown to increase coronary blood flow approximately 2.5-fold above basal levels for 2 to 8 minutes' duration. Preliminary data derived from a phase II trial in 122 patients have demonstrated a low side-effect profile and a high concordance with standard adenosine imaging. Additional clinical trials for this agent are possible.[80]

SUMMARY

Pharmacologic MPI is a vital part of today's nuclear cardiology practice. Vasodilator agents (adenosine and dipyridamole) are the agents of choice with pharmacologic MPI, caused by their long track record of safety and excellent diagnostic and prognostic utility. However, frequent side effects and nonserious adverse reactions do impact on their tolerability. Dobutamine is the agent of choice for patients with bronchospastic airway disease, since conventional vasodilatory agents are contraindicated. The addition of exercise to dipyridamole and adenosine infusion protocols improves patient tolerance, decreases the incidence of adverse events, improves image quality, and may also enhance diagnostic sensitivity. Novel selective A2A receptor agonists opened new horizon for pharmacologic-stress MPI, with the potential for reducing patients symptoms, enhancing safety, simplifying stress protocol, and improving nuclear laboratory efficiency. Advances in pharmacologic stress testing are likely to further extend and enhance the role of MPI in the care of patients with cardiovascular disease.

REFERENCES

1. *Data on File.* Malvern, PA: Arlington Medical Resources; 2004:3.
2. Hendel RC, Jamil T, Glover DK. Pharmacologic stress testing: New methods and new agents. *J Nucl Cardiol.* 2003;10:197.
3. Thomas GS, Miyamoto MI. Should simultaneous exercise become the standard for adenosine myocardial perfusion imaging? *Am J Cardiol.* 2004;94:3D.
4. Cerqueira MD. The future of pharmacologic stress: selective A2A adenosine receptor agonists. *Am J Cardiol.* 2004;94:33D.
5. Calnon DA, Glover DK, Beller GA, et al. Effects of dobutamine stress on myocardial blood flow, 99mTc sestamibi uptake, and systolic wall thickening in the presence of coronary artery stenoses: Implications for dobutamine stress testing. *Circulation.* 1997;96:2353.
6. Wu JC, Yun JJ, Heller EN, et al. Limitations of dobutamine for enhancing flow heterogeneity in the presence of single coronary stenosis: Implications for technetium-99m-sestamibi imaging. *J Nucl Med.* 1998;39:417.

7. Elhendy A, Valkema R, van Domburg RT, et al. Safety of dobutamine-atropine stress myocardial perfusion scintigraphy. *J Nucl Med.* 1998;39:1662.

8. Elhendy A, van Domburg RT, Bax JJ, et al. Safety, hemodynamic profile, and feasibility of dobutamine stress technetium myocardial perfusion single-photon emission CT imaging for evaluation of coronary artery disease in the elderly. *Chest.* 2000;117:649.

9. Tsutsui JM, Elhendy A, Xie F, et al. Safety of dobutamine stress real-time myocardial contrast echocardiography. *J Am Coll Cardiol.* 2005;45:1235.

10. Geleijnse ML, Elhendy A, Fioretti PM, et al. Dobutamine stress myocardial perfusion imaging. *J Am Coll Cardiol.* 2000;36:2017.

11. Coma-Canella I. Sensitivity and specificity of dobutamine–electrocardiography test to detect multivessel disease after acute myocardial infarction. *Eur Heart J.* 1990;11:249.

12. Sizemore C, Lewis JF. Clinical relevance of chest pain during dobutamine stress echocardiography in women. *Clin Cardiol.* 1999;22:715.

13. Mairesse GH, Marwick TH, Vanoverschelde JL, et al. How accurate is dobutamine stress electrocardiography for detection of coronary artery disease? Comparison with two-dimensional echocardiography and technetium-99m methoxyl isobutyl isonitrile (mibi) perfusion scintigraphy. *J Am Coll Cardiol.* 1994;24:920.

14. Daoud EG, Pitt A, Armstrong WF. Electrocardiographic response during dobutamine stress echocardiography. *Am Heart J.* 1995;129:672.

15. Geleijnse ML, Elhendy A, van Domburg RT, et al. Prognostic value of dobutamine-atropine stress technetium-99m sestamibi perfusion scintigraphy in patients with chest pain. *J Am Coll Cardiol.* 1996;28:447.

16. Calnon DA, McGrath PD, Doss AL, et al. Prognostic value of dobutamine stress technetium-99m-sestamibi single-photon emission computed tomography myocardial perfusion imaging: Stratification of a high-risk population. *J Am Coll Cardiol* 2001;38:1511.

17. Schinkel AF, Elhendy A, van Domburg RT, et al. Prognostic value of dobutamine-atropine stress (99m)Tc-tetrofosmin myocardial perfusion SPECT in patients with known or suspected coronary artery disease. *J Nucl Med.* 2002;43:767.

18. Huang PJ, Yen RF, Chieng PU, et al. Do beta-blockers affect the diagnostic sensitivity of dobutamine stress thallium-201 single photon emission computed tomographic imaging? *J Nucl Cardiol.* 1998; 5:34.

19. Cosin-Sales J, Maceira AM, Garcia-Velloso MJ, et al. Safety and feasibility of atropine added to submaximal exercise stress testing with Tl-201 SPECT for the diagnosis of myocardial ischemia. *J Nucl Cardiol.* 2002;9:581.

20. Verani MS. Adenosine thallium 201 myocardial perfusion scintigraphy. *Am Heart J.* 1991;122:269.

21. Navare SM, Kapetanopoulos A, Heller GV. Pharmacologic radionuclide myocardial perfusion imaging. *Curr Cardiol Rep.* 2003;5:16.

22. Fung AY, Gallagher KP, Buda AJ. The physiologic basis of dobutamine as compared with dipyridamole stress interventions in the assessment of critical coronary stenosis. *Circulation.* 1987;76:943.

23. Feldman RL, Nichols WW, Pepine CJ, et al. Acute effect of intravenous dipyridamole on regional coronary hemodynamics and metabolism. *Circulation.* 1981;64:333.

24. Nishimura S, Kimball KT, Mahmarian JJ, et al. Angiographic and hemodynamic determinants of myocardial ischemia during adenosine thallium-201 scintigraphy in coronary artery disease. *Circulation.* 1993;87:1211.

25. Zheng XM, Williams RC. Serum caffeine levels after 24-hour abstention: Clinical implications on dipyridamole (201)Tl myocardial perfusion imaging. *J Nucl Med Technol.* 2002;30:123.

26. Kubo S, Tadamura E, Toyoda H, et al. Effect of caffeine intake on myocardial hyperemic flow induced by adenosine triphosphate and dipyridamole. *J Nucl Med.* 2004;45:730.

27. Lette J, Tatum JL, Fraser S, et al. Safety of dipyridamole testing in 73,806 patients: the Multicenter Dipyridamole Safety Study. *J Nucl Cardiol.* 1995;2:3.

28. Henzlova MJ, Cerqueira MD, Mahmarian JJ, et al. Stress protocols and tracers. *J Nucl Cardiol.* 2006;13:e80.

29. Ranhosky A, Kempthorne-Rawson J. The safety of intravenous dipyridamole thallium myocardial perfusion imaging. Intravenous Dipyridamole Thallium Imaging Study Group. *Circulation.* 1990;81:1205.

30. Brown KA, Heller GV, Landin RS, et al. Early dipyridamole (99m)Tc-sestamibi single photon emission computed tomographic imaging 2 to 4 days after acute myocardial infarction predicts in-hospital and postdischarge cardiac events: Comparison with submaximal exercise imaging. *Circulation.* 1999;100:2060.

31. Treuth MG, Reyes GA, He ZX, et al. Tolerance and diagnostic accuracy of an abbreviated adenosine infusion for myocardial scintigraphy: A randomized, prospective study. *J Nucl Cardiol.* 2001;8:548.

32. Villegas BJ, Hendel RC, Dahlberg ST, et al. Comparison of 3- versus 6-minute infusions of adenosine in thallium-201 myocardial perfusion imaging. *Am Heart J.* 1993;126:103.

33. O'Keefe JH Jr, Bateman TM, Handlin LR, et al. Four-versus 6-minute infusion protocol for adenosine thallium-201 single photon emission computed tomography imaging. *Am Heart J.* 1995;129: 482.

34. Bokhari S, Ficaro EP, McCallister BD Jr. Adenosine stress protocols for myocardial perfusion imaging. *J Nucl Cardiol*. 2007;14:415.

35. Cerqueira MD, Verani MS, Schwaiger M, et al. Safety profile of adenosine stress perfusion imaging: results from the Adenoscan Multicenter Trial Registry. *J Am Coll Cardiol*. 1994;23:384.

36. Marshall ES, Raichlen JS, Tighe DA, et al. ST-segment depression during adenosine infusion as a predictor of myocardial ischemia. *Am Heart J*. 1994;127:305.

37. Abbott BG, Afshar M, Berger AK, et al. Prognostic significance of ischemic electrocardiographic changes during adenosine infusion in patients with normal myocardial perfusion imaging. *J Nucl Cardiol*. 2003;10:9.

38. Gulati M, Pratap P, Kansal P, et al. Gender differences in the value of ST-segment depression during adenosine stress testing. *Am J Cardiol* 2004;94:997.

39. Klodas E, Miller TD, Christian TF, et al. Prognostic significance of ischemic electrocardiographic changes during vasodilator stress testing in patients with normal SPECT images. *J Nucl Cardiol*. 2003;10:4.

40. Dahlberg S, Leppo J. Risk stratification of the normal perfusion scan: Does normal stress perfusion always mean very low risk? *J Nucl Cardiol*. 2003;10:87.

41. Chow BJ, Wong JW, Yoshinaga K, et al. Prognostic significance of dipyridamole-induced ST depression in patients with normal 82Rb PET myocardial perfusion imaging. *J Nucl Med*. 2005;46:1095.

42. Vaduganathan P, He ZX, Raghavan C, et al. Detection of left anterior descending coronary artery stenosis in patients with left bundle branch block: Exercise, adenosine or dobutamine imaging? *J Am Coll Cardiol* 1996;28:543.

43. O'Keefe JH Jr, Bateman TM, Silvestri R, et al. Safety and diagnostic accuracy of adenosine thallium-201 scintigraphy in patients unable to exercise and those with left bundle branch block. *Am Heart J*. 1992;124:614.

44. Burns RJ, Galligan L, Wright LM, et al. Improved specificity of myocardial thallium-201 single-photon emission computed tomography in patients with left bundle branch block by dipyridamole. *Am J Cardiol*. 1991;68:504.

45. Taillefer R, Ahlberg AW, Masood Y, et al. Acute beta-blockade reduces the extent and severity of myocardial perfusion defects with dipyridamole Tc-99m sestamibi SPECT imaging. *J Am Coll Cardiol*. 2003;42:1475.

46. Sharir T, Rabinowitz B, Livschitz S, et al. Underestimation of extent and severity of coronary artery disease by dipyridamole stress thallium-201 single-photon emission computed tomographic myocardial perfusion imaging in patients taking antianginal drugs. *J Am Coll Cardiol*. 1998;31:1540.

47. Ignaszewski AP, McCormick LX, Heslip PG, et al. Safety and clinical utility of combined intravenous dipyridamole/symptom-limited exercise stress test with thallium-201 imaging in patients with known or suspected coronary artery disease. *J Nucl Med*. 1993;34:2053.

48. Casale PN, Guiney TE, Strauss HW, et al. Simultaneous low level treadmill exercise and intravenous dipyridamole stress thallium imaging. *Am J Cardiol*. 1988;62:799.

49. Cramer MJ, Verzijlbergen JF, van der Wall EE, et al. Comparison of adenosine and high-dose dipyridamole both combined with low-level exercise stress for 99Tcm-MIBI SPET myocardial perfusion imaging. *Nucl Med Commun*. 1996;17:97.

50. Stern S, Greenberg ID, Corne R. Effect of exercise supplementation on dipyridamole thallium-201 image quality. *J Nucl Med*. 1991;32:1559.

51. Pennell DJ, Mavrogeni SI, Forbat SM, et al. Adenosine combined with dynamic exercise for myocardial perfusion imaging. *J Am Coll Cardiol*. 1995;25:1300.

52. Mahmood S, Gupta NK, Gunning M, et al. 201Tl myocardial perfusion SPET: adenosine alone or combined with dynamic exercise. *Nucl Med Commun*. 1994;15:586.

53. Jamil G, Ahlberg AW, Elliott MD, et al. Impact of limited treadmill exercise on adenosine Tc-99m sestamibi single-photon emission computed tomographic myocardial perfusion imaging in coronary artery disease. *Am J Cardiol*. 1999;84:400.

54. Hashimoto A, Palmar EL, Scott JA, et al. Complications of exercise and pharmacologic stress tests: Differences in younger and elderly patients. *J Nucl Cardiol*. 1999;6:612.

55. Holly TA, Satran A, Bromet DS, et al. The impact of adjunctive adenosine infusion during exercise myocardial perfusion imaging: Results of the Both Exercise and Adenosine Stress Test (BEAST) trial. *J Nucl Cardiol*. 2003;10:291.

56. Thomas GS, Prill NV, Majmundar H, et al. Treadmill exercise during adenosine infusion is safe, results in fewer adverse reactions, and improves myocardial perfusion image quality. *J Nucl Cardiol*. 2000;7:439.

57. Elliott MD, Holly TA, Leonard SM, et al. Impact of an abbreviated adenosine protocol incorporating adjunctive treadmill exercise on adverse effects and image quality in patients undergoing stress myocardial perfusion imaging. *J Nucl Cardiol*. 2000;7:584.

58. Samady H, Wackers FJ, Joska TM, et al. Pharmacologic stress perfusion imaging with adenosine: Role of simultaneous low-level treadmill exercise. *J Nucl Cardiol*. 2002;9:188.

59. Brown KA. Exercise-dipyridamole myocardial perfusion imaging: The circle is now complete. *J Nucl Med*. 1993;34:2061.

60. Hurwitz GA, Powe JE, Driedger AA, et al. Dipyridamole combined with symptom-limited exercise for myocardial perfusion scintigraphy: Image characteristics and clinical role. *Eur J Nucl Med*. 1990;17:61.

61. Laarman GJ, Niemeyer MG, van der Wall EE, et al. Dipyridamole thallium testing: noncardiac side effects, cardiac effects, electrocardiographic changes and hemodynamic changes after dipyridamole infusion with and without exercise. *Int J Cardiol*. 1988; 20:231.

62. Muller-Suur R, Eriksson SV, Strandberg LE, et al. Comparison of adenosine and exercise stress test for quantitative perfusion imaging in patients on beta-blocker therapy. *Cardiology*. 2001;95:112.

63. Wilson RF, Wyche K, Christensen BV, et al. Effects of adenosine on human coronary arterial circulation. *Circulation*. 1990;82:1595.

64. Miyamoto MI, Rockman HA, Guth BD, et al. Effect of alpha-adrenergic stimulation on regional contractile function and myocardial blood flow with and without ischemia. *Circulation*. 1991;84:1715.

65. Heusch G, Baumgart D, Camici P, et al. Alpha-adrenergic coronary vasoconstriction and myocardial ischemia in humans. *Circulation*. 2000;101:689.

66. Thomas GS, Miyamoto MI, Morello AP III, et al. Technetium 99m sestamibi myocardial perfusion imaging predicts clinical outcome in the community outpatient setting. The Nuclear Utility in the Community (NUC) Study. *J Am Coll Cardiol*. 2004;43:213.

67. Lakkis NM, He ZX, Verani MS. Diagnosis of coronary artery disease by exercise thallium-201 tomography in patients with a right ventricular pacemaker. *J Am Coll Cardiol*. 1997;29:1221.

68. Gaspardone A, Crea F, Tomai F, et al. Muscular and cardiac adenosine-induced pain is mediated by A1 receptors. *J Am Coll Cardiol*. 1995;25:251.

69. Martin PL, Ueeda M, Olsson RA. 2-Phenylethoxy-9-methyladenine: an adenosine receptor antagonist that discriminates between A2 adenosine receptors in the aorta and the coronary vessels from the guinea pig. *J Pharmacol Exp Ther*. 1993;265:248.

70. Belardinelli L, Shryock JC, Snowdy S, et al. The A2A adenosine receptor mediates coronary vasodilation. *J Pharmacol Exp Ther*. 1998;284:1066.

71. Linden J, Thai T, Figler H, et al. Characterization of human A(2B) adenosine receptors: Radioligand binding, Western blotting, and coupling to G(q) in human embryonic kidney 293 cells and HMC-1 mast cells. *Mol Pharmacol*. 1999;56:705.

72. Auchampach JA, Jin X, Wan TC, et al. Canine mast cell adenosine receptors: Cloning and expression of the A3 receptor and evidence that degranulation is mediated by the A2B receptor. *Mol Pharmacol*. 1997;52:846.

73. Gao Z, Li Z, Baker SP, et al. Novel short-acting A2A adenosine receptor agonists for coronary vasodilation: Inverse relationship between affinity and duration of action of A2A agonists. *J Pharmacol Exp Ther*. 2001;298:209.

74. Shryock JC, Snowdy S, Baraldi PG, et al. A2A-adenosine receptor reserve for coronary vasodilation. *Circulation*. 1998;98:711.

75. Lieu HD, Von Mering GO, Gordi T, et al. Regadenoson, a selective A2A adenosine receptor agonist causes dose-dependent increases in coronary blood flow velocity in humans. *J Nucl Cardiol*. 2007;14:514.

76. Hendel RC, Bateman TM, Cerqueira MD, et al. Initial clinical experience with regadenoson, a novel selective A(2A) agonist for pharmacologic stress single-photon emission computed tomography myocardial perfusion imaging. *J Am Coll Cardiol*. 2005;46:2069.

77. Iskandrian AE, Bateman TM, Belardinelli L, et al. Adenosine versus regadenoson comparative evaluation in myocardial perfusion imaging: Results of the ADVANCE phase 3 multicenter international trial. *J Nucl Cardiol*. 2007;14:645.

78. Hodgson JM, R.J. B, Dib N, et al. A randomized, parallel group study of the coronary hyperemic and systemic hemodynamic responses to the novel pharmacological-stress agent, binodenoson. *J Nucl Cardiol*. 2003;10:S91; abstract 12.3.

79. Udelson JE, Heller GV, Wackers FJ, et al. Randomized, controlled dose-ranging study of the selective adenosine A2A receptor agonist binodenoson for pharmacological stress as an adjunct to myocardial perfusion imaging. *Circulation*. 2004;109:457.

80. Hendel R, Taillefer R, Widner P, et al. Preliminary experience with BMS068645, a selective a2a adenosine agonist, for pharmacologic stress myocardial perfusion imaging. *Circulation*. 2005;112:474.

SECTION 4

SPECT MYOCARDIAL PERFUSION IMAGING TECHNIQUES

CHAPTER 9

Protocols and Acquisition Parameters for SPECT Myocardial Perfusion Imaging

April Mann

INTRODUCTION

When performing single photon emission computer tomography (SPECT) myocardial perfusion imaging, there are several technical parameters that should be considered. Image quality and diagnostic accuracy are dependent on the use of an appropriate myocardial perfusion imaging protocol, a properly functioning system, and the acquisition techniques that are applied. If the acquisition is performed inappropriately, it may result in poor-quality images and misdiagnosis. In order to optimize image quality, it is necessary to ensure patient comfort, utilize appropriate imaging protocols, perform appropriate camera setup, utilize appropriate acquisition parameters, and recognize potential sources of internal and external attenuation and artifacts. This chapter will review various imaging protocols, camera quality control, and acquisition parameter techniques.

IMAGING PROTOCOLS

There are four commonly used imaging protocols for stress myocardial perfusion imaging.[1-3] These include 1- and 2-day 99m-technetium-labeled isotope protocols, dual-isotope (201-thallium rest/ 99m-technetium-labeled stress) protocol, and 201-thallium stress/delay protocol. The protocol of choice for each laboratory should be based on several factors, including physical characteristics of the isotope; dosimetry and physical/biological half-lives; biodistribution of adjacent organs to the heart; the patient population being studied (inpatient vs. outpatient); logistical considerations of the laboratory; the clinical questions being addressed; the availability of personnel including physician, nurse, and technologist; radiopharmaceutical availability; camera type and technical limitations; patient convenience; and costeffectiveness.[2] Given these considerations, it is important to then maintain consistency with a chosen protocol. This will allow better recognition of abnormalities/artifacts based on deviation from standards. It is important to recognize, however, that optimizing image quality, diagnostic accuracy, and patient outcomes are the main goals to be achieved with every protocol.

Stress/Delay 201-Thallium Protocol

Although the oldest of the accepted imaging protocols, stress/delay 201-thallium (201-Tl) studies are currently used the least.[2,4] The introduction of Tc-99m-labeled imaging agents in the 1990s offered better imaging characteristics and far less artifacts than that of the 201-Tl protocol.[2,5,6] Isotope characteristics of 201-Tl that should be considered are that (1) radiation dosimetry limits the dose administered (2.0–4.5 mCi), (2) the myocardial half-life is 2 to 3 hours, (3) 201-Tl has significant myocardial redistribution, (4) the physical half-life is 73 hours, and (5) the imaging energy of 201-Tl is 68 to 80 KeV.[2] Because of low count statistics and imaging energy, it is imperative that images are acquired for an appropriate amount of time in order to achieve an adequate amount of counts. This will decrease the possibility of attenuation artifacts and poor-quality studies.

To perform this protocol, 201-Tl is injected during either peak exercise [at least 85% maximum predicted heart rate (MPHR)] or pharmacologic stress. As a result of the early redistribution characteristics, the image acquisition needs to begin almost immediately postinjection (5–7 minutes). Caution should be taken when image acquisition begins this early postexercise, as "upward creep" (increased respiratory motion) may be present and degrade image quality. Because of almost complete redistribution of 201-Tl, the patient returns 4 hours postinjection to undergo delay imaging with no second injection. Total time for this protocol (other laboratory factors including camera backlog, etc., are not included) is approximately 5 hours (Figure 9-1).

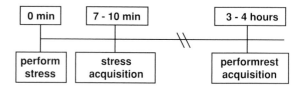

One Day Protocol
Single Isotope - Thalliium

Figure 9-1.   Thallium stress/delay protocol.

Advantages of this protocol include the presence of 201-Tl if myocardial viability is a clinical question and only one injection is required. Disadvantages include the unfavorable imaging characteristics of 201-Tl, long procedure times, and image quality with ECG-gated SPECT, which may be questionable.

Two-Day (Tc-99m) Protocol

The 2-day technetium protocol can be performed using either Tc-99m sestamibi or Tc-99m tetrofosmin. Unlike 201-Tl, neither of these tracers has significant myocardial redistribution properties. Therefore, imaging times poststress can be more flexible, and the image acquisition may be repeated if significant motion or other technical sources of artifact are present. However, a second injection for stress and rest is required. Also, since the image acquisition does not need to be performed immediately poststress injection, "upward creep" is significantly less than with the 201-Tl-only protocol. Isotope characteristics of the Tc-labeled tracers are (1) physical half-life of 6 hours, (2) image energy of 140 keV, (3) radiation dosimetry allows 25 to 45 mCi to be administered, and (4) no myocardial redistribution. With this protocol, optimal count statistics can be acquired for both image sets (stress/rest), since the maximum dosage (25–45 mCi) of the Tc-99m-labeled tracer is used (as compared to the 1-day protocol), resulting in the best image quality.

To perform this protocol, a stress injection is performed during peak exercise (at least 85% MPHR) or pharmacologic stress, and images are

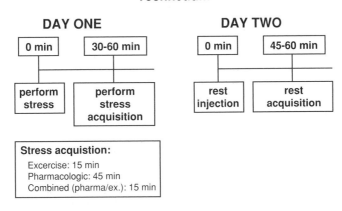

Figure 9-2. Two-day (Tc-99m) protocol.

acquired 15 to 60 minutes postinjection. If exercise is performed, image acquisition may begin 10 to 15 minutes postinjection. If pharmacologic stress is performed, image acquisition must be delay up to 60 minutes postinjection to allow adequate live clearance and maximize myocardial uptake. The patient returns on a subsequent day to undergo the rest portion of the procedure. A rest injection is performed and images are acquired approximately 45 to 60 minutes postinjection. The delay in acquisition time again is to allow for adequate liver clearance and maximize myocardial uptake. Total time for this protocol (other laboratory factors including camera backlog, etc., are not included) on both days is approximately 1.5 to 2 hours (Figure 9-2). Stress and rest image sequence can vary since the protocol is performed for more than 2 days. Rest/stress tracer dosages should be consistent with ASNC imaging guidelines.[1] It has also been suggested in order to achieve maximum count statistics with the Tc-labeled tracers, it may be helpful to dose patients based on body weight (Table 9-1).

Advantages of the 2-day protocol include optimal image quality for both the stress and the rest study, ECG-gated SPECT may be performed on both sets of images because of better count statistics and the option for stress-only imaging is possible. In this case, if the stress image is completely normal then rest imaging is not necessary. Disadvantages include patient inconvenience, longer wait time for results, and increased physician decision-making if a stress-only protocol is followed.

Stress-Only Imaging When performing a 2-day protocol, it may be possible to perform stress-only imaging. If the stress study is performed first and is completely normal, there is no reason to perform the rest study. Until recently, this has proven to be somewhat challenging as a result

Table 9-1

Example of Weight-Based Dosing Chart for Tc-Labeled Tracers

Weight	Two Day	One Day
<160 lb	25.0 mCi	10/30 mCi
160–170 lb	27.5 mCi	11/33 mCi
170–180 lb	29.2 mCi	12/35 mCi
180–190 lb	30.0 mCi	12/36 mCi
190–200 lb	32.5 mCi	13/39 mCi
200–210 lb	34.0 mCi	14/41 mCi
210–220 lb	35.7 mCi	14/42 mCi
220–230 lb	37.3 mCi	14/43 mCi
240–250 lb	38.9 mCi	14/44 mCi
<250 lb	40.0 mCi	15/45 mCi

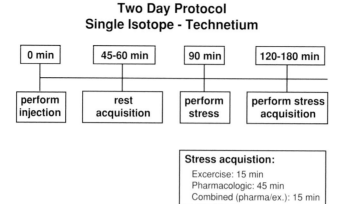

Figure 9-3. One-day (Tc-99m) protocol.

of attenuation artifacts. With ECG-gated SPECT and area of decreased activity with normal wall motion and thickening could be either myocardial ischemia or attenuation artifact. This was not easily sorted out, and the patient was required to return for rest images. The validation of attenuation corrections algorithms has now made this a more feasible option.[7]

One-Day (Tc-99m) Protocol

Currently, the 1-day technetium imaging protocol is the most popular of the Tc-99m protocols in many laboratories because of the improved patient convenience and throughput. Similar to the 2-day protocol, this can also be performed with 99m sestamibi or Tc-99m tetrofosmin. The rest is most often performed first, and it is important to always maintain at least a 1:3 ratio with tracer dosages (first dose three times the second dose, e.g. 10/30 mCi), in order to achieve optimal counts statistics and avoid artifacts caused by counts from the first injection that may lead to missed ischemia. A stress/rest sequence may be performed; however, this is not recommended because the highest-quality image should be the stress.

To perform this protocol, a rest injection is given and images are acquired approximately 45 to 60 minutes postinjection to allow adequate liver clearance and maximize myocardial uptake. The patient is then prepared for the stress test, a stress injection is performed during peak exercise (at least 85% MPHR) or pharmacologic stress, and images are acquired 15 to 60 minutes postinjection. If pharmacologic stress is performed, image acquisition must be delayed up to 60 minutes postinjection, to allow for adequate live clearance and maximize myocardial uptake. Total time for this protocol (other laboratory factors including camera backlog, etc., are not included) is approximately 2.5 to 3 hours (Figure 9-3). Rest/stress tracer dosages should be consistent with ASNC imaging guidelines and, similar to the 2-day protocol, may be based on patient body weight (Table 9-1).[1]

The advantages of the 1-day protocol include patient convenience, faster result turnaround time than the 2-day protocol, and ease of interpretation and identification of left ventricular cavity dilation (single-isotope comparison). A disadvantage of this protocol is that one image set is of lesser quality and this may result in artifacts. Further, the presence of the rest dose may mask ischemia on the stress images.

Dual-Isotope (201-Tl/Tc-99m Protocol)

Although the Tc-99m imaging protocols have many advantages, the concept of the dual isotope

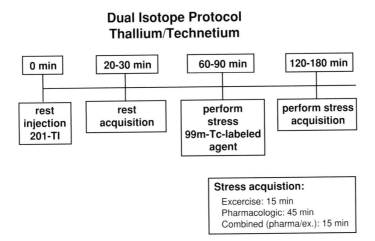

Figure 9-4. Dual isotope protocol.

protocol was introduced by Dr. Daniel Berman and colleagues to assess perfusion and myocardial viability in a single study.[8] This protocol requires more attention to detail when acquiring images and interpreting studies as two different isotopes with different imaging characteristics are being used.

To perform this protocol, an injection of 201-Tl is given at rest and images are acquired 10 to 20 minutes postinjection. Unlike the Tc-labeled tracers, there is no liver activity present and the imaging characteristics of 201-Tl make it possible to start the rest images sooner with this protocol. Following the rest acquisition, the patient is prepared for the stress test, and an injection of a Tc-99m-labeled tracer is given at peak exercise (at least 85% MPHR) or pharmacologic stress. Stress images are acquired 15 to 60 minutes poststress injection. As with the other protocols, if pharmacologic stress is performed, image acquisition must be delayed up to 60 minutes postinjection to allow for adequate live clearance and maximize myocardial uptake. Total time for this protocol (other laboratory factors including camera backlog, etc., are not included) is approximately 2 to 2.5 hours (Figure 9-4). Tc-labeled agent dosages should be consistent with the ASNC imaging guidelines and may be based on weight (Table 9-1).[1]

Advantages of this protocol are efficiency and quicker patient throughput. Since 201-Tl is being used, further assessment for myocardial viability can be performed if necessary, and there are abundant prognostic data available in the literature with the use of the dual-isotope protocol. Disadvantages are that it is more difficult to evaluate transient cavity dilation and fixed vs. partially reversible defects for determination of attenuation artifact or coronary artery disease because of the differences in isotope characteristics. Stress-only imaging cannot be performed with this protocol, and rest ECG-gated SPECT imaging may be questionable with 201-Tl.

CAMERA CONSIDERATIONS

There are currently two common types of systems used today to perform SPECT myocardial perfusion imaging. These are the single- and dual-head systems. Typically, the dual-head camera has become the system of choice, since it requires half the time to acquire the same amount of projections as the single head. This had led to increased patient comfort and less artifact caused by patient motion.

Before any image acquisition takes place, it is necessary to ensure that the equipment is

Table 9-2

Recommended Frequency for Gamma
Camera Quality Control Procedures

Test	Frequency
Energy peaking	Daily
Uniformity	Daily
Sensitivity	Daily or weekly
Resolution and linearity	Weekly
Center of rotation	Weekly
SPECT phantom evaluation	Quarterly
Preventive maintenance	Every 6 months

From Mann et al.[8]

functioning properly and the appropriate collimator is chosen for the protocol being performed. There are several required and recommended equipment quality control procedures that should be performed on each imaging system.[8,9,10] The recommended frequency of the procedures may vary between equipment manufacturers; however, all are important to ensure proper system performance (Table 9-2). These tasks consist of daily, weekly, and quarterly system testing and should include preventive maintenance by a qualified service engineer at least every 6 months to ensure proper performance of the system. Even if these tests are not required or recommended specifically by the manufacturer, it is necessary to perform them in order to ensure a properly functioning system and be in compliance with ASNC guidelines and Intersocietal Commission for the Accreditation of Nuclear Medicine Laboratory (ICANL) standards.

Daily Quality Control

Energy Peaking Energy peaking (photopeak analysis) should be performed daily to verify that the camera is counting photons using the correct energy.[9,11] Each imaging system should be checked before use to ensure that the camera-peaking electronics are functioning properly, that the energy window has not drifted, and that the energy spectrum is of the appropriate shape.

During the procedure, the pulse height analyzer's energy window should be manually or au-

tomatically placed over the correct photopeak energy. It is recommended that no greater than a 2% energy window be used in order to obtain the most accurate peak energy.[9,12] If the test is performed intrinsically, a point source should be placed at least 1.5 m away from the surface of the camera detector. If performed extrinsically, a sheet source should be used. In either case, the source should be enough to flood the entire field of view (FOV).

Verifying the photopeak daily will help prevent artifacts that may occur as a result of inappropriate photons entering the acquisition and degrading image quality. An off-centered photopeak may also result in poor counts statistics, which will also result in a poor-quality image.[9,11,13] If a dual-isotope protocol is being performed on some older imaging systems, it may be necessary to perform this procedure between each acquisition of 201-Tl and Tc-99m isotopes.

Uniformity Flood A daily uniformity flood should be performed to analyze system performance and to ensure that the sensitivity response of the system is uniform across the detector surface.[9-14] This is performed by exposure of the detector surface to a radioactive source. The recommended method is to perform this procedure intrinsically using a Tc-99m point source of approximately 100 to 500 μCi in 0.5 mL or less of volume. The point source should be placed in the center and at a distance of approximately five useful fields of view (UFOVs) away from the detector surface. An acquisition should be performed for approximately 2 to 5 million counts, using a 20% energy window.[9,10] This may also be performed extrinsically using a 57-cobalt sheet source. The extrinsic method is performed frequently on dual-head camera systems because the acquisition can be performed on both detectors at the same time. It is important to remember, however, that during the uniformity analysis of extrinsic floods the outer 10% to 20% of the FOV should not be considered because of possible edge packing.[9,10]

After the acquisition of the flood field uniformity, the image should be evaluated visually, and

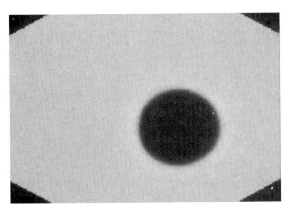

Figure 9-5. Illustration of a uniformity flood that had a cluster of photomultiplier tubes not functioning. (From Mann et al.[8]).

a computerized analysis should be performed to measure the performance of the system. Central FOV and UFOV parameters should be <5%. This analysis should be performed following manufacturers' protocols and will be specific to each imaging system. If nonuniformities are detected, the system should not be used until service is performed. Severe artifacts, such as malfunctioning photomultiplier tubes, will be easily detected (Figure 9-5). Smaller abnormalities may be more difficult to detect, however. These small, undetected nonuniformities may produce artifacts within pa-

tient acquisitions and result in a misinterpretation of the study.[10,12,14,15]

Weekly Quality Control

Center of Rotation A center of rotation (COR) should be performed weekly in order to ensure and maintain the detector's electronic matrix alignment.[9,10,12,14,15] This is the x-axis position of the actual axis of rotation, as seen by the image matrix.[10] If a COR error occurs, it may produce what has been characterized as a "doughnut"-shaped or "tuning fork" artifact (Figure 9-6).[9] This artifact may appear similar to an artifact caused by patient motion on the perfusion images. This error becomes more pronounced if the deviation widens, particularly greater than two pixels in a 64 × 64 matrix. Smaller deviations may not produce an artifact but could result in decreased spatial resolution and image contrast.[9,10]

Several manufacturers have recommended camera-specific protocols to follow when performing COR procedures. Most recommend using a 500 to 750 μCi point source placed off-centered in the FOV at approximately 4 to 8 inches away from the detector surface.[9,10] The acquisition is then performed using similar parameters as a standard SPECT. An analysis of this acquisition should be performed, and for any misalignment of greater

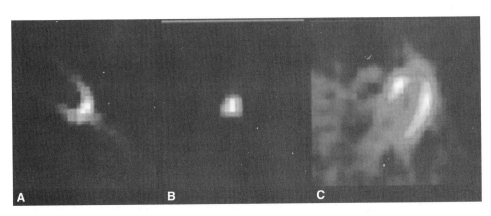

Figure 9-6. (**A**) Tuning fork artifact, (**B**) normal COR image, and (**C**) apical artifact a result of COR deviation. (From Mann et al.[8]) (See color insert.)

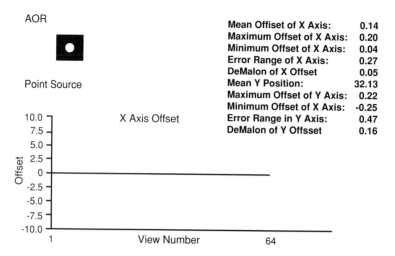

Figure 9-7.   Example of a COR analysis. Mean × offset should be less than 0.5 and evaluation of the graph should be performed for any deviation as well. (From Mann et al.[8])

than 0.5 pixels of the *x*-axis the COR should be recalibrated (Figure 9-7).

System Resolution and Linearity Test
System spatial resolution and linearity evaluation should be performed weekly. This procedure is performed to document spatial resolution over time, as well as evaluate the detector's ability to produce straight lines.[9,10] This procedure should be performed intrinsically using a radioactive point source and a test phantom. This evaluation should not be performed extrinsically because the patterns of the lead bars in the phantom and the lead septa of the collimator may interfere with one another causing artifacts.

There are several bar phantoms available commercially, which may be used for this test. The most commonly used are the parallel-line-equal-spaced (PLES), orthogonal hole, and four-quadrant phantoms.[9,10] The four-quadrant phantom has four sections of differing thickness lead bars that are equally spaced. If this type of phantom is used routinely, it should be placed over the detector surface so that each differing-size lead bar is in a different position from the previously performed test (rotated 90 degrees from the previously placed position). This will allow the

most tightly spaced bars of the phantom to appear over the entire surface of the detector every fifth acquisition. This will provide the most thorough evaluation of the entire detector surface over time.[9,10]

Acquisition parameters for the resolution and linearity test should be similar to those used to perform a daily uniformity flood. Upon completion, the image should be evaluated visually to assess the straightness of the lines produced by the bar phantom and for how well each different-size lead bar is visualized (Figure 9-8). The test should be stored in an electronic format for comparison of system resolution over time. As a decrease in resolution appears (loss of visualization of individual bars) maintenance should be performed. Manufacturers may supply software to evaluate linearity and resolution that should be used when available.

Quarterly Quality Control

SPECT Phantom   The National Electrical Manufacturers' Association (NEMA) recommends that SPECT phantoms be performed quarterly.[11,13] This allows evaluation of an imaging system's performance and limitations by providing a comparative means to judge previous

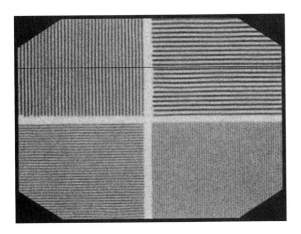

Figure 9-8. Four-quadrant bar phantom image.

performance with the most recent phantom acquisition.[9,10] Commercially available multipurpose Plexiglas and water-filled SPECT phantoms have attenuation and scattering properties similar to that of tissue, thus simulating clinical conditions in a three-dimensional view. This provides a realistic comparison of system performance similar to that in the clinical setting. Therefore, acquisition parameters used should be similar to that of standard SPECT.

Collimation When choosing a collimator for use with SPECT myocardial perfusion imaging, there are several factors that need to be considered. First, it is helpful to understand what the purpose of a collimator is. Collimators are lead shields with multiple holes used to cause *selective interference* of gamma rays not traveling in a selected direction, reduce scatter, and improve image quality. They are necessary to locate the line of emission of photons for tomographic reconstruction.[14]

There are several types of collimators available for myocardial perfusion imaging. Selection is based on the type of study and radiopharmaceutical being used. The general all-purpose (GAP), also referred to as a low-energy all-purpose (LEAP) collimator, is the most common. Two other common types are the low-energy high-resolution (LEHR) and fan beam (converging)

collimators. The GAP/LEAP collimator is used predominantly for 201-Tl imaging, and the LEHR collimator is used with most Tc-99m perfusion studies.[1,14,15] The fan beam (converging) collimator is used with older triple-head systems.

The GAP/LEAP collimator is considered a lower-resolution collimator and is associated with a shorter bore (hole) length, larger hole diameter, and thicker septa compared to the LEHR collimator.[1,9,15] These differences result in better resolution but a decrease in sensitivity (count statistics). Therefore, it may be necessary to image longer with the LEHR collimator. Caution should also be taken when choosing a collimator because if the sensitivity is too high, lesion contrast may be decreased, and this may lead to a decrease in clinical sensitivity. If resolution is too high, then the images may become noisy, and this may result in a decrease in clinical specificity. Therefore, it is necessary to verify the manufacturer's and imaging guideline recommendations in order to choose the most appropriate collimator for the protocol type and imaging system being used. Collimator names may also vary based on the manufacturer, so care must be taken to understand specific collimator performance specification[9] by the vendor. Inappropriate collimator choice can result in a poor-quality image acquisition.

Preventive Maintenance Preventive maintenance is very important in ensuring proper imaging system performance. Even with a good-quality control program, camera electronics may shift over time and will need to be recalibrated by a properly trained service engineer based on camera-specific recommendations. ICANL standards and ASNC imaging guidelines recommend that preventive maintenance be performed twice a year (every 6 months) following the manufacturer's specifications.

ACQUISITION CONSIDERATIONS

An important way to assure optimal image quality with all of the protocols for SPECT myocardial perfusion imaging is to use proper imaging techniques. There are several technical aspects that should be considered when determining what the proper camera setup should be for stress/rest image acquisition. Acquisition parameter considerations should include acquisition mode, collimation, scan radius, number of projections (angular sampling), counts statistics, matrix size, orbit and orbit type and patient positioning, ECG-gated SPECT, and attenuation correction.[1,3,7,16–22] These parameters must be well understood in order to produce high-quality, interpretable images.

Patient Positioning

Achieving a high-quality and technically accurate myocardial perfusion study is dependent on the correct positioning of the patient throughout the acquisition period. This is true for both the relationship of the patients to the detector and their comfort on the imaging table. Positioning the patient as comfortably as possible before the acquisition begins will eliminate anxiety and minimize artifacts caused by patient motion.

As described later, image radius may affect spatial resolution. Therefore, the detector should be placed as close to the patient as possible throughout the acquisition.[3,14] The patient's arms should be placed above the head in a comfortable position, allowing the detector to pass more closely to the chest wall and avoid the possibility of attenuation. If this is not possible, however, the arms may be positioned at the side in order to decrease the temptation of movement or shifting during the acquisition.[23] It is acceptable to allow the detector to brush against the patient occasionally, provided that the contact does not cause the patient to move or shift, or produce anxiety or discomfort. If this is the case, it is imperative to inform the patient that this may occur prior to the start of the acquisition in order to decrease anxiety and patient motion.

In order to avoid truncation (omitting part of the heart from the FOV), the heart should be placed in the center of the FOV, and it is very important that positioning is reproducible between the stress and rest images. This will help reduce artifacts that may occur during image processing.

All of these considerations contribute to improved technical accuracy of the acquisition process and, ultimately, improved image quality.

Acquisition Modes

One important parameter for SPECT myocardial perfusion imaging is the acquisition mode being used. There are three basic types: (1) step and shoot, (2) continuous acquisition, and (3) continuous step and shoot. Step and shoot is the most common method used for perfusion imaging.[1] This method acquires an image set with the camera head(s) at a given angle (projection). When the projection is acquired, the camera head proceeds to the next given angle (projection). During the movement of the camera head(s) between angles (projections), no data are acquired. This pause in the acquisition, referred to as "dead time," increases imaging time in proportion to the number of projections being acquired.[1,15]

A second mode is continuous acquisition, which acquires data through the entire set orbit.[1,14,15] During this acquisition mode, the "dead time" is eliminated, and more counts can be obtained for the same amount of imaging time. Thus, the necessary counts can be acquired, and the study can be completed in less time. However, this may result in blurring of the images because of motion artifact. The increased sensitivity of this mode is considered by some to outweigh the blurring created.[1,14–16,24]

The third mode of acquisition is continuous step and shoot. This acquisition method is a combination of the two others described. During this mode, the camera head(s) acquires an image set at a given angle (projection). When the projection is acquired, the camera head proceeds to the next given angle (projection). During the movement of the camera head(s) between angles (projections), data continue to be acquired. This eliminates the "dead time," thus shortening the acquisition.[15,17] Therefore, the same advantage is gained as the continuous-mode acquisition. When considering which method is best for the imaging, it is important to understand the limitations of the specific camera being used for acquisition. All modes may vary slightly between camera vendors. Therefore, it may be necessary to follow the manufacturers' recommendations in order to achieve optimal image quality.

Acquisition Radius

Following the basic principles of nuclear medicine, the closer the detector surface is to the patient, the more count statistics will be achieved, resulting in improved image quality. Applying that principle to SPECT myocardial perfusion imaging, the scan radius should be as close to the patient as reasonably possible. Spatial resolution decreases as the collimator detector is moved further from the source. If the radius is too large, excessive blurring of the images may occur, resulting in contrast and resolution loss and spatial distortion.[1,14] This may result in a decrease in clinical sensitivity and specificity.

Projections (Angular Sampling)

The number of projections (angular sampling) and time per projection are very important considerations for SPECT myocardial perfusion imaging.[1,3,14,17,24] In order to acquire a high-quality image set, the study must contain the appropriate count density. Perfusion defects may be created simply as a result of poor count statistics. To ensure that each is optimal, it is necessary to customize the acquisition parameters to the protocol being performed and the imaging system being used. The manufacturer's system recommendations and various published imaging guidelines may be used as a reliable reference.[1] It should be noted that these guidelines are used to set minimal standards for accreditation and should be followed in order to meet these requirements.

It is also important to understand that the number of projections (angular samples) should be optimized to the collimator and matrix size.[1,3,14] Undersampling can lead to a loss in resolution and oversampling can result in loss in countdensity. For 180-degree image acquisition [45-degree right anterior oblique (RAO) to 45-degree anterior oblique (LAO)], 32 projections result in an image being acquired approximately every 6 degrees. When this is increased to 64 projections, images are acquired approximately every 3 degrees. The result is more myocardial surface area being imaged and greater count statistics being obtained. Therefore, when performing SPECT myocardial perfusion imaging with Tc-99m-labeled agents, 64 projections should be acquired. As a result of the redistribution characteristics of 201-Tl, however, it is recommended that only 32 projections be acquired.[1]

Detector Orbits

There are two types of orbits commonly used with SPECT myocardial perfusion imaging. These are circular and elliptical (body contouring) orbits.[1,14] A circular orbit is defined by a fixed radius or distance of the detector from the axis of rotation.[1,14] Since the detector remains at this fixed distance throughout the acquisition, at some points it will be farther away from the myocardium than others. Therefore, spatial resolution is decreased because of the distance of the detector from the myocardium.[1,14] Elliptical orbits follow the contour of the patient's body, allowing the camera to be close to the patient, especially in the anterior view. This allows for increased spatial resolution.

The primary differences between these two orbits are spatial resolution and image quality based on the distance of the detector to the myocardium at a given angle. Most common methods of image reconstruction, however, do not take into consideration the changes in spatial resolution that result from an elliptical orbit. This can produce imaging artifacts resulting from the variation in source to detector differences.[1,8,17,18] Although there is an overall loss in spatial resolution associated with the circular orbit, this is considered to be preferable to the resolution-related artifact caused by using an elliptical orbit.[1,14] Therefore, the circular orbit continues to be the most commonly used with perfusion imaging. However, some manufacturers have improved the elliptical orbits of individual systems, and it may be feasible with certain systems to use this orbit.

180- Vs. 360-Degree Acquisition

Another consideration for SPECT myocardial perfusion imaging is whether to perform 180- or 360-degree angular orbit. Since the heart is located anteriorly and to the left side of the patient's body, it is possible to increase the quality of the projection data by limiting the acquisition range to a 180-degree RAO to LPO.[1,14] The 180-degree acquisition most commonly used begins at 45-degree RAO. Increased defect or lesion contrast and improved signal-to-noise ratios have been reported with this type of acquisition.[21] The recommendation of which to apply is generally dependent on the type of imaging system being use. Performing a 360-degree acquisition with a single- or dual-head system will increase the amount of time needed to complete the study.[1,14] It may be beneficial with these systems to use the extra time to acquire more count statistics per projection. Currently with myocardial perfusion imaging, the 180-degree acquisition is preferred.

ECG-Gated SPECT

ECG-gated SPECT imaging has become a routine procedure in nuclear cardiology laboratories as a result of the additional valuable information added to the interpreting physician. Gated SPECT imaging provides assessment of ventricular function independent from perfusion defects, and functional information can be gained from both the left and the right ventricles. It has also been shown to increase specificity and confidence by helping to differentiate breast and diaphragmatic attenuation artifacts from true perfusion defects.[25]

ECG-gated SPECT acquisition is similar to standard SPECT, and the same acquisition parameters should be considered. In addition, the patient should be attached to a standard three-lead (leads I, II, and III) monitoring device interfaced to the camera system. Gated SPECT imaging divides the cardiac cycle into equal time intervals or segments, referred to as temporal frames, and data are collected while the tomographic images are being acquired. Each projection in the tomographic study contains data corresponding to all intervals in the cardiac cycle. The R wave of each ECG complex marks the start of a new interval. The cardiac cycle is generally divided into eight temporal frames per cardiac cycle, and each interval represents a point on the ECG and volume curve (Figure 9-9). The acquisition may also be performed for 16 frames/cardiac cycle for better representation of the end diastole (ED) and end systole (ES). It is then necessary to increase the time/projection in order to acquire optimal count statistics.

When performing gated SPECT imaging, caution should be taken when performing an acquisition on a patient with an abnormal heart rhythm (R-R interval).[25–28] This irregular rhythm may result in the misrepresentation of ED and ES, causing a perfusion artifact as well as an underestimation of the left ventricular ejection fraction (LVEF).[25–28] While some systems have the capability to prevent this problem during the acquisition, others do not. Therefore, it is important to understand the limitations of the imaging system being used, and in some instances gated SPECT should not be performed. Depending on the type of system being used, it may also be feasible to gate both the rest and the stress images. If this is performed with a low-dose study, caution should be taken to ensure appropriate count statistics.

Attenuation Correction

A more recent acquisition consideration is attenuation correction. Attenuation artifacts have been proven to have a negative effect on the proper interpretation of stress myocardial perfusion imaging. Solutions to reduce or eliminate these artifacts have included the use of prone and ECG-gated SPECT imaging. However, both of these solutions have proven to be selective (prone for inferior perfusion abnormalities, gated for fixed perfusion abnormalities) and are unable to completely resolve attenuation artifacts.

Attenuation correction hardware/software algorithms, similar to those used for PET imaging, have been considered to be a more appropriate solution for the resolution of attenuation artifacts. These hardware/software applications have been

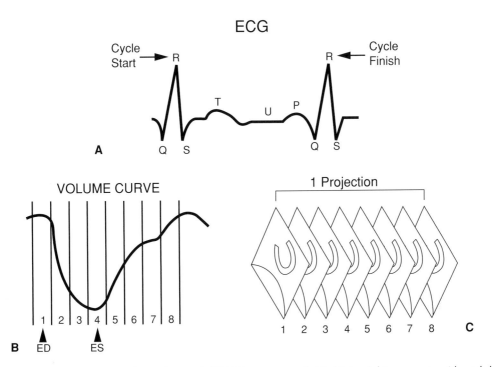

Figure 9-9. (**A**) ECG complex with R-R interval. (**B**) Volume curve divided into eight segments with end diastole and end systole. (**C**) One projection containing eight temporal frames.

available for more than 10 years. However, previous attempts to resolve attenuation artifacts with these methods resulted in improved specificity but in some cases reduced sensitivity, particularly in the RCA territory because of overcorrection in the inferior wall. This reduced sensitivity strongly impacted the use of attenuation correction in clinical situations. More recently, advances in attenuation correction algorithms have proven more accurate and reliable artifact resolution.[7]

The currently available applications are either line source (scanning, multiple array, or point) or computed tomography (CT) based, and both have been proven and documented to be more accurate and successful than previously released versions. When performing acquisitions with attenuation correction, it is important to understand the requirements and limitations of the specific hardware/software being used. It is also necessary to follow the manufacturer's recommendations for

acquisition parameters and quality control requirement to assure optimal image quality and system performance.

CONCLUSION

To assure optimal image quality and diagnostic accuracy with SPECT myocardial perfusion imaging, it is fundamentally important to use proper imaging techniques and understand the various protocols and imaging acquisition parameters. Protocol selection should be based on laboratory logistics and the type of equipment being used. It may also be necessary to research different protocols through literature review and site visits. Always keep consistency with a protocol and imaging parameters and determine what will work best for the laboratory. Lastly, it is imperative never to compromise image quality or patient outcomes by short cutting procedures or techniques.

REFERENCES

1. Hansen C, et al. Myocardial perfusion and function SPECT. In: DePuey EG, ed. ASNC Imaging guidelines for nuclear cardiology procedures: A report of the American Society of Nuclear Cardiology Quality Assurance Committee. *J Nucl Cardiol*. 2006;13(6):e97–e120.

2. Taillefer R. Radionuclide myocardial perfusion imaging protocols. In: Heller GV, Hendel RC, eds. *Nuclear Cardiology: Practical Applications*. New York, NY: McGraw Hill; 2004.

3. Watson D. Acquisition, processing and quantification of nuclear cardiac images. In: Iskandrian AE, Verani MS, eds. *Nuclear Cardiac Imaging Principles and Applications*. 3rd ed. New York, NY: Oxford University Press; 2003.

4. Pohost GM, Zir LM, Moore RH, et al. Differentiation of transiently ischemic from infracted myocardium by serial imaging after a single dose of thallium-201. *Circulation*. 1977;55:294–302.

5. Taillefer R, Dupras G, Sporn V, et al. Myocardial perfusion imaging with a new tracer, technetium-99m-hexamibi (methoxy isobutyl isonitrile): Comparison with thallium 201-imaging. *Clin Nucl Med*. 1989;14:89–96.

6. Taillefer R, Lambert R, Dupras G, et al. Clinical comparison between thallium,-201 and Tc-99m-methoxy isobutyl isonitrile (hexamibi) myocardial perfusion for the detection of coronary artery disease. *Eur J Nucl Med*. 1989;15:280–286.

7. Singh B, Bateman T, Case J, Heller G. Attenuation Artifact, attenuation correction and the future of myocardial perfusion SPECT. *J Nucl Cardiol*. 2007;14:153–164.

8. Mann A. Quality control for myocardial perfusion imaging. In: Heller GV, Hendel RC, eds. *Nuclear Cardiology: Practical Applications*. New York, NY: McGraw Hill; 2004.

9. Nichols K, et al. Instrumentation quality assurance and performance. *J Nucl Cardiol*. 2006;13:e25–e41.

10. Nichols KJ, Galt JR. Quality control for SPECT imaging. In: DePuey EG, Garcia EV, Berman DA, eds. *Cardiac SPECT Imaging*, 2nd ed. Philadelphia, PA: Lippincott, Williams and Wilkins; 2001.

11. National Electrical Manufacturer's Association. *Performance Measurements of Scintillation Cameras*. Standards publication no. NU1-1994. Washington, DC: National Electrical Manufacturer's Association; 1994.

12. Early PJ, Sodee DB. Quality assurance. In: *Principles and Practice of Nuclear Medicine*. St. Louis, MO: C.V. Mosby; 1985.

13. National Electrical Manufacturer's Association. National Electrical Manufacturer's Association recommendations for implementing SPECT instrumentation quality control. *J Nucl Med Technol*. 1999;27:67–72.

14. Cullom SJ. Principles of cardiac SPECT imaging. In: DePuey EG, Garcia EV, Berman DA, eds. *Cardiac SPECT Imaging*, 2nd ed. Philadelphia, PA: Lippincott, Williams and Wilkins; 2001.

15. Baron JM, Choraguai P. Myocardial single-photon emission computed topography quality assurance. *J Nucl Cardiol*. 1996;3:157–166.

16. Galt JR, Garcia EV. Advances in instrumentation for cardiac SPECT. In: DePuey EG, Garcia EV, Berman DA, eds. *Cardiac SPECT Imaging*. 2nd ed. Philadelphia, PA: Lippincott, Williams and Wilkins; 2001.

17. Maniawski PJ, Morgan HT, Whackers FJTH. Orbit-related variation in spatial resolution as a source of artifactual defects in thallium-201 SPECT. *J Nucl Med*. 1991;32(5):871–875.

18. Garcia EV, Cooke CD, Van Train KF, et al. Technical aspects of myocardial SPECT imaging with technetium-99m sestamibi. *Am J Cardiol*. 1990;66(13):23E.

19. Go RT, MacIntyre WJ, Houser TS, et al. Clinical evaluation of 360° and 180° data sampling techniques for transaxial SPECT thallium-201 myocardial perfusion imaging. *J Nucl Med*. 1985;26:695–706.

20. Hoffman EJ. 180° compared with 360° sampling in SPECT. *J Nucl Med*. 1982;23:745–746.

21. Maublant JC, Peycelon P, Kwiatkowski F, et al. Comparison between 180° and 360° data collection in technetium-99m MIBI SPECT of the myocardium. *J Nucl Med*. 1989;30:295–300.

22. Eisner RL, Nowak DJ, Pettigrew R, et al. Fundamentals of 180° reconstruction in SPECT imaging. *J Nucl Med*. 1986;27:1717–1728.

23. Toma DM, White MP, Mann A, et al. Influence of arm positioning upon rest/stress Tc-99m sestamibi tomographic imaging. *J Nucl Cardiol*. 1999;6:163–168.

24. Breszk JA, Hawman EG. Evaluation of SPECT angular sampling effects: Continuous vs. step and shoot. *J Nucl Med*. 1987;28:1308–1314.

25. DePuey G, Rozanski A. Using gated technetium-99m-sestamibi SPECT to characterize fixed myocardial defects as infarct or artifact. *J Nucl Med*. 1995;36:952–955.

26. White MP, Mann A, Saari MA. Gated SPECT imaging 101. *J Nucl Cardiol*. 1998;5:523–526.

27. Cullom SJ, Case JA, Bateman TM. Electrocardiographically gated myocardial perfusion SPECT: Technical principles and quality control considerations. *J Nucl Cardiol*. 1998;5:418–425.

28. Nichols K, Dorbala S, DePuey EG, et al. Influence of arrhythmias on gated SPECT myocardial perfusion and function quantification. *J Nucl Med*. 1999;40:924–934.

CHAPTER 10

Myocardial SPECT Processing

Russell D. Folks

INTRODUCTION

In this chapter, we discuss the processing steps that occur between image acquisition and interpretation. After a general introduction, each step in the typical sequence is covered: filtering, reconstruction, reorientation, and quantitative analysis. Aspects of quantitation including segmentation, parameter selection with its attendant challenges, myocardial sampling, and normal file comparison are discussed. Sources of discrepancy between visual and quantitative analysis of myocardial SPECT are noted. The chapter concludes with a summary of how users can optimize their understanding and use of processing software.

A myocardial SPECT study consists of a set of images acquired at various angles as the camera rotates around a patient's chest. These images are appropriately referred to as planar projections, since they are two-dimensional projections of the three-dimensional patient. The set of images is sometimes called the "raw data" for the study. Although important information can be gained by inspecting the raw images, some processing is necessary in order to fully visualize and understand the information contained in the images.

In the most general sense, any computerized image processing uses software that performs a sequence of steps, using specified parameters, to produce output in some agreed-upon format. In the case of SPECT processing, we are manipulating image information in order to produce new images and data that summarize the amount and location of radiotracer uptake and show how that uptake changes over time. By these broad definitions, filtering, image reconstruction, and quantitation are all methods of processing images.

To obtain accurate results from cardiac SPECT processing, all the following should be carefully done:

- Patient selection, to ensure study protocol and stress are appropriate to the patient.
- Instrument quality control.

- Image acquisition. No correction program or processing technique can fully and adequately fix all of the problems that could occur because of a poor acquisition.

A deficiency in any of the above items means that the final results will be less accurate and less useful than they could be.

Before reconstruction, some preprocessing can be done, such as correction for technetium decay, or summation of gated projections into a pseudo-ungated study for analysis of perfusion. Motion correction can also be applied at this point. On some computer systems, motion correction can be automatically applied to each image set. It can also be selectively applied after visual inspection of the projections, which is probably the better approach. There are several motion-correcting algorithms; some work best for subtle motion while others are good for gross motion. Correction software can produce unwanted changes in the images, particularly if a correction for lateral shift is included. If the software makes fractional pixel shifts then, in effect, a filtering step has been applied. Images shifted in this way often have a different texture or smoothness than the unshifted versions. If an image set exhibits motion, and the acquisition cannot be repeated, it may be necessary to try more than one motion correction program, if available, in order to get the best results. After motion correction, the original and final projections should always be compared, to make sure that the quality of the images has been improved, rather than degraded, by the correction.

IMAGE FILTERING

Several concepts related to image filtering will be needed to understand the details of the tomographic reconstruction process.

Resolution

As shown in Figure 10-1, a curve can be drawn to represent how a point (or line) source of radioactivity is seen by a detector. If the imaging system were perfect, this profile curve would have a sharp

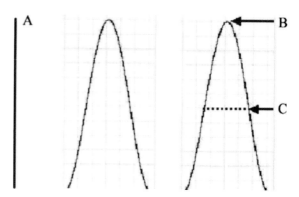

Figure 10-1.   If a line source of radioactivity (**A**) is imaged by a nuclear medicine detector, a profile perpendicular to the line can be drawn across the image of the line. This produces a plot that represents the activity seen from one side of the detector to the other. This is referred to as the line-spread function (or the point-spread function, if a point is imaged instead of a line). If the imaging system were perfect, the plot would be of the same width as the line source. The plot has width, or spread, that is greater than the line itself in part because resolution of the detector is limited. The plot is an approximation of the line. The detector response can be characterized by the maximum value of the plot (**B**), which can be compared to the count density of the line source, and by the full width at half the maximum (**C**), which is a measure of spread, and by inference a measure of resolution.

rise with the same width as the point being imaged. Because resolution is limited, the imaging system cannot detect the true edges of the point, and so the curve has some spread. The curve is therefore known as the point-spread function, often abbreviated PSF. The standard way of describing the degree of spread in the curve is to measure its width at half the maximum height. The full width at half maximum (FWHM) is a way of characterizing the resolution of an imaging system. The lower the FWHM, the smaller the object that can be accurately imaged.[1]

Frequency

Important in understanding image filtering is the concept of frequency. Frequency can be thought of as the rate of change in information content as one moves across an image. If pixel values change frequently, then the image is said to have high-frequency information. If the image is mostly made up of uniform pixel values, with little fluctuation, this is low-frequency information. Nuclear medicine images can be composed of any combination of frequencies. Those images that have mostly high-frequency content, we typically consider to be visually "noisy." Those that are mostly low frequency, we describe them as "blurry." Applying a filter to an image certainly changes the pixel values, but the filter can also be thought of as operating on the *frequencies* in the image. The filtering process, when thought of in this way, is sometimes referred to as filtering "in frequency space" or "in the frequency domain."[2] Frequency is given in units that express the number of changes in pixel values per unit of distance within the image. For SPECT image resolutions, the units are, for example, cycles per centimeter. Figure 10-2 shows idealized images of different frequencies.

We can treat the entire image as a collection of frequencies, but is there any advantage to doing so? There would be an advantage if we could express those frequencies as a collection of simpler elements, because then filtering would be a sim-pler mathematical task. Decomposing the original curve into simpler components is exactly what is accomplished by a mathematical step called the Fourier transform.[3] The simpler elements are combinations of sines and cosines, curves that always have the same shape. Figure 10-3 illustrates the concept. Once we have these simple curves, they can be manipulated. The amplitude of some can be increased, the amplitude of others decreased. The phase can be shifted. Since each simple curve is a specific frequency component that is contained in the original image, we can be sure that, when the simple curves are added back together after manipulation, they will produce a new curve that is the frequency representation of a new image. This is an image that has been altered in a predictable way from the original image—in other words, "filtered."

Filter Definition

A filter is defined by an equation, which can be plotted for a range of frequencies. Depicting a filter visually in this way succinctly indicates how it will affect the various frequencies in the image. We can tell which frequencies will be reduced or removed, and which will be left unchanged. The simplest filter that is used for SPECT is the ramp filter, so named because of the ramp-like appearance of its plot. Other filters in common use for SPECT include the Hanning and Butterworth, both of which can be specified by numeric parameters that describe how they work. The Hanning filter is characterized by a parameter known as *cut-off frequency*, the frequency at which the filter is defined to be zero. The Butterworth filter is characterized by two parameters, both relating to the shape of the filter plot's downward course from its peak to zero. The *critical frequency* is the point at which the filter begins its roll-off to zero, that is, the point at which the filter kernel (plot) changes slope. The *power* characterizes the steepness of the roll-off. Some software vendors use the term *order* instead of power. The power is twice the order. Filter cutoff and critical frequency are expressed in units that include a reference to frequency.

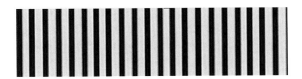

Figure 10-2. Two hypothetical images. The lower image contains more transitions from signal (light gray) to no signal (black) and therefore has higher-frequency information than the upper image.

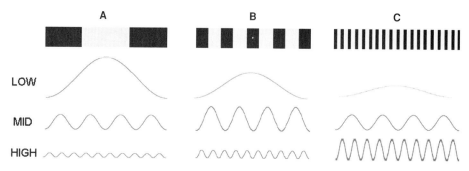

Figure 10-3.   Three images containing information of predominantly low frequency (**A**), mid-range frequency (**B**), and high frequency (**C**). In the frequency domain, the simpler components that make up each image are sine and cosine curves, as suggested by the curves below each image. Only three frequencies are shown, for simplicity. LOW, MID, and HIGH each represent a single, specific frequency, so the number of "peaks" in that curve is always the same, regardless of whether it is a component of image **A**, **B**, or **C**. However, the amplitude (height) of the curve is different for each image because amplitude represents the relative contribution of that frequency to the image. Thus, low-frequency image **A** has a large low-frequency component curve and a very small high-frequency component. Image **C** has plenty of high frequencies but not much low-frequency information, so its high-frequency component is of higher amplitude than its low-frequency component. Real-world images are much more complex, but their frequencies can still be broken down into components such as these, by means of the Fourier transform.

Depending on the camera manufacturer, filter units may by given as cycles per centimeter, cycles per pixel, or fraction of the *Nyquist* frequency. The Nyquist frequency is the highest frequency that can be faithfully displayed in a digital image, given the limitations of the imaging system. The Nyquist frequency is always 0.5 cycles per pixel.

As we have noted, images contain structures composed of various frequencies, and different kinds of information are conveyed by different frequencies. Low frequency, corresponding to pixel values that are not rapidly changing, is associated with much of the diagnostic information in the image. In myocardial SPECT, for example, we are concerned with the large and mostly uniform normal ventricular wall, and with discrete areas of perfusion deficit, where counts are lacking. Image detail, which includes the edges of structures, is composed of high-frequency information. Noise is also high frequency. Intermediate frequencies convey information about image contrast, as well as some diagnostic information.

If we undertake to determine the optimum filter for a given imaging situation, we should take into account several factors,[4] including the following:

- The energy of the isotope being imaged.
- The amount of scatter that is anticipated.
- The collimator that is used.
- The kind of information we hope to obtain from the images. If the goal is to detect the simple presence or absence of radiopharmaceutical uptake in a certain area, that is very different from the case where we need to determine the relative uptake in many small, adjacent regions, or to discern the exact shape of an area of uptake.

In order to optimize an image for interpretation, we would prefer to maximize important detail and edges, preserve contrast, and eliminate noise. Important image components are present in all parts of the frequency range; therefore, it is not possible to obtain ideal images purely by filtering. By using filters to eliminate certain frequencies that might contain unnecessary or redundant information, we will always be throwing away other information that we might wish to keep. The goal

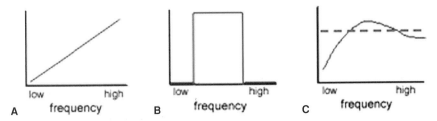

Figure 10-4.   Representation of the behavior of several possible filters. The area under the plot represents frequencies that remain in the image after the filter is applied. For the ramp filter **A**, the lower the frequency, the more of that frequency that is removed. Since high frequencies are passed through, this is called a high-pass filter. Filter **B** is a band-pass filter, because a range (band) of frequencies is allowed through. Filter **C** is called a restoration filter, because certain frequencies (indicated by the part of the plot above the dashed line) are enhanced beyond their magnitude in the original image. Thus, information that was lost is restored to the image.

of filtering, in a practical sense, is to strike the best compromise between smoothness and detail in the image.

The degree to which filtering can improve images will be limited by the quality of the acquisition. To obtain optimal images, there must be sufficient counts in each image, and there must be sufficient angular sampling, or number of projections. If angular sampling is too low, the reconstruction process will introduce artifacts, regardless of the filter used.

Frequencies that are preserved after the filtering operation are said to have been *passed* by the filter. Filters used in SPECT reconstruction and processing, regardless of type, definition, or name, can be classified according to which part of the frequency spectrum they pass, as illustrated in Figure 10-4. High-pass filters allow higher frequencies to be maintained in the image and preferentially remove or diminish (filter out) lower frequencies. Low-pass filters do the opposite. Band-pass filters preserve a certain range, or band, of frequencies and remove or diminish frequencies outside this band. Passing a certain range of frequencies using a filter can have the effect of emphasizing or de-emphasizing image details such as edges. Figure 10-5 shows, conceptually, why this happens.

There are some filters that do more than preserve or remove existing frequencies. These filters are defined so that they augment certain frequencies, with the goal of restoring image information

that has been lost or obscured because of scatter, poor resolution, or noise. Such filters are, therefore, known as *restoration* filters, the Metz filter being one common example. To restore what was lost, you must first know what was lost. Thus, the

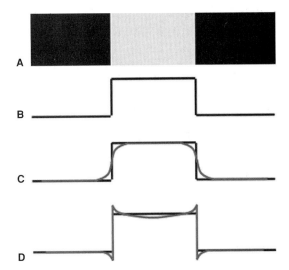

Figure 10-5.   (**A**) The simplest image and (**B**) the image represented as a count profile. In this image, there is a single-frequency "cycle," or transition from no signal (black) to signal (light gray) back to no signal. (**C**) Curve shows the same plot in black, and a red overlay indicating the result of applying a low-pass filter. The transition (the edges) has been blurred. (**D**) Curve shows the result of applying a high-pass filter. The edges are preserved, with some loss of the peak.

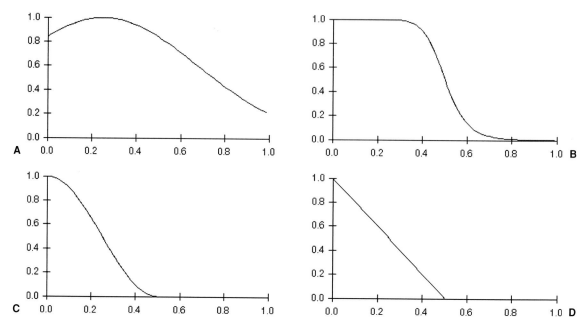

Figure 10-6.   Four different filters. Although the cutoff or critical value is 0.4 for each one, they are defined differently, so they each "pass" a different range of higher frequencies. The filters are Gaussian (**A**), Butterworth (**B**), Hanning (**C**), and Parzen (**D**).

effectiveness of a restoration filter, like any filter, depends greatly on knowing the imaging conditions listed above, as well as on careful tuning of filter parameters.[5,6] Other considerations include the type of camera that is used to acquire the images, and the imaging protocol. One example is the use of a multidetector system for SPECT. When these systems were first introduced, it was thought that they would be used to produce images of much greater count density, since two or three cameras were acquiring data simultaneously. In practice, however, the introduction of multidetector systems has led to protocols in which total imaging time is decreased, in order to enhance laboratory efficiency. Images acquired using a multidetector system may need to be filtered differently than those from a single-detector system, even if the total imaging time is the same.[7]

Figure 10-6 gives examples of the frequency plots, or filter kernels, for several different filters. Once a filter has been chosen, its parameters must be set. This is a critical step. Figure 10-7 shows how the same filter with different parameters can result in images of very different texture. Fortunately, the user does not have to make all of these decisions on a case-by-case basis, since the developers of today's commercial software packages for cardiac SPECT have recommended filter settings for various types of SPECT studies. In the great majority of instances, these settings should be used. Occasionally, if the reconstructed images are of unusually poor quality as a result of patient size or other technical factors, the filter settings can be adjusted in order to accomplish what the recommended filter was designed to produce: images with consistent texture and contrast. Filters should be adjusted with care by changing the power first, and then the critical frequency if necessary.

IMAGE RECONSTRUCTION

If we examine the SPECT projection set in a cine loop we see that, at certain angles, a particular

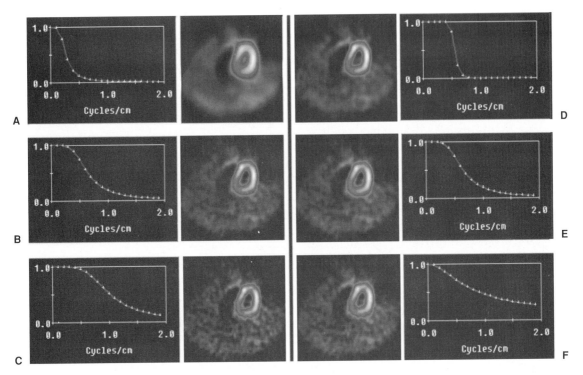

Figure 10-7.   The same transaxial image slice, with six different variations of a Butterworh filter applied. In the left column, the power is constant at 5, and critical frequencies vary: 0.22 (**A**), 0.52 (**B**), and 0.82 (**C**). In the right column, the critical frequency is constant at 0.52, and the power varies: 20 (**D**), 5 (**E**), and 2.5 (**F**). The critical frequency makes more difference in the appearance of the image. (**A**) and (**C**) are quite different in image texture, although the critical frequency is different by less than a factor of 4. (**D**) and (**F**) are similar even though the power differs by a factor of 8. The expected difference in effect of two filters can be approximated by noting the difference in the area under the two filter curve definitions. (See color insert.)

anatomic structure might be positioned behind another, while the two structures are separated from each other at other angles. Because the SPECT study is composed of views of the object from many angles, it seems logical that all of the pixel count data needed to construct a three-dimensional view of the patient is contained in the projection set. Reconstruction is the process of converting raw projection data, usually covering at least a 180-degree arc, into a set of tomographic slices. This is the step in which two-dimensional data become three dimensional and is accomplished purely by mathematical manipulation of the data.

Reconstruction Methods

It is necessary for the reconstruction algorithm to know the uniformity of response across the usable area of the detector, in order to know how much weight to give to counts in various places within a projection. Thus, an energy- and collimator-specific uniformity correction must be used, which requires acquisition of a high-count flood. The reconstruction algorithm must also know the mathematical center of the acquisition arc. If that center differs from the physical center around which the detector rotates, then a correction must be applied during reconstruction. To identify the physical center, a *center-of-rotation correction* is calculated for the camera by means of a 360-degree tomographic acquisition of a point source. This acquisition is not energy specific. The center should be checked on a regular basis, so that reconstruction will be accurate.

There are several classes of algorithms that can be used for reconstruction. *Analytic* methods have that name because mathematical equations can be written to describe the process, and an exact solution to a series of these equations can be found. As implemented in nuclear medicine, these methods require certain assumptions about the nature of SPECT images and ignore important properties of the images, in the name of usability and simplicity. Nevertheless, analytic methods are efficient, computationally fast, and straightforward to implement. The necessary assumptions and limitations are well understood. An analytic method that utilizes filtered back-projection (discussed below) is currently the most commonly implemented reconstruction method for SPECT images. The conceptual steps in this method are shown in Figure 10-8.

Iterative reconstruction is routinely used in PET and is becoming more widely used in SPECT. Iterative methods are based on a conceptual model of SPECT imaging that is fundamentally different from that used in filtered back-projection. This

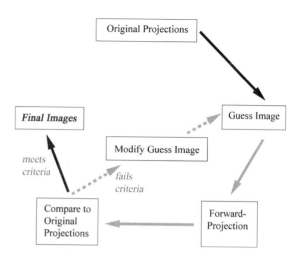

Figure 10-9. Diagram of the steps in iterative reconstruction. Solid arrows indicate the steps that are always performed. Gray arrows indicate the steps that are repeated (iterated), in order to refine the guess image until the solution achieves a certain level of correctness. In some implementations, the initial guess image is derived from a reconstruction performed with filtered back-projection.

model is intended to describe the reality of the imaging process more closely[8] and includes a different set of assumptions about the data.[9] Consequently, iterative methods are more complex than filtered back-projection, and the computations involved require more time. In this type of reconstruction, preliminary images are generated and then modified by repeating, or iterating, a sequence of processing steps. Iterative methodology provides a convenient mathematical framework for manipulating the image data in additional ways during reconstruction and so has become the method of choice when SPECT is combined with corrections for attenuation, scatter, and resolution. The conceptual steps in iterative reconstruction are shown in Figure 10-9.

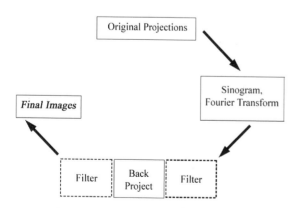

Figure 10-8. Diagram of the steps in the filtered back-projection method of reconstruction. Filtering (dashed boxes) can occur before back-projection, or after, or both.

Filtered Back-Projection

We will use the technique of filtered back-projection to explore some theoretical concepts in SPECT reconstruction.

The basic problem of reconstruction has to do with count overlap. We have a set of planar projections, which make up a complete SPECT acquisition. A given projection is composed of many pixels containing counted photons. Each photon has traveled along a straight line from a given point inside the patient, into the detector (discounting scatter). We can know the location at which the photon interacted with the crystal but cannot know at what depth the photon originated.[10] So the projection image is made up of counts that all originated at some undetermined depth within the patient. The image we see is composed of all these counts, projected onto a single plane. This is why the term *planar projection* is used to describe the raw data obtained from a SPECT acquisition.

A transaxial slice (also called a transverse slice by some software vendors) contains counts that are, in a plane, perpendicular to the planar projection set. Therefore, as the reconstruction algorithm builds one transaxial slice at a time, it uses counts from a single row of the projections (Figure 10-10). During acquisition, a single point source inside a patient may contribute a photon to many

different projection images, that is, the same point in the object is sampled by the camera from many angles. As data from more angles is used during reconstruction, the transaxial slice becomes more complete and is a more refined representation of the counts in that "slice" through the patient. This implies that there is a threshold of *angular sampling* or a certain lower limit to the number of projections that must be acquired in order to produce reconstructed images of acceptable quality.

Consider an example photon, which, as mentioned above, arises in a patient being imaged and interacts with a scintillation detector. The photon is assumed to have originated somewhere along a straight line that extends from the place at which it entered the detector, through the object. Thus, we can define a *line of acquisition*, as the straight line consisting of all the possible originating locations of the photon, as shown in Figure 10-11. The angle of the line of acquisition, with respect to the detector face, is limited by the collimator. In the reconstruction process, the line of acquisition of a detected photon is converted into a line of counts in the reconstructed image, a

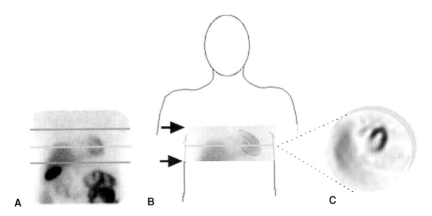

Figure 10-10.   A SPECT acquisition consists of a series of planar projection images. An anterior projection is shown in image (**A**). In a myocardial study, the area of interest is around the heart, so, during reconstruction, this area is identified (gray lines in **A**) either automatically or manually. The complete SPECT acquisition represents a three-dimensional object, the patient's chest, shown in image (**B**), with the same area of interest indicated by arrows. The green line represents an arbitrarily chosen row of pixels, which happens to pass through the heart and the top of the liver. The counts in this row, together with the same row from all other projections, are used to construct a transaxial slice, shown as image (**C**). Transaxial slices are reconstructed from counts in each row that lies between the arrows, and this stack of slices comprises the volume of data that are relevant to the heart.

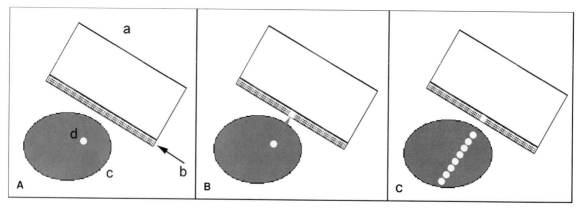

Figure 10-11. Panel (**A**) shows a camera (a) with its crystal (b), a source to be imaged (c), containing a point (d), which gives rise to a photon. In panel (**B**), the photon travels straight into the detector (arrow), interacting with the crystal (white box). Up to this point, as far as the reconstruction software is concerned, the source of the photon could be anywhere along a line that stretches through the source, as indicated by the line of white dots in panel (**C**). In other words, the direction in which the point source lies is known because the line of incidence of its photon is known, and only its depth is unknown. Its actual position could be any of the dots in (**C**) and is determined only when data from multiple projections are used in reconstruction. From this we can also see why scatter is such a problem: changing the direction of the incident photon violates the basic "straight line" assumption of the reconstruction algorithm, reducing the precision with which we can locate the point that produced the photon.

process known as *back-projecting* the detected photon. Photons originating at the same point in the patient as our example photon are similarly back-projected from each camera angle, each time creating a line (or ray) of counts. In the reconstructed slice, these rays of counts from multiple planar projections cross at the actual point of origin of the photons. In this way, the photons' origin is located within the reconstructed image.[4] When all planar projections have been used, a complete transaxial slice is obtained. Real-world images consist of many point sources, but each point is dealt with in the same way as our example point.

The back-projection method tends to produce streaks in the final images, the result of the summing of pixel columns from different acquisition angles that contain inconsistent information. In addition, the assumptions that are part of the back-projection method do not fully match the reality of SPECT. For example, scatter is a significant factor, and photons that arrive at the detector are not just from a single plane in the patient. There is interference between adjacent pixels of different activity.

Some of these factors tend to cause blurring of the reconstructed image and, although this is a natural result of the back-projection algorithm, we would like to reduce it if possible. For this purpose, a filtering step is added, hence the term *filtered back-projection*.

To understand the effect of filtering, recall the point-spread function. The function can be drawn to represent what is seen by the camera from any given acquisition angle. As discussed above, a filter can be applied to preserve high-frequency information, such as object edges. When a filter is applied during reconstruction, the result is that the edge of the response curve is enhanced. The enhancement includes negative areas immediately surrounding the curve peak (as was shown in Figure 10-4). These negative areas occur in the response profile for each angle that contributes to the reconstruction. The reconstructed point, defined by the summation of back-projected rays, is treated like an edge, and the net effect is that this point becomes more discreet and is, thus, a better representation of the original point in space. The rays themselves are blurred out within the rest of the image. SPECT projections are often subjected to a ramp filter as a first step in reconstruction. It is the ramp filter that introduces the negative component to the back-projected rays, enhancing edges in the process. Unfortunately, high-count areas in the image tend to provide well-defined edges. When these are enhanced during filtering, the adjacent areas from which counts are removed are larger than usual, which tend to produce areas of low or negative counts in the image. This problem is characteristic of filtered back-projection, and, because it arises from a filtering step, it is referred to as the *ramp filter artifact*.

There are several ways filtering can be accomplished for SPECT reconstruction:

- Planar projection images can be filtered before being reconstructed (*prefiltering*).
- Transaxial slices can be filtered after begin generated (*postfiltering*).
- Filtering can be applied both before and after reconstruction.

For SPECT, filtering must occur in all three dimensions, to avoid introducing artifacts, but each dimension does not have to be filtered in the same step as the others. For a reconstructed image slice, its two dimensions X and Y are filtered in one step because this is most efficient. The third dimension Z is the dimension that extends through the set of slices, as shown in Figure 10-12, and this dimension can be filtered in a separate step. All of this flexibility as to when and how to filter gives rise to commonly used terms such as *3-D postfilter* to describe both the type of the filter and the point in processing at which it is applied.

Iterative Reconstruction

Out of a number of iterative approaches to reconstruction, there are two that are both commercially available and in common use for SPECT today. Maximum likelihood expectation maximization (MLEM) is the older of the two, having been first applied to emission tomography in 1982.[11] Ordered-subsets expectation maximiza-

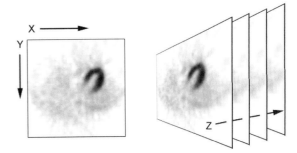

Figure 10-12. Reconstruction generates a set of transaxial slices. A single one of these slices has dimensions of length and width (X, Y), and the set of slices has a third dimension Z, which is through the entire set. In the images on the right, the patient's head is to the right, and the front of the patient's chest is pointing up.

tion (OSEM) was described in 1994.[12] Since OSEM is really a special case of MLEM, the two approaches have a number of features in common. One of these is the exclusion of negative pixel values from the reconstruction. This is important because we know that our original images, which we will submit to reconstruction, should have no negative pixel values, so we would prefer that no negative values be introduced by the reconstruction itself. As we have seen, this constraint does not hold for filtered back-projection. Since the integrity and appearance of the final images vary with the number of iterations and with other parameters as well, depending on the method, one key to the success of this type of reconstruction is the ability to determine the best set of parameters. As an MLEM reconstruction proceeds, the algorithm uses the difference between the original projections and a set of projections created from the reconstructed images to determine how to make mathematical adjustments for the next iteration. In the terminology of statistics, the original projections are the measured data, and the reconstructed images are a function of that data. MLEM seeks the function, out of all possible functions, which has the greatest probability of having been derived from the data that were measured. This probability aspect is what gives rise to the "maximum likelihood" part of the name.

MLEM uses data from all of the acquired projections, during each iteration. If it were possible to use only some of the projections, there would be fewer calculations per step, with a potential speed improvement. OSEM is a method that tries to realize this advantage. In order to use fewer projections at a time, it has to be determined how to divide or group the available projections, and in what order to use them. To begin, for a given set of projection images, there are a number of potential subsets: projections from the start of the study, from the middle of the study, etc. For each OSEM iteration, one subset of projections is used at a time, rather than the full set. There are different ways to organize the subsets, in terms of which ones are used first, but the principle is that each subset of projections uses data that are separated as much as possible, in terms of acquisition angle, from the following subset. In this way, the subsets are used in a specific order, the order being defined so as to introduce the maximum new information with each step. This methodology of "ordering subsets" gives OSEM part of its name.

We have noted that the number of iterations is variable for MLEM reconstruction. For OSEM, both the number of iterations and the number of subsets must be initially set. In general, MLEM and OSEM converge to a final result at the same rate when both parameters are counted. For example, MLEM with 20 iterations will be as "correct" as an OSEM with two iterations and 10 subsets, but the OSEM will require substantially less time.[9]

Iterative methods have been shown to result in reconstructed images that are less noisy than those that are the product of filtered back-projection.[13] Iterative reconstruction can also be of practical use in non-attenuation-corrected SPECT in certain circumstances. If there is high-count extracardiac activity, which appears to cause either streak artifacts that impact myocardial counts or low-count or negative areas caused by the ramp filter artifact when filtered back-projection is used, artifact can sometimes be reduced by performing iterative reconstruction.

Manual Reconstruction

When SPECT reconstruction is performed, it is usually limited to that part of the image volume that includes the heart. So the user's only task is to define the limits of this part of the volume, typically by placing lines above and below the heart on the projection images. The reconstructed volume should include all of the heart and exclude most of the rest of the image, in order to produce a transaxial file that is of manageable size.

IMAGE REORIENTATION

Transaxial slices, the product of SPECT reconstruction, are perpendicular to the long axis of the patient's body and represent the three-dimensional set of counts that are relevant to the heart (assuming that the entire image volume has not been reconstructed). Reorientation is the step of rearranging the pixel counts in transaxial slices so that they are oriented along the long and short axis (SA) of the left ventricle, the most advantageous orientation for viewing the heart. Reconstruction and reorientation are distinct steps. Reconstruction is the generation of three-dimensional images, as slices transverse to the long axis of the body, starting from planar projection images. Reorientation follows reconstruction and is a reordering of the count data in the transaxial slices. This step is analogous to extracting counts from the three-dimensional data set, along certain planes that are parallel, or perpendicular, to the long axis of the heart. Figure 10-13 shows the relative orientations of the body and the heart, for reference. Reorientation is sometimes referred to as a rotation of the data in the transaxials. Mathematically, the reorientation step can be described as two sequential rotations of the counts in the three-dimensional transaxial data set.

Automatic vs. Manual Reorientation

Several automated methods for reorientation have been reported.[14–18] These approaches have certain general elements in common:

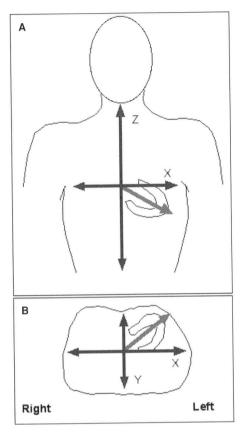

Figure 10-13. The heart is positioned in the chest at an angle that is oblique to the long (**A**) and short (**B**) axes of the body. The body's axes are indicated by blue arrows and the heart's axes by red arrows. To obtain slices of the heart that follow its own long and short axes, we perform consecutive rotations of the transaxial data, also known as "image reorientation." We begin with slices that are oriented along the body's long axis and end with slices that are oriented along the heart's long axis. In the process, we change the coordinate system that will be used to analyze myocardial counts quantitatively; our worldview becomes local to the heart.

- Identifying the location of the LV, based on assumptions of its usual location and shape.
- Distinguishing the LV from surrounding non-LV areas.
- Using the assumed, characteristic shape of the LV as a starting point for either finding

its axes or fitting it to a template for further analysis.

The elements in this list are similar to the mental steps a human user follows in performing similar tasks. The advantage of the automated method is that it is completely reproducible: for a given input, the algorithm will always produce the same output.

If automatic software is available for reorientation, it should be used, because it treats images in a consistent manner. Even if this software appears to work, however, the user should review the reoriented images for correctness. As for any automatic software, it is up to the user to understand what the software is doing and override it if necessary. For reorientation, that means knowing how to properly select the necessary angles, and how improper angle selection affects the images.

The heart is a three-dimensional structure and, in all aspects of myocardial SPECT processing, we are dealing with three dimensions. When performing manual reorientation, the goal is to draw a line on the image so as to bisect the ventricle as exactly as possible. The line represents a plane along which counts will be extracted from the image volume—the line is the edge of the plane. The first plane is defined on the transaxial image, in order to produce images that are oriented along the heart's vertical long axis (VLA). A VLA slice image is produced when all counts on the defined plane are extracted from the transaxial slice stack. Additional VLA slices are obtained by extracting counts from planes parallel to the first one and separated by one or more pixels. Using the mid-VLA slice as a guide, another plane is defined, which will be used to extract the horizontal long-axis (HLA) counts. From the HLA plane, a perpendicular plane is automatically extracted to form the SA images.

The accuracy with which the VLA plane is defined will limit the accuracy of later planes. This is an example of a general principle: the earlier in the processing stream in which a step is performed (or a decision is made, or an error is introduced), the greater number of effects the step can have on later steps, the greater the magnitude of those effects is

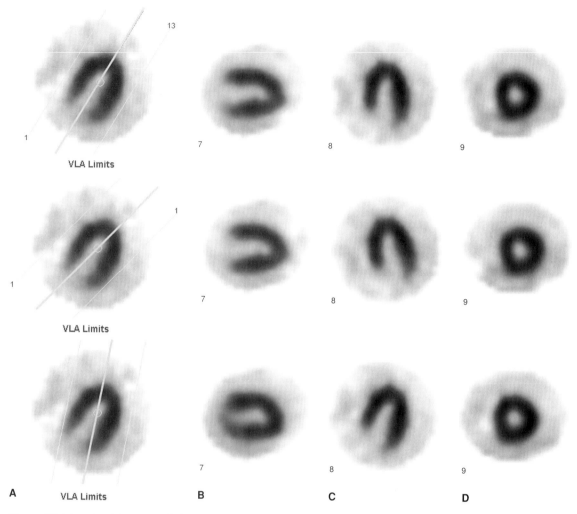

Figure 10-14.   A mid-transaxial slice (column **A**), on which angles are defined for extraction of the vertical long-axis plane (column **B**). The top row shows an acceptable angle. In row 2, the angle is too clockwise, passing to the right of the apex. Compared to the acceptable angle in the top row, this has little effect on the VLA, produces some change in the SA in column **D** (look at the right ventricle), and produces a noticeable shift in the position of the HLA in column **C**. In row 3, the angle is too counterclockwise, passing to the left of the apex. The result is a noticeable difference in VLA and HLA, compared to the top row, while the SA is less affected than it was in row 2. The degree of effect will be different for different heart sizes and shapes.

likely to be. Figure 10-14 shows that variation in the VLA angle can have noticeable effects on the other images, even if the optimal HLA/SA plane is used. Fortunately, today's software makes it relatively easy to monitor the reorientation process, because the long-axis images are usually realigned

to horizontal and vertical planes for review. Thus, both VLA and HLA images should appear to be symmetrical around horizontal and vertical lines, respectively. If they are not so, if they appear to be "leaning," then the reorientation planes should be adjusted. Figure 10-15 shows the effects of varying

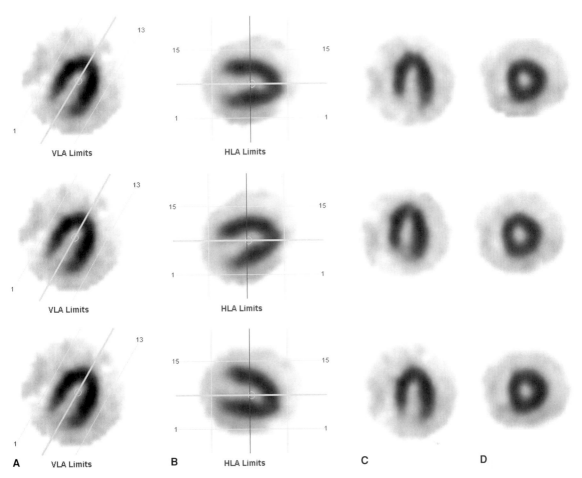

Figure 10-15. A mid-transaxial slice with proper VLA plane (column **A**) and three different attempts at defining a plane for extraction of the HLA (column **B**). In the top row, the plane is appropriate, while in row 2 it is too clockwise, passing below the true apex. In row 3, the angle is too counterclockwise, passing above the true apex. The effects are subtle on the SA slices, but more noticeable on the HLA.

the HLA plane angle. Note that the effects of these changes are more subtle than for changes in the VLA plane, particularly on the SA. This might be expected, since the HLA plane is one step later in the processing stream than the VLA plane.

The main effect of suboptimal reorientation is a change in the apparent location or size of a perfusion defect. Defining an incorrect VLA plane may make it impossible to accurately localize an apical perfusion defect. In reorientation, consistency is crucial. Stress and rest (and any additional sets

acquired as part of the same study) should usually have the same planes defined. There are two exceptions to this general rule: (1) the patient was positioned differently on the imaging table and (2) there has been a profound change in the ventricular size (Figure 10-16) or radiopharmaceutical uptake pattern, as in the case of a large, reversible perfusion defect. In any case, special care must be taken with reconstruction and reorientation, to optimize the ability of software—or of the physician—to make a comparison between stress

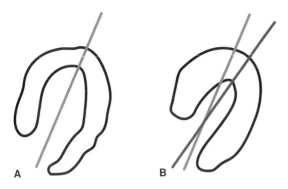

Figure 10-16.   These outlines are derived from a real exercise stress (**A**) and rest (**B**) transaxial slice in the same patient. The stress VLA reorientation plane is shown in gray on both images. Because of a change in ventricular shape and apparent thickness, the rest plane (black line) is defined differently than that for stress.

and rest. The best approach when defining reorientation planes manually is to think of the heart in three dimensions, and to determine the best angles using multiple slices, not just the center slice that is initially presented by the display program. That center slice may include a large defect and may, thus, have the least amount of visible myocardium from which to judge angles. Or it may be distorted because of a defect in another wall or because of physiologic remodeling of the heart that has occurred in response to disease. This multislice approach is relatively immune to the confusion that can result from ventricular aneurysms, large defects, and unusual myocardial shapes. See Figure 10-17 for a few examples of myocardial shapes.

Once images have been reoriented into VLA, HLA, and SA slice sets, we have the input necessary for quantitative analysis.

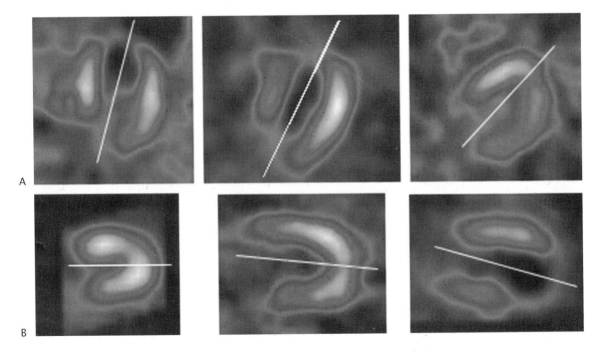

Figure 10-17.   Examples of mid-transaxial slices (row **A**) and mid-vertical long-axis slices (row **B**), in six different patients, showing some of the variety in heart position, size, shape, and defect pattern that can be seen. Reorientation planes are indicated by white lines. Consistency in choosing these planes is the key to providing appropriate images for interpretation or quantitative analysis.

QUANTITATIVE ANALYSIS

Before describing the specific steps in quantitative analysis of myocardial SPECT, a few general ideas should be considered.

Often the words "quantitation" and "quantification" are used interchangeably. Quantification, a somewhat more general term, refers to the process of representing some image feature using numeric values, whether measured or simply assigned. Quantitation refers to the use of calculations, measurements, or other analytic processes, which result in numeric values that characterize an image feature.

Quantitation is not strictly necessary in order to derive a meaningful conclusion from a myocardial SPECT study. The oblique slice images themselves can be visually interpreted, to assess myocardial perfusion. Before quantitative software became widespread, this was the standard practice, and a number of physicians continue to follow this routine. Perfusion can be quantified without the use of complicated software, by dividing the myocardium into segments, and assigning a numeric value to each segment to represent the perfusion seen visually on the slices. In this case, the analysis of the images takes place in the mind of the reader, rather than in computer software algorithms. A typical division scheme is shown in Figure 10-18. This technique is straightforward to implement and understand.

One of the main reasons for doing any kind of analysis of myocardial perfusion SPECT images, whether the analysis is visual or software aided, is to characterize myocardial blood perfusion. There are many comparisons that can be done:

- one major myocardial wall compared to another in the same study;
- stress compared to rest;
- an individual patient compared to a predefined normal pattern;
- the perfusion pattern in a given study, compared to a study in the same patient performed at another time.

There are several quantitative programs that have become commercially available in recent years.[19–23] Clinicians who have more than one of these analysis packages, and apply them to the same patient data, may see calculational differences and will want to know how to interpret one set of numbers with respect to the other, and to understand the causes of differences.[24]

Normal file comparison, with its related calculations and parametric images, requires additional software and places the burden of understanding the use of that software on both the technologist and the physician. Nevertheless, this and other sophisticated types of quantitative analysis carry a number of potential advantages.

Quantitation can help to define the limits of normalcy in a consistent way for a given population. It helps differentiate artifact from pathology, by displaying data in different ways and by providing automated quality control features. Because the quantitative result is reproducible for a certain input, it aids interpretation by providing an objective "second reading" of the study. Thus, the physician's attention can be drawn not only to obvious features but to parts of the study that are subtle but significant, helping to ensure that the interpretation is comprehensive. Interpretation can be done with greater confidence if there is objective evidence to back up the reader's opinion of the visual count distribution. Quantitation of myocardial images improves overall diagnostic yield and enhances reliability, accuracy, confidence, and reproducibility of interpretation.[21,25] Results of analysis can be expressed in many forms, allowing the interpreter access to an objective quantification

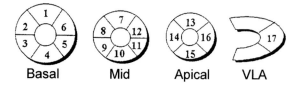

Figure 10-18. Typical scheme for dividing the LV myocardium into segments. When a system becomes standardized as this one has, references to segments are routine and easily understood, and comparison between studies is easy.

of features such as defect extent, severity, mass, reversibility, and function. The output of analysis programs can be connected to external decision support systems such as expert systems,[26] neural networks,[27] and case databases,[28] with potential further improvement in interpretation efficiency and confidence. Finally, the sophistication, which quantitative tools bring to the processing and interpretation of images, helps nuclear cardiology compete with other modalities, all of which are continuing to advance and provide new tools.

For myocardial SPECT, quantitative image processing in the most general sense is the process of reorganizing a subset of pixels from relevant slice images into a set of data, which can then be analyzed objectively, with the results summarized in a succinct way. The results can be qualitative in the form of images, quantitative as numeric values, or a combination of both. To be sure that the selected subset of pixels is an accurate representation of the LV myocardium, the first task is to identify the LV within the available images. This is essentially the process of limiting which image pixels will be subjected to further analysis and is sometimes referred to as "segmentation."

Cardiac Segmentation

In current commercial software, the heart is segmented automatically, with various algorithms coming into play to ensure consistency and handle unusual count patterns. Although this step often works well, the user should understand the software, the imaging system, and cardiac anatomy well enough to review LV localization and make adjustments if necessary. If the heart position and size are determined manually, then the accuracy of further analysis depends entirely on the user performing this step correctly. The normal LV shape is irregular and can vary considerably from one patient to the next. It can also vary in the same patient over time, or between the stress and resting states. Quantitative programs assume a specific simple left ventricular shape, either an ellipse or a cylinder with one hemispherical cap. Starting with this assumption of a standard shape, the LV can

be accurately located in space if we can specify its center, radius, and length. Software automatically finds these parameters and is usually very accurate. These parameters should probably not be changed unless there is a clear error, in order to maintain reproducibility.[29,30]

After automatically finding the location of the heart, the software displays its result to the user by placing various widgets (circles, lines, crosshairs, etc.) on the image. Pixels under the circle or line are included in the analysis. For example, if the apex and base limits are indicated by lines at slices 4 and 13, then the heart has been determined to have 10 slices. Slice 4 is the first slice and slice 13 is the last one. In software sold today, widgets are typically smaller than the width of one image pixel (which is not true in older systems). It is also important to remember that computer systems always smooth and interpolate images when these are zoomed for display. The actual image pixels are much larger (and fewer) than it may appear. There are several display configurations for reviewing cardiac segmentation in different commercial software packages (Figure 10-19), but the goal of identifying the heart and excluding noncritical structures is the same.

The location of the LV is characterized by its center of mass. This center becomes the starting point for searching for LV sample pixels, making it arguably the most important parameter. The chosen center should be valid for all slices and should therefore be reviewed on all slices, since the normal ventricular lumen can change shape from apex to base. The presence of multiple perfusion defects, or a single, large defect, can also distort LV shape and may cause inaccurate center placement.

LV size is characterized by a radial extent (also referred to as "ventricular radius of search," "search limit," etc.) and a longitudinal extent, or length. The radial extent defines the farthest point to which an algorithm will search in an attempt to find the edge of the heart. Anatomically, myocardial length is from the first apical slice that definitely includes myocardium to the last slice at the base, adjacent to the aortic valve plane. A properly chosen base slice will have a septal side that seems

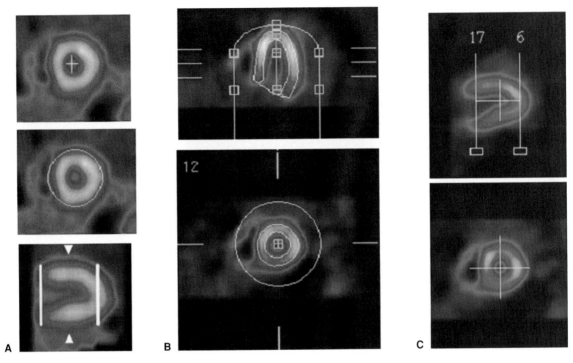

Figure 10-19. Columns **A**, **B**, and **C** represent the initial parameter finding widgets associated with three commercial programs used for quantitative myocardial SPECT analysis. The interfaces are different, but the tasks are the same: to identify the left ventricle while excluding nonessential areas of the image.

to be missing. The basal interventricular septum is nonmuscular membrane and extends a little farther down on this side. There is muscle on the lateral side, though, which is why this slice is included.

Factors That Affect Parameter Selection

Noncardiac areas of significant radiotracer uptake should be excluded from quantitative analysis. Of all the structures around the heart, the gastrointestinal tract and associated organs are most likely to contain enough counts to be problematic for image processing and review. Counts may be high in any of the following areas:

- Liver and spleen. These are large organs, with substantial blood supply, that accumulate technetium-based myocardial tracers.

- Gallbladder, which concentrates the radiopharmaceutical and excretes it into the small bowel.
- Small bowel, which may be anywhere from the 3 to the 8 o'clock positions, relative to the SA. The location of a hot spot usually changes with time.
- Stomach, because of reflux of counts from the small bowel.
- Esophagus, with counts seen in the lower part because of gastroesophageal reflux, or higher in the mediastinum because of hiatal hernia.

Small bowel is the most likely area to be a problem for image analysis because the counts can be high relative to the myocardium, and because it can be physically close to the inferior LV wall. High counts in bowel, adjacent to even a single SA

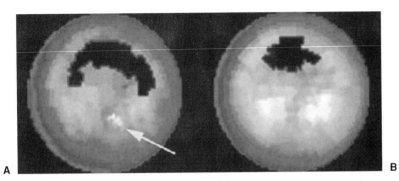
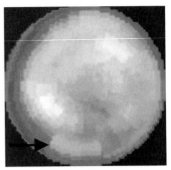

Figure 10-20.   Panel **A** shows a polar map with a "fatal" artifact because of hot bowel (gray arrow). When the radial limit is tightened, the hot spot disappears, and, since it was hotter than myocardium, the entire map is renormalized correctly. Note the difference between the artifactual map and the corrected one, shown as the rightmost image in panel **A**. The perfusion defect extent has also changed. Panel **B** shows a "nonfatal" bowel artifact (black arrow), which does not affect normalization.

slice, can cause a characteristic hot-spot artifact on polar plots, which may interfere with clinical interpretation by changing the normalization of the entire plot. If more than one slice is affected, the polar map artifact becomes wedge shaped, as a result of distortion inherent in this type of display. Even if the normalization is not affected, there can still be a hot spot that may mask a real perfusion defect or make the defect appear smaller or less severe than it is. Figure 10-20 shows two examples of the effect of bowel.

As with any type of image processing, the best way to deal with hot bowel is to take an organized approach to setting the parameters. One recommendation is to start by bringing the radius of search in tighter, more so than usual. Review the radius on all slices, to make sure that valid myocardium is not being excluded from analysis. If bowel cannot be excluded by tightening the radial limit, then adjust the center away from the hot bowel, but keeping it within the ventricular lumen. In the difficult case, you can increase the radius, and then move the center away from bowel, so that the arc is sufficiently wide to encompass the entire LV. Consider whether to adjust the second study (stress or rest) to match the one with bowel. It is not recommended to change the apex/base slice selection to eliminate bowel hot spot, since quan-

titation may be affected. However, if the bowel is very hot and confined to the apex, the apical slice could be shifted by one in order to prevent a critical artifact. The other suggestions should be tried first, and the apex changed as a last resort.

In some cases, it may not be possible to eliminate the problem, and quantitation may be compromised. In this case, the slice images alone may be used for interpretation, although the myocardial wall adjacent to the hot bowel may still be uninterpretable. The best approach is to recognize bowel uptake before acquisition, give the patient water to drink, have them walk around, or just wait a few minutes before acquiring the images, if possible.

SAMPLING THE MYOCARDIUM

The purpose for segmenting the heart and defining its precise extent is so that the pixels within the myocardium can be analyzed. This involves the process of myocardial sampling, which consists of several steps that are simple in concept:

- dividing the left ventricle into areas;
- searching each area;
- identifying a representative count from each area, which is referred to as the "sample" for that area;

- combining these sample counts in an organized way for analysis.

Note that these steps, which are carried out automatically for complex computerized analysis, are the same steps the human user performs for the simpler visual analysis shown in Figure 10-18.

The left ventricle is already divided into areas, in the form of SA slices, but it is further subdivided during sampling. A software algorithm searches from the defined ventricular center outward, to some defined limit within the image (i.e., the radial extent). Somewhere along this search ray a pixel count is identified and taken to be representative of that search. This is typically the maximum count found in that particular direction, although it may also be a sequence of pixels identified between the defined edges of the myocardial wall.[19,21,22] In the most commonly used methodology, the searches proceed around the circumference of the slice, and all of the sampled counts found for the slice are combined into a sequential set of values that characterizes the tracer uptake in the slice. For these reasons, we refer to the process as generating *circumferential profiles*.[31] An example profile is shown in Figure 10-21. The profiles themselves can be directly interpreted by the physician, or the set of them can be converted into images, which are plotted in polar coordinates. This conversion is summarized in Figure 10-22. Circumferential profile analysis has been used to analyze myocardial perfusion images for many years and originated in attempts to quantitate the radiotracer uptake in planar thallium images.[32] From early on, it was recognized that user decisions made during manual processing might affect the results.[33] In this respect, automatic algorithms have an advantage over a totally manual process, even if further quantitative steps are not performed beyond generation of the profiles.

Circumferential profiles consist of counts compared to angle, plotted in rectangular coordinates as shown in Figure 10-21. Circumferential profiles can also be combined into a stack, apex to base, and the count values converted into colors. These color values can be plotted in polar coordi-

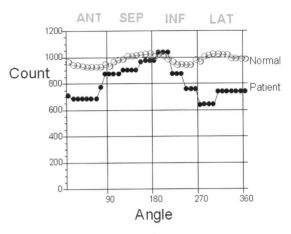

Figure 10-21. Example of a circumferential profile for one short-axis slice. This is a plot of counts vs. angle as one moves in a circle around the slice. There are 40 sampled points in the patient slice (black plot), which proceed sequentially around the myocardial walls, labeled at the top of the axis. The normal values for these samples are shown in the white plot. Areas where the patient plot is significantly below normal indicate perfusion deficit in that area. An important part of establishing a normal database is determining the threshold of a significant defect.

nates, which is the source of the term *polar map*, also sometimes called a bull's-eye map. Although widely used, this methodology has certain drawbacks, including the distortion inherent in the display, as well as the *partial volume effect*. This effect arises from the limited resolution of the imaging system. For example, if a SPECT system acquires images into an image matrix with pixels of size 1 cm, then the system is capable of localizing detected photons only to within an accuracy of 1 cm. Photons originating in anatomic structures smaller than that, or from structures (such as the heart) that have moved, may contribute photons to the same 1 cm. Any photon that is detected then represents an average of several sources; i.e., it represents only part of the tissue volume.

One alternative to the circumferential profile method is to first treat the myocardium as a whole by fitting it to a template. Then, comparisons to expected normal distributions can be made.[34,35]

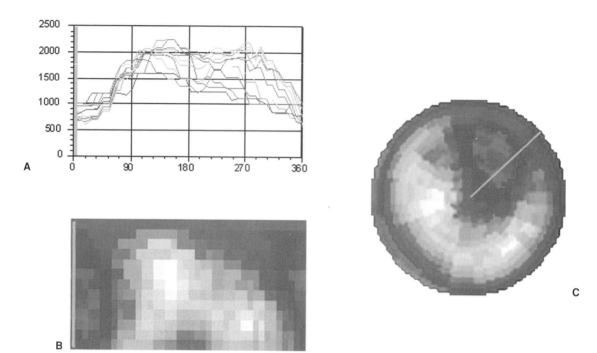

Figure 10-22.   Circumferential profiles for all short-axis slices of a patient study (**A**). The green line represents the starting point of sampling, which is 45 degrees right anterior oblique. When the counts from these profiles are converted into colors, and stacked, they form an array (**B**). The top row is the apex; the bottom row is the base. Here the ventricular counts are plotted in rectangular coordinates, giving equal area to each slice. This creates distortion in the shape of the ventricle being represented, especially at the apex, which is overrepresented, being stretched out across the top of the array. The counts in the array can also be plotted in polar coordinates (**C**), to form the familiar polar map, or bull's-eye map, roughly equivalent to looking at the heart from the apical end while still seeing the entire ventricle. Here there is a different kind of distortion. The apex is given less area than it should be, and the base is given more area than it should be. (See color insert.)

Normal File Comparison

Sampling is an efficient way to analyze the pixel count pattern in the images, from which we infer myocardial perfusion. Commercial software provides the capability to compare the sampled counts to expected normal values, whether we are dealing with profiles, polar maps, or three-dimensional distributions. In the polar map methodology, the normal distribution is represented by a set of values that are the means from a number of patients with low likelihood of significant coronary artery disease. The file of means is of some fixed size, in terms of the number of SA slices. In one program, for example, a normal file consists of 12 slices. This

implies that, for comparison to an individual patient who can have an arbitrary number of SA slices depending on heart size, an algorithm must determine which patient profile is to be compared to which mean normal profile. Inherent in the normal file is a definition of how different the patient profile must be from the corresponding normal profile before the difference is considered significant. The threshold for abnormality may be fixed[20,36] or may vary from one region of the LV myocardium to another,[21] and, because it is predefined, areas of the patient LV that have counts that fall below the threshold can be designated as significant defects and flagged in a different color on the polar

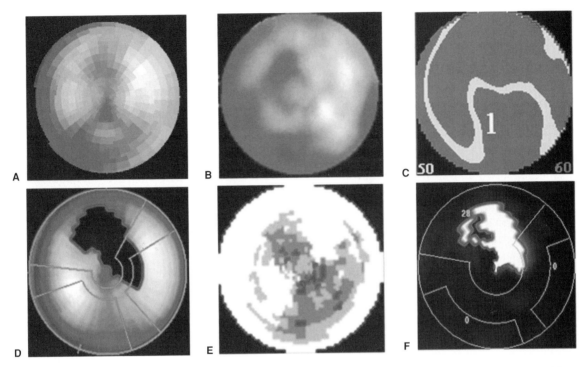

Figure 10-23.   Different types of polar map displays of myocardial perfusion, taken from various commercial programs. These plots, from six different patients, show raw perfusion (**A**); raw smoothed perfusion (**B**); quantized perfusion, in which counts have been grouped by value (**C**); raw perfusion with defect extent indicated in black and coronary territories overlaid (**D**); defect severity indicated by the number of standard deviations below mean normal (**E**); and thresholded reversibility, shown in white, with overlaid coronary territories (**F**). (See color insert.)

map.[37] In some commercialized techniques, the thresholds of abnormality have been determined from multiple sets of patients with a variety of defect patterns, involving intensive analysis of various combinations of defect location and extent.[38,39] A simplified technique has also been reported, which uses a novel normalization scheme in a collection of normal studies, working out thresholds for abnormality without the need for an abnormal test group.[36] Figure 10-23 shows different types of polar map displays that can be created.

Sources of Discrepancy

One of the major uses of quantitation in SPECT is to provide an objective result. The physician is, therefore, concerned about any discrepancy between quantitative results and the impression derived from visual assessment of the images. A number of factors can cause a quantitative defect to be present that was not appreciated visually on the slice images, or vice versa.

Attenuation, being always present, must be taken into account. There is a complex combination of hardware and software that can be used to compensate for attenuation in certain camera/computer systems. Quantitation of attenuation-corrected studies involves certain assumptions that may be given more or less weight by the software than they would be given by a physician. The physician can also draw on extensive knowledge of anatomy and physiology, whereas current software has no way to do this.

Patient motion is a factor over which we have limited control. Before acquisition, the patient can be cautioned not to move, and if need be, projections can be shifted manually or automatically to compensate for unavoidable motion. Again, the human interpreter can often "read around" the image artifact that may occur, but normal file comparison software cannot.

Whatever data are in the polar maps are also in the slice images. The converse is not true, since the polar maps are constructed from a subset of the pixels in the slices. The parameters of processing, discussed above, control which subset of pixels is analyzed; thus, parameter selection affects the appearance of the polar maps, as well as the comparison to normal. Parameter definition is a factor over which we do have control. For more than 10 years, there has been a trend toward automation in myocardial SPECT processing, which improves efficiency and reproducibility. All of the major camera vendors offer software with automation features. Reconstruction/reorientation software has been shown to be both accurate and reproducible.[17,18] Automatic parameter selection is also accurate while being more reproducible than the human operator. The several leading commercial analysis packages differ in their details and may also differ somewhat in the values calculated and reported for perfusion and function.[24,40] Differences in results are caused, in part, by parameter selection, but also to internal program details such as how sampling is done, how coronary territories are defined, how the comparison to normal is managed, and whether the algorithms for determining defect size and severity were optimized for sensitivity or specificity. The range of patients in the normal database also will have an effect, although probably less than the other factors listed here. Care should be taken in comparing studies done in the same patient at different times, if processing was done with different software.

TECHNOLOGIST CONTRIBUTION

The users of SPECT processing software are most often nuclear medicine technologists but can also be radiologic technologists, physicians, physician assistants, or other personnel. One of the unfortunate consequences of automation is the idea that computer operators need no longer do anything but provide input (acquired data) and receive output (processed images). This is not the case. Operators still need to be knowledgeable as to what the software is doing, how the various processing steps depend on each other, and how accuracy and reproducibility are affected by input image quality, patient anatomy and pathology, and the number and kind of corrections that are applied to the data. There are a number of practical suggestions that can be followed in order to make the best use of processing software. The knowledgeable user will try to accomplish as many of the following as possible:

- Know how camera quality control problems affect image quality.
- Understand the challenges of SPECT: attenuation, limited resolution, motion, and ECG-gating inconsistencies.
- Understand the general methodologies used by various kinds of image-correction software, such as attenuation correction, with its attendant need for stringent quality control. Motion correction should probably not be applied to every acquired data set, and in any case the corrected file should be compared to the uncorrected version, to be sure that image quality has improved.
- Be aware of standards in image handling, such as the filter settings recommended by the software creator, the American College of Cardiology format for image display[41] (VLA: apex to the left, HLA: apex to the top, SA: right ventricle to the left), and image-processing guidelines supplied by professional organizations such as the American Society of Nuclear Cardiology.[42,43]
- Be aware that, for cardiac image processing, the "state of the art" is a moving target and that the term "state of the art" is often loosely used.
- Experiment with different processing parameters, when possible. Change the reconstruction angles, for example, or the apex slice,

and try to understand the effects that follow. Most computer hardware and software are fast enough and sophisticated enough to allow this to be done easily.

- When using software from different vendors, consider the task that is to be done, rather than focusing on the particular tools or user interface the software provides.

- Observe clinical study interpretations, in order to know what the important image features are and how images are used clinically. This enables the person responsible for processing to be aware of all of the available images and to pre-interpret studies before they are sent to the physician who will produce the final report. Problems can often be detected and corrected before images are sent for interpretation.

CONCLUSION

In this chapter, we have discussed the various kinds of image processing that are most commonly performed on myocardial SPECT studies. We began with image filtering, which is necessary to understand in order to appreciate the details of reconstruction. Filtered back-projection and iterative methods were discussed as the two most commonly implemented reconstruction methods for SPECT. Image reorientation was covered as the means for generating the slice data, which are the primary resource for interpreting the SPECT study. The necessary precursors to quantitative processing include not only reoriented images, but also the uniformity matrix and center of rotation, which denote physical conditions under which data acquisition takes place. Quantitation of perfusion can take many forms and can be simple or complex. The general principles were noted, including the concepts of cardiac segmentation, sampling, and comparison of the patient study to a normal database. The potential advantages of appropriately performed quantitation were listed, as were factors that complicate the process. These factors include extracardiac radiotracer accumulation and limitations in image display types and software sophistication, which lead to discrepancies between quantitative and visual results.

ACKNOWLEDGMENT

The author thanks John N. Aarsvold, PhD, for extensive comments and discussion in the preparation of this chapter. Additional thanks are due to Dr. Ernest V. Garcia, PhD, and C. David Cooke, MSEE, for reviewing the manuscript and providing helpful advice.

REFERENCES

1. Faber TL, Folks RD. Computer processing methods for nuclear medicine images. *J Nucl Med Technol*. 1994; 22:145–162.

2. Galt JR, Hise HL, Garcia EV, Nowak DJ. Filtering in frequency space. *J Nucl Med Technol*. 1986;14:152–160.

3. Groch MW, Erwin WD. SPECT in the year 2000: Basic principles. *J Nucl Med Technol*. 2000;28:233–244.

4. Zubal IG, Wisniewski G. Understanding Fourier space and filter selection. *J Nucl Cardiol*. 1997;4:234–243.

5. King MA, Schwinger RB, Penney BC. Variation of the count-dependent Metz filter with imaging system modulation transfer function. *Med Phys*. 1986;13:139–149.

6. King MA, Miller TR. Use of a nonstationary temporal Wiener filter in nuclear medicine. *Eur J Nucl Med*. 1985;10:458–461.

7. DePuey EG, Melancon S, Masini D. Comparison of single-detector and 90°-angled two-detector cameras for technetium-99m-sestamibi cardiac SPECT. *J Nucl Med Technol*. 1995;23:158–166.

8. Bruyant PP. Analytic and iterative reconstruction algorithms in SPECT. *J Nucl Med*. 2002;43:1343–1358.

9. Lalush DS, Wernick MN. Iterative image reconstruction. In: Wernick MN, Aarsvold JN, eds. *Emission Tomography*. San Diego, CA: Elsevier; 2004:443–472.

10. Germano G. Technical aspects of myocardial SPECT imaging. *J Nucl Med*. 2001;42:1499–1507.

11. Shepp LA, Vardi Y. Maximum likelihood estimation for emission tomography. *IEEE Trans Med Imag*. 1982;1:113–121.

12. Hudson HM, Larkin RS. Accelerated image reconstruction using ordered subsets of projection data. *IEEE Trans Med Imag*. 1994;13:601–609.

13. Leong LK, Kruger RL, O'Connor MK. A comparison of the uniformity requirements for SPECT image

reconstruction using FBP and OSEM techniques. *J Nucl Med Technol*. 2001;29:79–83.

14. Zuo-Xiang H, Maublant JC, Cauvin JC, Veyre A. Reorientation of the left ventricular long-axis on myocardial transaxial tomograms by a linear fitting method. *J Nucl Med*. 1991;32:1794–1800.

15. Slomka PJ, Hurwitz GA, Stephenson J, Cradduck T. Automated Alignment and sizing of myocardial stress and rest scans to three-dimensional normal templates using an image registration algorithm. *J Nucl Med*. 1995;36:1115–1122.

16. He Z-X, Maublant JC, Cauvin JC, Veyre A. Reorientation of the left ventricular long-axis on myocardial transaxial tomograms by a linear fitting method. *J Nucl Med*. 1991;32:1794–1800.

17. Germano G, Kavanagh PB, Su H-T, et al. Automatic reorientation of three-dimensional, transaxial myocardial perfusion SPECT images. *J Nucl Med*. 1995;36:1107–1114.

18. Mullick R, Ezquerra NG. Automatic determination of left ventricular orientation from SPECT data. *IEEE Trans Med Imaging*. 1995;14:88–99.

19. Germano G, Kavanagh PB, Berman DS. An automatic approach to the analysis, quantitation and review of perfusion and function from myocardial perfusion SPECT images. *Int J Card Imaging*. 1997;13:337–346.

20. Ficaro EP, Kritzman JN, Corbett JR. Development and clinical validation of normal Tc-99m sestamibi database: Comparison of 3D-MSPECT to CEqual. *J Nucl Med*. 1999;40:125P.

21. Garcia EV, Cooke CD, Van Train KF, et al. Technical aspects of myocardial SPECT imaging with Technetium-99m Sestamibi. *Am J Cardiol*. 1990;66(Suppl):23E–31E.

22. Liu YH, Sinusas AJ, DeMan P, Zaret BL, Wackers FJT. Quantification of SPECT myocardial perfusion images: Methodology and validation of the Yale-CQ method. *J Nucl Cardiol*. 1999;6:190–204.

23. Faber TL, Cooke CD, Folks RD, et al. Left ventricular function and perfusion from gated SPECT perfusion images: An integrated method. *J Nucl Med*. 1999;40:650–659.

24. Santana CA, Folks RD, Rivero A, et al. Comparison of the extent of the myocardial perfusion defect using three different totally automatic programs for the quantification of myocardial perfusion SPECT. *J Nucl Med*. 2004;45:221P.

25. Wackers FJT. Science, art, and artifacts: How important is quantification for the practicing physician interpreting myocardial perfusion studies? *J Nucl Cardiol*. 1994;1:S109–S117.

26. Garcia EV, Cooke CD, Folks RD, et al. Expert system (PERFEX) interpretation of myocardial perfusion tomograms: Validation using 655 prospective patients. *J Nucl Med*. 1999;40:126P.

27. Hamilton D, Riley PJ, Miola UJ, Amro AA. A feed forward neural network for classification of bull's-eye myocardial perfusion images. *Eur J Nucl Med*. 1995;22:108–115.

28. Khorsand A, Haddad M, Graf S, Moertl D, Sochor H, Porenta G. Automated assessment of dipyridamole Tl-201 myocardial SPECT perfusion scintigraphy by case-based reasoning. *J Nucl Med*. 2001;42:189–193.

29. Santana CA, Rivero A, Folks RD, et al. Diagnostic performance of totally automatic vs. manual processing for the quantification of myocardial perfusion SPECT. *J Nucl Cardiol*. 2004;11:S4.

30. Folks RD, Santana CA, Rivero A, Faber TL, Garcia EV. Effect of quantitative parameters on calculation of transient ischemic dilatation index in dual isotope SPECT. *J Nucl Med*. 2004;45:485P.

31. Ficaro EP, Corbett JR. Advances in quantitative perfusion SPECT imaging. *J Nucl Cardiol*. 2004;11:62–70.

32. Burow RD, Pond M, Schafer AW. "Circumferential profiles" a new method for computer analysis of thallium-201 myocardial perfusion images. *J Nucl Med*. 1979;20:771–777.

33. Siegel HJ, Chen DCP, Jacobs L, Melchiore G. The impact of operator decision on quantitative circumferential profile analysis of myocardial thallium-201 scintigraphy: A systematic evaluation. *J Nucl Med Technol*. 1989;17:58–60.

34. Itti E, Klein G, Rosso J, et al. Assessment of myocardial reperfusion after myocardial infarction using automatic 3-dimensional quantification and template matching. *J Nucl Med*. 2004;45:1981–1988.

35. Goris ML, Holtz B, Thirion JP, Similon P. Factors affecting and computation of myocardial perfusion reference images. *Nucl Med Commun*. 1999;20:627–635.

36. Slomka PJ, Nishina H, Berman DS, et al. Automated quantification of myocardial perfusion SPECT using simplified normal limits. *J Nucl Cardiol*. 2005;12:66–77.

37. Gabor FV, Datz FL, Christian PE, Gullberg GT, Morton KA. Computer-assisted diagnosis of cardiac perfusion studies. *J Nucl Med Technol*. 1991;19:238–244.

38. Maddahi J, Van Train KF, Prigent F, et al. Quantitative single photon emission computerized thallium-201 tomography for the evaluation of coronary artery disease: Optimization and prospective validation of a new technique. *J Am Coll Cardiol*. 1989;14:1689–1699.

39. Van Train KF, Areeda J, Garcia EV, et al. Quantitative same-day rest-stress technetium-99m sestamibi SPECT: Definition and validation of stress normal limits and criteria for abnormality. *J Nucl Med*. 1993;34:1494–1502.

40. Nichols KJ, Santana CA, Folks R, et al. Comparison between ECTb and QGS for assessment of left ventricular function from gated myocardial perfusion SPECT. *J Nucl Cardiol.* 2002;9:285–293.

41. Committee on advanced cardiac imaging and technology cocc, American Heart Association, Cardiovascular Imaging Committee ACoC, Board of Directors cc, Society of Nuclear Medicine. Standardization of cardiac tomographic imaging. *J Nucl Med.* 1992;33:1434–1435.

42. Port SC, ed. Imaging guidelines for nuclear cardiology procedures, Part 2. *J Nucl Cardiol.* 1999;6:G49–G84.

43. DePuey EG, Garcia EV, eds. Updated imaging guidelines for nuclear cardiology procedures, Part 1. *J Nucl Cardiol.* 2001;8:G5–G62.

CHAPTER 11

Technical Considerations in Quantifying Myocardial Perfusion and Function

Edward P. Ficaro

James R. Corbett

INTRODUCTION

Myocardial perfusion imaging (MPI) is one of the primary noninvasive imaging modalities for the assessment of cardiac heart disease (CHD). For the past 20 years, perfusion imaging has been accomplished primarily with single-photon emission computed tomography (SPECT), but recently perfusion imaging with positron emission tomography (PET) has seen increased clinical utilization. A major factor in the widespread use of MPI for the detection of coronary disease is the availability of automated, highly accurate algorithms and review methods for quantifying myocardial perfusion and function. Automated, computer algorithms provide highly reproducible estimates of cardiac parameters that can be used to assess the progression of and/or the response to the medical management of disease. Limits of normalcy or abnormality thresholds are easily defined using quantitative methods. Automated methods are generally more suitable than visual interpretations for

determining abnormal thresholds because their estimates have less variability in the calculated mean values, resulting in better-defined thresholds between normal and abnormal. Lastly, automated quantitative algorithms are well suited to replace tedious repetitive manual calculations or measurements on large amounts of image data, effectively reducing unwieldy analyses to a few key parameters that can be calculated almost instantaneously and used in the final diagnostic interpretations of the patient studies. For example, consider a cine review of the left ventricular (LV) volume throughout the cardiac cycle, where the physician is visually estimating the change in volume between end diastole (ED) and end systole (ES) to provide an estimate of left ventricular ejection fraction (LVEF). Today, algorithms are widely available to find the endocardial surface of the left ventricle throughout the cardiac cycle, determine the point of ED and ES, and output the LVEF. Similar automated analysis can be achieved for regional wall motion, wall thickening, and regional myocardial tissue classification (i.e., normal, ischemic, and scar). By correlating these quantitative cardiac parameters, the physician is better able to assess the extent of cardiac disease and also identify and eliminate or compensate for artifacts that are common in all imaging modalities.

Today, quantification of both LV perfusion and function is routinely performed with gated myocardial perfusion tomographic imaging.[1] While there are several automated software packages available[2-8] for the quantification and review of myocardial perfusion images, there are technical variables that can confound the algorithms in these packages resulting in suboptimal or erroneous estimates. The objective of this chapter is to review the factors that are important for the accurate quantification of both myocardial perfusion and LV systolic function.

MYOCARDIAL PERFUSION

The regional intensity of the tracer uptake in the heart provides an index of myocardial blood flow. The parameters of interest from emission computed tomographic (ECT) perfusion images, i.e., SPECT or PET, are

- identification of regional perfusion defects;
- quantification of the extent and severity of perfusion defects; and
- classification of regional perfusion defects as ischemic or scar.

Regional perfusion defects are determined by comparing the individual patient's data to a known normal distribution (normals database) generated from SPECT studies acquired from low-likelihood normal volunteers and patients. In order to determine such normal distributions and make clinical comparisons therefrom, a standardized result template that minimizes the effects of individual variations in subject/patient cardiac anatomy and intrathoracic cardiac orientation is required. The circumferential profile (CP) reduces a 2D image into a line profile.[9,10] In constructing a CP, the algorithm samples the myocardial tracer intensity profile along a ray emanating from the center of a selected SA slice. At predefined steps (angular increments) circling clockwise about the left ventricle, myocardial intensity profiles are recorded. From the myocardial intensity profiles along each ray, the max myocardial intensity is recorded as a function of angle reducing the perfusion pattern in each 2D short-axis image to a "circumferential" line profile.

To handle the 3D volumetric images of the heart that both SPECT and PET provide, the polar map template is used to sample the 3D volume of the left ventricle.[11] In constructing a polar map, CPs are constructed for each slice in the 3D volume from the LV apex to the base. Each CP is mapped onto a polar map in concentric rings of increasing diameter, with the apex at the center and the most basal ring having the greatest diameter. The center of the polar map representing the apex is generally sampled from long-axis images to minimize the partial volume effect that occurs when SA images are sampled. To account for differences in the axial dimension of the heart between patients, the axial sampling length (slice thickness or polar map ring width) is normalized so that each patient's polar map consists of the same number of sampling points. With this approach, the polar map is the standard template for representing the 3D volume of the left ventricle. By effectively eliminating the anatomical variations of the left ventricle, the polar map provides the capability for interstudy comparisons and the construction of normal databases. Various polar map normalization methods (e.g., each ring separately to its peak intensity and entire map to peak intensity in the heart) have been proposed and validated.

A comparison of the patient's polar map distribution to a normal distribution provides the extent of the perfusion abnormality in percent of the LV volume affected.[12,13] Defect severity is generally reported as the mean number of standard deviations that the defect area is below the normal mean. To associate defects with specific coronary territories, a regional overlay template representing the three vascular territories, left anterior descending (LAD), left circumflex (LCx), and right coronary artery (RCA), is used. Receiver operating curve (ROC) analyses have defined defect extent thresholds of 12% or greater for the LAD and LCx and 8% or greater for the RCA as indicative of abnormal myocardial perfusion/probable coronary stenoses in those vascular territories.[14]

In addition to tabulated defect extent values, various polar map displays are available to aid in the interpretation of the tomographic slices.[15] The "blackout" polar map sets those sectors in the polar map that are abnormal (e.g., $>2.5\sigma$ below the normal mean) to the color black, while maintaining the intensities/colors of normal sectors. The blackout map provides a visual representation of defect locations and sizes. A second map, defect severity or z-score map, maps the defect abnormalities in units of standard deviations below the normal mean. Both of these maps in combination with the vascular overlay template provide extent and severity values in each vascular territory.

To quantify defect "reversibility," a reversibility map is calculated by normalizing the rest map to the stress map based on the ratio of intensities at the location within the map of peak stress intensity.[16] The reversibility map is then the difference from subtracting the stress map from the normalized rest map. Similar to normal perfusion databases, normal reversibility databases are constructed to define the thresholds differentiating normal, ischemia, and scar. Ischemic sectors in the map are defined as those defect sectors in the stress map whose corresponding reversibility value is greater than the ischemic threshold (e.g., mean $+ 2.5\sigma$). The fraction of the defect that is ischemic is the number of ischemic sectors divided by the total number of sectors in the defect (ischemic fraction). The fraction of the defect that is fixed or scar is equal to the number of fixed sectors divided by the total number of sectors in the defect (1 – the ischemic fraction). A graphic display of this data can be seen incorporated with the blackout map where "scar" sectors are coded black and "ischemic" sectors are coded white (or cross-hatched), while normal sectors maintain the reconstructed intensities of the sampled 3D LV volume.

Several commercial software packages are available to automatically resample the LV image volume to a polar map[2,4,6] or a series of circumferential line profiles (CPs)[7] that can be compared to a normal distribution for the identification of perfusion abnormalities. Several technical factors can influence the accuracy of the resampling process that should be checked prior to reporting the results of the quantification. The factors to be discussed are (1) volume reorientation where the heart volume is reoriented to the long axis of the LV, (2) the center and axial limits used to construct the CPs, (3) the patients used to define the normal database distribution, (4) the thresholds for defining abnormal, and (5) the impact of advanced reconstruction algorithms on perfusion quantification.

Volume Reorientation

The cardiac images reconstructed from the acquired raw projection images, referred to as transverse images, are oriented orthogonal to the long axis of the body and generally include the entire volume of the heart. For display and cardiac review, the transverse reconstructed image volumes are reoriented orthogonal to the long axis of the left ventricle (short-axis images (SA)) and parallel to the long axis of the left ventricle (horizontal long-axis (HLA) and vertical long-axis (VLA) images). The reorientation includes angular rotations about the x- and y-axis. Because stress and rest volumes are viewed in comparative displays, it is important that the reorientation angles for the stress and rest image volumes be consistent. This is best achieved in an environment where the stress and rest images are reoriented side by side at the same time. There are algorithms available for automatically reorienting the heart along the long axis,[17,18] but these automatically reoriented images should be visually verified for the accuracy of the estimated reslice angles. Because patients may not be positioned in exactly the same way for both stress and rest imaging, the reslice angles for the stress and rest images may vary slightly. If the patient is positioned differently for stress and rest imaging and the same reslice angles are used for

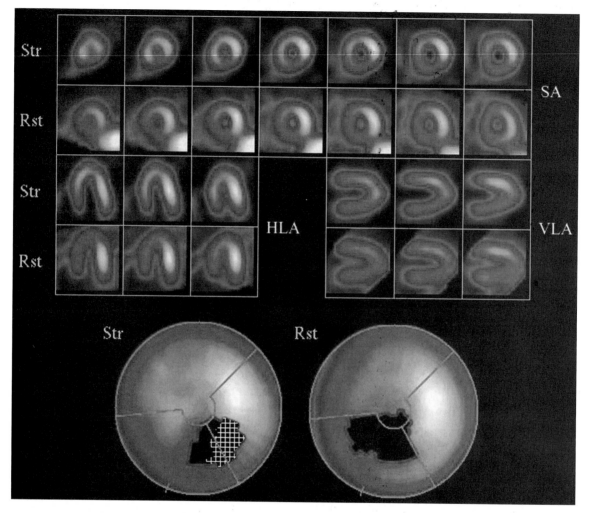

Figure 11-1.   Effect of misalignment between stress and rest studies. There is approximately a 10-degree tilt (counterclockwise) in the HLA stress images compared to the rest images. As a result, the defect in the polar map for the stress study is shifted from the inferoseptal to the inferolateral location. This shift changes the classification of the defect from fixed to partially reversible. SA, short axis; HLA, horizontal long axis; VLA, vertical long axis.

both image sets or the reslice angles are inaccurately chosen differently when the patient is positioned exactly the same way for both stress and rest studies, the position and shape of defects may not match optimally on polar map analysis. Slight inaccuracies in the reorientation angles between stress and rest images can significantly change the

location and classification of identified defects (ischemic vs. scar) (Figure 11-1).

Quantitative estimates of perfusion defect size and type are also affected by reorientation errors. This is seen in Figure 11-2, where stress and rest images were resliced with up to 10-degree differences in the reslice angles and compared to

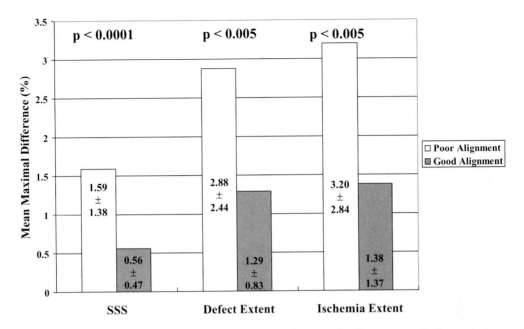

Figure 11-2. The effect that misalignment between stress and rest studies has on quantitative perfusion estimates. The "poor alignment" consists of studies where the angular differences in the reorientation angles differ by 5 to 10 degrees, compared to the "good alignment" where the angles are defined in a paired setting. With poor alignment, significant increases in variability for all three parameters are seen. SSS, summed stress score.

the stress and rest images where the reorientation angles were matched. In a clinical study at the University of Michigan, where this was analyzed quantitatively,[19] the summed stress scores (SSS), stress defect extent, and ischemic extent were all significantly affected, showing increases in error and variability when reorientation angles were not properly chosen.

Limits for Constructing Polar Maps

The LV center and the axial limits (base and apex) are important parameters either in constructing a series of CPs (e.g., basal, mid, distal, and apex) for display or for generating a series of CPs for each SA image of a study to be incorporated into a polar map. When the center position is incorrect, defects located near the offset center point will be larger than their actual size, while defects that are located away from the center point will be underestimated in size. This is a product of the an-

gular sampling that is used to construct the CPs. The base and apex provide the limits of the LV that will be sampled. The basal position should be selected to be consistent with the limit used to construct the normals databases. Typical basal limit locations are (1) beginning of the membranous septum, (2) mid membranous septum, and (3) the last near-complete SA slice for the anterior-lateral wall when progressing from apex toward the base. Figure 11-3 shows the effect of correct center and basal limits (Figure 11-3A), incorrect centering (Figure 11-3B), and incorrect basal limits (Figure 11-3C) used to construct polar maps. This patient has a nearly perfectly matched fixed defect comprising approximately 30% of the LV when the proper limits are used for the quantification. When the center position (middle) is offset toward the defect in the stress study (Figure 11-3B), the defect size increases from 31% to 37%, and the part of the defect (9%) denoted by cross-hatching is considered reversible or ischemic. In

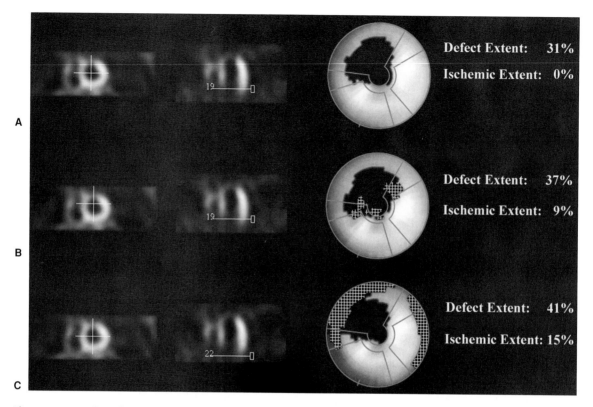

Figure 11-3.   The effect of incorrect limits used to create polar maps for comparison to a normals database. The correct limits are used in row (**A**), and the stress perfusion blackout map is displayed with its corresponding statistics. Incorrect centering was introduced in row (**B**), where the center is offset toward the anterior wall creating a larger defect that is partially reversible (denoted by cross-hatching in blackout polar map). In row (**C**), the basal position is extended too far toward the left atrium, creating artifactual defects in the basal anteroseptal and lateral walls and incorrectly increasing the overall defect size and reversibility fraction.

Figure 11-3C, where the basal limit is extended toward the left atrium by three slices too far (approximately 2 cm), the defect incorrectly extends to the basal bands of the anteroseptal and lateral walls, caused by a mismatch of limits with the appropriate normals database. The overall defect size increases from 31% to 41%, and the ischemic portion increases from 0% to 15%. These figures clearly demonstrate the necessity for proper quality control of the processing and quantification parameters critical to maintain accurate quantitative estimates of defect extent, especially important when assessments for the extent and progression of disease are required.

Database Construction and Thresholds

In the examples presented in Figure 11-3, the perfusion abnormalities are quantified by comparing the patient's polar map to a normal distribution defined by a database of subjects with normal cardiac perfusion. The normal distribution is defined by constructing a normal database from volunteers or patients with low pretest likelihood ($\leq$5%) for coronary heart disease.[20] By imaging normal patients with a low likelihood for CHD, mean and variance limits for normal perfusion in polar map format can be defined. In the absence of an algorithm to correct for soft-tissue attenuation, the normal distribution will be dependent on body habitus. This effect is most commonly seen comparing databases from men and women,[12] where the normal male database distribution in the inferior wall is 10% to 15% lower than that seen in the normal female distribution because of more prominent diaphragmatic attenuation in males. Similarly, the anterior wall is reduced in intensity for women compared to men because of breast attenuation. Similar differences can be seen between ethnic populations that differ significantly in average body mass index. As a result, it is important to consider the physical characteristics of the subjects that were used to construct the database in comparison to the general clinical patient population and individual patient being studied. Significant differences between the body habitus characteristics of patients and the subjects used to construct normal databases can result in incorrect quantification of defect size and severity. Figure 11-4 illustrates the effects on normalcy when female patients with varying breast size are compared with (1) a database of female patients with relatively small breasts (B-cup or smaller) and (2) a database of female patients with varying breast sizes (A to D-cup).

Varying the abnormality threshold can offset differences between clinical patient populations and database populations. The abnormality threshold is defined as a preset number of standard deviations (σ) below the mean, typically 2.0σ or 2.5σ. Some quantitative software packages permit regionally varying thresholds based on ROC analyses to account for large and small variances in database populations.[21–23] It is also important to understand the relationship between abnormality thresholds and diagnostic accuracy for the detection of coronary heart disease. Increasing the number of standard deviations (e.g., from 2.5σ down to 3.0σ) decreases the absolute abnormality threshold, resulting in decreased sensitivity and increased specificity. Likewise, decreasing the number of standard deviations (e.g., 2.5σ down to 2.0σ) increases the absolute threshold, resulting in increased sensitivity and decreased specificity.

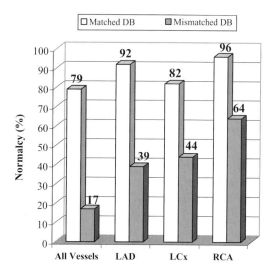

Figure 11-4. Effect on normalcy rates for a low-likelihood female patient population compared to a database from subjects with differing body habitus, i.e., breast size (mismatched DB) and subjects with similar body habitus (matched DB). The patient population had varying breast sizes consistent with the "matched" normals database. The "mismatched" database consisted only of females with small breasts. Use of the mismatched database resulted in significantly lower normalcy rates, which were most apparent in the LAD and LCx territories, which are most affected by breast soft-tissue attenuation. LAD, left anterior descending artery; LCx, left circumflex artery; RCA, right coronary artery.

Under most situations, there is a trade-off in sensitivity and specificity when thresholds are adjusted.

Advanced Reconstruction Algorithms

Since the introduction of SPECT imaging, image reconstruction using the filtered backprojection (FBP) algorithm has been the standard. While iterative reconstruction algorithms were described and utilized in the areas of research since the early 1980s, these algorithms were not used routinely in clinical practice as a result of increased computation time and resources (i.e., memory) required compared to FBP. However, while FBP is significantly faster than iterative methods, it does not model the counting statistics and introduces significant bias and noise in reconstructed images, especially low-count studies. Iterative algorithms have the capability of modeling several factors that routinely degrade the information content of the image, including photon attenuation (absorption and scatter), collimator response, and boundary information. The capability of these algorithms to model photon attenuation combined with the increased computational speed of modern desktop workstations has resulted in the clinical utilization of iterative statistical algorithms in recent years.

For perfusion SPECT imaging, iterative algorithms, especially those that model and correct

for photon attenuation, significantly improve the accuracy of reconstructed tracer distributions in the myocardium. Several studies have shown improved homogeneity in normal myocardium compared to FBP[24,25] and resultant increased accuracy for the detection of CHD.[24,26] Attenuation-corrected (AC) databases have been shown to be equivalent between genders, which is not true for databases generated from uncorrected FBP studies.[24,25] As a result, FBP and iterative AC databases cannot be interchanged; clinical patient studies must be matched and analyzed with normals databases generated with normals data that were similarly processed and reconstructed. Recent studies also suggest that databases generated with data processed with iterative algorithms, which do not account for photon attenuation but do account for collimator response and photon scatter, are significantly different from databases generated from standard FBP-reconstructed normal studies (Figure 11-5). This is an area of ongoing investigation.

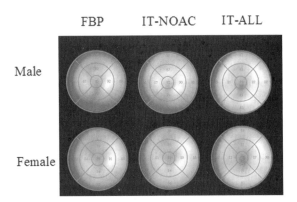

Figure 11-5. Comparison of male and female normals database distributions for different reconstruction algorithms. The filtered backprojection (FBP) databases are significantly different for males and females and are also significantly different from distributions derived from iterative algorithms. The middle column databases (IT-NOAC) generated using an iterative algorithm that modeled scatter and collimator response but not photon absorption are different than FBP databases. The maps for IT-ALL were reconstructed with an iterative algorithm that corrected for photon absorption as well as scatter and collimator response. These distributions are statistically equivalent in males and females. The differences between databases generated using different reconstruction algorithms demonstrate the importance of matching clinical patient data and the appropriate normals database similarly processed. (See color insert.)

MYOCARDIAL FUNCTION

The following parameters are routinely estimated by most quantitative software packages from gated myocardial perfusion SPECT studies:

- LV volumes throughout the cardiac cycle
- LVEF
- Regional LV wall motion
- Regional LV wall thickening
- Transient ischemic dilation (TID)

The key component in the quantitative analysis of gated perfusion SPECT images is finding the endocardial and epicardial surfaces of the left ventricle. After the surfaces have been estimated for each interval in the gating cycle, the chamber volumes subtended by the endocardial surface are determined. From the estimated volumes, the peak volume is designated as the end-diastolic volume (EDv) while the smallest volume is designated the end-systolic volume (ESv). Knowing the EDv and ESv values, the LVEF is defined as 100%*

(EDv − ESv)/EDv. Many algorithms have been proposed for estimating LV systolic function, but four commercially available programs bear mentioning: QGS from Cedars-Sinai, Emory Cardiac Toolbox (ECTb) from Emory University, Corridor4DM (4DM) from the University of Michigan, and Wackers-Liu CQ (WLCQ) from Yale University. Each of these programs uses sophisticated algorithms for automatic quantification of LV function. While there are many similarities in the modeling algorithms used by these programs, there are key differences, which are outlined in Table 11-1. The surface locator is the engine that estimates the endocardial and epicardial surfaces. For each of the algorithms the mid-myocardial surface is determined by finding the maximum intensity along line profiles through the LV myocardium. For areas where there are severe perfusion defect intensities, each of the software programs utilizes different multidimensional interpolators to fill in surface locations poorly defined by the severely reduced and statistically noisy image data. The abilities of these algorithms to accurately render the LV wall in the presence of large perfusion defects and high levels of extracardiac activity vary. This should be understood by the operator.

The primary areas where these software programs differ are in modeling wall thickening from ED to ES and the motion of the mitral valve plane that defines the basal extent of the LV. For wall thickening, 4DM and QGS use geometric (Gaussian) models and empirically correct for resolution effects. The geometric fitting that is employed by these algorithms is quite robust, but they are more susceptible to issues that affect resolution (e.g., image filtering and noise). The ECTb and WLCQ programs are count-based algorithms, where thickening through the cardiac cycle is derived from the partial volume effect or the Fourier size–intensity relationship.[27,28] This relationship is based on the fact that the resolution of SPECT imaging as measured by the full-width-at-half-maximum (FWHM) is greater than the myocardial wall thickness. As a result, the intensity of the LV wall counts will vary linearly, with wall thickness generally increasing as the wall thickens during systole, as the partial volume effect is decreased and count recovery is increased, and then decreasing during diastole as the wall thins with increasing partial volume effect. Of course should the LV wall thin during systole in areas of ischemia or ischemic injury, the partial volume effect will increase and the magnitude of count recovery will paradoxically decrease from ED to ES. While the count-based model is less affected by changes in image resolution compared to geometric models, these algorithms are more affected by gating problems because of arrhythmias, which can create intensity artifacts through the cardiac cycle.[29] The modeling of the location of the mitral valve plane location throughout the cardiac cycle is also a source of differences between the software programs. While the absolute valve plane location has an affect on LV volumes for each specific temporal phase of the cardiac cycle, the displacement of valve plane location between ED and ES affects EF estimates. Algorithms that constrain the valve plane to a single slice or less will tend to artifactually lower the EF estimates, especially for normal hearts; this will be discussed in more detail later in this section.

Despite the many challenges faced by these algorithms, there have been several studies demonstrating good-to-excellent correlation of the estimated systolic function estimates with those from first-pass radionuclide angiography,[30–32] equilibrium radionuclide angiography,[33–35] contrast ventriculography,[3,36,37] echocardiography,[33,36,38–40] and cardiac magnetic resonance.[2,41–45] In contrast to each of the other imaging modalities, these algorithms have the advantages of being fully automated, producing nearly instantaneous results, with interstudy variability of five to six ejection fraction units or less.[25,46,47] Quantification of LV function has also been shown to be accurate for Tl-201, I-123, and a few PET tracers.[38,39,48–50] However, while the functional estimates from each of the software programs correlate well with each other,[42,44,45,51–53] there are significant differences that requires caution when monitoring serial assessments of LV function with different quantitative programs.

Table 11-1

Key Algorithmic Differences Between the Four Commercial Algorithms for Quantifying Left Ventricular Function from Myocardial Perfusion SPECT Images

Software	Surface Locator	Surface Interpolator for Perfusion Defects	Wall Thickening	Valve Plane Estimator
4DM	• Gaussian fit to intensity line profile through myocardial wall • Peak location of fit is adjusted to the location of peak activity • Mid-myocardial surface is assigned to peak location	• Spline interpolators coupled between three dimensions and time (for gated studies)	• Initial wall thickness estimated from Gaussian fit • Average wall thickness at ED is scaled to 10 mm, and mass is estimated • Remaining frames are scaled to conserve mass	• 50% threshold of heart activity to identify location of valve plane at each temporal frame • Movement is smoothed with a periodic spline interpolator • Displacement of valve plane between ED and ES is constrained to be between 5 and 20 mm
QGS	• Asymmetric Gaussian fit to intensity line profile through myocardial wall • Maxima represents peak location • Mid-myocardial surface is assigned to peak location	• Nearest neighbor interpolation (4 × 4 neighborhood)	• Initial wall thickness estimates from Gaussian fit • Wall thickness estimates are scaled by empirical resolution correction factor derived from phantom SPECT data • Thickness estimates are refined to conserve mass throughout the cardiac cycle	• 25% threshold of heart activity to identify location of valve plane at each temporal frame • The valve plane is further constrained to having an area above 10% of the mid-myocardial surface area
ECTb	• Maximum activity determined from intensity line profile through myocardial wall • Mid-myocardial surface is assigned to location of maximum activity	• In-plane interpolation (7 × 7 median filter)	• Frame with maximum volume subtended by mid-myocardial surface is ED frame • Wall thickness for ED frame is set to a uniform 10 mm • Wall thickening through cardiac cycle is computed from linearity of count density and myocardial thickness (partial volume)	• Location is determined at each interval using a combination of 30% and 65% thresholds
WL CQ	• Maximum activity determined from intensity line profile through myocardial wall • Mid-myocardial surface is assigned to location of maximum activity	• Median location from surrounding surfaces	• A myocardial thickness of 12 mm is assigned to the frame where the median count density occurs in the cardiac cycle • Wall thickening throughout the cardiac cycle is based on the linearity of count density and myocardial thickness (partial volume)	• Location of last basal slice containing septum + 10 mm offset toward atrium

With these programs, quantification is not limited to global systolic function. From the estimated LV endocardial surfaces at ED and ES, regional wall motion can be estimated from the radial surface displacement between ED and ES. Regional wall motion maps can be displayed in 2D polar map format or overlaid on 3D displays of the LV surfaces. Regional wall motion can be visually assessed by viewing the 2D image slices with or without the surface overlays in cine mode or by viewing the 3D volume in cine mode. Regional wall thickening is estimated from either the geometric difference, i.e., radial separation between the endocardial and epicardial LV wall surfaces at ES compared to ED, or the relative difference in the perfusion count intensities between ES and ED using the Fourier size–intensity relationship. Quantitative evaluations of regional wall motion and thickening provide useful assessments of regional wall function and are useful for assessments of regional wall viability. This information, when used in parallel with the perfusion data, can aid in identifying attenuation artifacts, i.e., fixed perfusion defects with normal wall motion and thickening. Lastly, TID is the ratio of the ungated endocardial volume at stress to the volume at rest. This parameter has been found to provide significant prognostic information in patients with known or suspected coronary heart disease.

There are several technical factors that affect the accuracy of commercial algorithms for the quantification of LV systolic function. The factors to be discussed here will be limited to (1) resolution issues, (2) filtering and pixel sizes, (3) valve plane position, and (4) miscellaneous variables related to temporal sampling and image noise.

Resolution Issues

The mean LV wall thickness in normal hearts is approximately 9 to 10 mm at ED and 16 to 18 mm at ES.[54–56] Accurate spatial sampling of the myocardial thickness requires, according to the sampling theorem, at worst, 5-mm resolution elements at ED, to provide a minimum of two sample points over the 10-mm LV wall thickness. However, the typical reconstructed resolution for gated cardiac SPECT images is between 12 and 15 mm FWHM for studies acquired with adequate count densities and reconstructed with optimal low-pass filters. This is an insufficient reconstructed resolution to accurately determine the true endocardial and epicardial borders of the LV myocardium. As a result, each of the commercially available surface detection algorithms compensates these resolution effects by either scaling the wall thickness to the normal mean value at ED (e.g., 10 mm) or applying an empirical correction factor based on the estimated reconstructed resolution of the image volume. Both approaches are approximations that do not account for regional differences in thickening or thinning of the myocardium that accompany many cardiac disease processes. Fortunately, because ejection fraction is a ratio of EDv and ESv, errors in wall thickness cancel, resulting in very accurate EF values. This fact is illustrated in Figure 11-6. In the top row, the endo- and epicardial surfaces of the left ventricle were determined from an edge detection operator (i.e., gradient or Laplacian filter). The estimated surfaces for the ED frame using a gradient operator are very close to the surfaces that would be drawn manually from a visual analysis. The problem is that the mean myocardial surface separation using this approach is 22 mm, more than twice the expected thickness for a normal heart. In the bottom row, the wall thickness has been scaled at the ED frame to a mean thickness of 10 mm. A comparison of the LVEF estimates for each method shows that the LVEF values are not significantly affected (20% vs. 21%), but the absolute LV volumes at ED and ES are very different (ED: 367 vs. 505 mL, ES: 296 vs. 401 mL). Gated magnetic resonance images for this same patient showed an ED volume of 480 mL more consistent with the volumes after scaling the LV wall thickness at ED to 10 mm. The overestimation in ED volume from the gated SPECT study is likely because of an underestimation of the mean LV wall thickness.

Because of the limited spatial resolution of gated cardiac SPECT imaging, the user should be aware of the model used for estimating wall

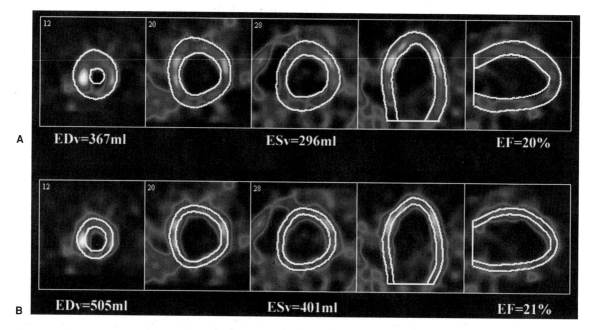

Figure 11-6. Resolution effects on wall thickness estimates. The surfaces in row (**A**) are determined from an edge detection gradient operator and reflect the poor resolution of SPECT images, resulting in an average myocardial wall thickness of 22 mm for the end-diastolic frame. In row (**B**), the wall-thickness estimates are scaled to provide a mean myocardial thickness of 10 mm. Scaling the surface locations significantly affects the end-diastolic volume (EDv) and end-systolic volume (ESv), but the ejection fraction (EF) is essentially unaffected as the errors in EDv and ESv cancel. (See color insert.)

thickening by the quantitative software package they are using. All of the current methods make assumptions that will not be strictly accurate for patients' hearts that deviate significantly from the typical normal myocardial thickness (e.g., hypertrophic cardiomyopathy or dilated cardiomyopathy resulting from myocardial infarcts). For patients who have regional or global hypertrophy or thinning, the user should be aware that the cardiac volumes and LVEF can be erroneous, depending on the size of the heart and the degree of hypertrophy or thinning.

The Small Heart, Filtering, and Voxel Size

Small hearts present a particularly difficult challenge relating to absolute accuracy and inter-study reproducibility of measurements from gated SPECT assessments of LV function. Because of the small LV volumes commonly seen in the studies of many patients with high LVEFs (>75%) and the relatively low spatial resolution of SPECT imaging discussed above, a change of only a few voxels within the endocardial surface, especially at ES, can have a significant impact on the calculated LVEF. For this reason, in the higher normal range, there have been seen, with all the available gated SPECT software quantification programs, increased variances in the calculated LVEF compared with gold-standard measures from other imaging modalities, e.g., contrast ventriculography and planar gated blood pool imaging. Although efforts are being made to improve on the accuracy and reproducibility of these measurements in the higher ranges of ejection fractions, it may not be realistic to expect much improvement with current imaging technology unless spatial resolution is significantly improved. However, it should be kept in mind that an ejection fraction of 75% or 85% or even 90% has no impact on patient prognosis. In the high normal range, the ejection fraction alone suggests an excellent outcome.

Of primary importance with gated SPECT MPI is the selection of the reconstructed voxel dimension and the post-reconstruction filter. Both of these parameters will affect the resolution of the LV in the obliquely reformatted short-axis images that are the typical input image format to the quantitative programs. The effects of voxel size and filter cutoff on determining LVEF from perfusion SPECT is well documented.[57–61] The effect of matrix size is illustrated by the data in Figure 11-7. In this figure, 14 patients who underwent both contrast ventriculography (CVG) and myocardial perfusion SPECT imaging were considered. The initial SPECT images were reconstructed with a voxel dimension of 6.6 mm, and the LVEF values were compared to those from CVG studies. There were significant differences (mean difference 14%) between LVEF values. These differences were most noticeable when the EDv was less than 100 mL and or the ESv was less then 40 mL. The differences in LV volumes were significantly reduced by reconstructing the SPECT images at the smaller voxel size of 4.8 mm. The smaller voxel dimensions decreased the mean difference between CVG and SPECT from 14% to 6%. However, there were still significant differences in EF for the smallest hearts; this is inherent to the relatively low spatial resolution of SPECT images and cannot be completely offset by decreasing the reconstructed voxel size.

Mitral Valve Plane Positioning

The location of the mitral valve plane determines the axial extent of the left ventricle. The mitral valve plane descends toward the apex as the LV shortens during ventricular systolic contraction and then returns to its starting position as the ventricle expands during diastole. Data from a number of sources and imaging modalities support this movement of the valve plane; in the normal human heart, the systolic descent of the mitral valve planes averages 8 to 12 mm from ED to systoles.[54,62–64] For a SPECT imaging, this distance represents one to two slices of plane motion when a slice thickness of 6 mm is reconstructed. Algorithms that constrain the motion of the mitral valve plane will tend to artifactually decrease the ejection fractions for healthier hearts, since the healthy, normal heart contracts more, both radially and axially, than is typical for hearts with impaired ventricular function. To illustrate the effects of modeling valve plane motion, a population of 120 patients who had both contrast ventriculography and myocardial perfusion SPECT imaging was considered. The SPECT studies were processed with 4DM where the valve plane was permitted to move between 5 and 20 mm of motion. For this model, the correlation between CVG and MPI was $r = 0.93$, with a root-mean-square error (RMSE) of 4.9 ± 4.0. The studies were reprocessed with the valve plane motion constrained to 6 mm or less. With this constraint applied, the correlation dropped slightly to 0.91 with an RMSE of 6.8 ± 5.1. In Figure 11-8, a Bland–Altman[65] plot of the difference in EF estimates from the two-valve plane models is plotted as a function of the CVG EF estimate. As seen in these data, the LVEF differences become progressively more negative with increasing ejection fraction. For a CVG EF of 50%, the mean underestimation of the LVEF would be approximately five units when valve plane motion is constrained. This would increase to seven units at an EF of 80% and decrease to three units at an EF of 20%. Differences in the handling of the valve plane can be a source of discrepancy between quantitative algorithms (e.g., QGS and 4DM)[66] and between imaging modalities or software that assume a fixed valve plane location (e.g., first pass and equilibrium radionuclide angiography). It is important for the user to understand this behavior when performing quality control on serial EF values, obtained using different algorithms on image data from the same or differing imaging modalities.

180

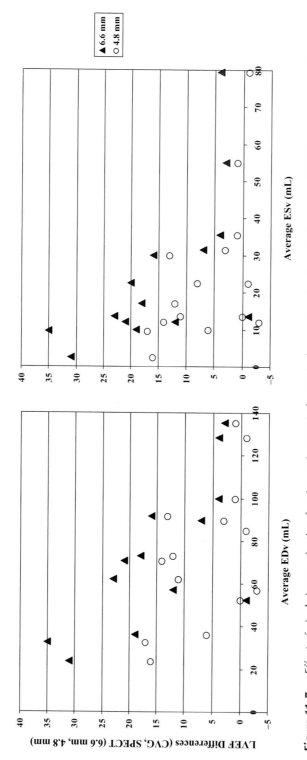

Figure 11-7. Effect of pixel size on ejection fraction estimates. Left ventricular ejection fractions derived from SPECT images with different pixel sizes (6.6 and 4.8 mm) are compared to values from contrast ventriculography (CVG). The difference between the SPECT and CVG estimates are plotted as a function of average EDv (**A**) and ESv (**B**). The differences in LVEF between SPECT and CVG become significantly large for EDV < 100 mL and ESv < 40 mL, and increase dramatically for smaller volumes. The LVEF differences are somewhat minimized by reconstructing with a smaller pixel size (4.8 vs. 6.6 mm).

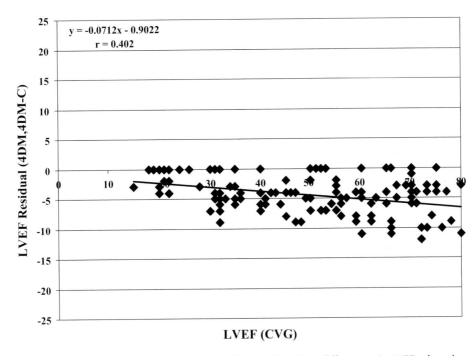

Figure 11-8. Effect of valve plane modeling. Bland–Altman plot of the differences in LVEF when the valve plane motion is constrained. The baseline LVEF models the valve plane motion between 5 and 20 mm. The constrained model reduces the range between ED and ES to be less than 6 mm of motion. The effect is a reduction in LVEF where the difference increases with increasing LVEF.

TID values are obtained from ungated images. These ungated images may be obtained from ungated imaging or time compression of gated studies. Since this is a measurement from ungated images, the consistency of valve plane localization on stress and rest or redistribution images is critical for accurate TID measurements. Should the valve plane be placed too far toward the apex on the rest images or too far back on the stress images, abnormal TID values may be obtained with unwarranted effects on estimations of patient prognosis.

Miscellaneous Factors

Several other factors play a role in an algorithm's accuracy in estimating systolic function. Eight or 16 time frames (temporal samples) are typically acquired over the cardiac cycle (R-R′ interval). The increased temporal sampling of 16-frame studies provides a more accurate estimate of the ESv. As a result, the LVEF values from studies with only eight frames will, on average, be approximately four to five EF units lower than the same study acquired with 16 frames.[5,67,68] It has been shown that Fourier filtering of the LV volume curve can reduce the difference between 8 and 16 frame studies,[69] and this option has been incorporated into several software packages.

Low-count, noisy images are problematic both qualitatively and quantitatively. Low-count studies suffer from low resolution because either they require more filtering or the images are noisy, resulting in lumpy myocardial intensity distributions that resemble diffuse speckled abnormalities. Low-resolution images, especially for small hearts, will often create artifactually high LVEF estimates, rarely low LVEF estimates.[58,59] Fluctuations in the count densities negatively impact the geometric fitting routines and likewise the thickening models based on count densities. To minimize the occurrence of images with suboptimal count density, acquisition and processing protocols should be created, which are consistent with the acquisition and processing parameters outlined in the ASNC imaging guidelines[70] for myocardial perfusion SPECT/PET tomography.

Iterative algorithms offer improved image resolution and decreased noise and, when attenuation correction is included, provide a more accurate intensity distribution. For most instances, functional estimates derived from images reconstructed with iterative algorithms will be consistent with estimates derived from images reconstructed from FBP. However, because the algorithms were designed and validated with FBP images, many of the thresholds and models were optimized for the distributions and resolutions expected from conventional FBP. Similar differences can be seen with some algorithms when PET images, with inherently better resolution and image statistics compared to SPECT images, are processed with a software algorithm that were designed for SPECT images. Once again, the user should be aware of the capabilities and validation of the algorithms prior to changing acquisition and/or processing protocols from the protocol recommended for the software.

CONCLUSION

SPECT and PET MPI are widely accepted noninvasive imaging modalities for the identification and assessment of coronary heart disease. The availability of highly automated and accurate quantitative software algorithms provide integrated processing and review environments, where clinical decisions regarding both myocardial perfusion and function can be made. It is important for the processing technologist and the reviewing physician to be aware of the technical issues that can con-

found the quantitative algorithms used in these software packages, which can result in suboptimal and sometimes erroneous parametric estimates. An understanding of the strengths and weaknesses of the quantitative software being used will provide the user a secondary objective reader, which can help increase diagnostic accuracy and reduce both intra- and interobserver (reader) variability in these important assessments of myocardial perfusion and function.

REFERENCES

1. Faber TL, Akers MS, Peshock RM, Corbett JR. Three-dimensional motion and perfusion quantification in gated single-photon emission computed tomograms. *J Nucl Med*. 1991;32(12):2311–2317.
2. Faber TL, Cooke CD, Folks RD, et al. Left ventricular function and perfusion from gated SPECT perfusion images: An integrated method. *J Nucl Med*. 1999; 40(4):650–659.
3. Ficaro EP, Quaife RA, Kritzman JN, Corbett JR. Accuracy and reproducibility of 3D-MSPECT for estimating left ventricular ejection fraction in patients with severe perfusion abnormalities. *Circulation*. 1999;100(18):I–26.
4. Ficaro EP, Kritzman JN, Corbett JR. Development and clinical validation of normal Tc-99m sestamibi database: Comparison of 3D-MSPECT to CEqual. *J Nucl Med*. 1999;40:125P (abstract).
5. Germano G, Kiat H, Kavanagh PB, et al. Automatic quantification of ejection fraction from gated myocardial perfusion SPECT. *J Nucl Med*. 1995;36(11):2138–2147.
6. Germano G, Kavanagh PB, Waechter P, et al. A new algorithm for the quantitation of myocardial perfusion SPECT. I: Technical principles and reproducibility [see comment]. *J Nucl Med*. 2000;41(4):712–719.
7. Liu YH, Sinusas AJ, DeMan P, Zaret BL, Wackers FJ. Quantification of SPECT myocardial perfusion images: Methodology and validation of the Yale-CQ method. *J Nucl Cardiol*. 1999;6(2):190–204.
8. Liu Y-H, Sinusas AJ, Khaimov D, Gebuza BI, Wackers FJT. New hybrid count- and geometry-based method for quantification of left ventricular volumes and ejection fraction from ECG-gated SPECT: Methodology and validation. *J Nucl Cardiol*. 2005;12(1):55–65.
9. Garcia E, Maddahi J, Berman D, Waxman A. Space/time quantitation of thallium-201 myocardial scintigraphy. *J Nucl Med*. 1981;22:309–317.
10. Meade R, Bamrah V, Horgan J, Ruetz P, Kronenwetter C, Yeh E. Quantitative methods in the evaluation of

thallium-201 myocardial perfusion images. *J Nucl Med.* 1978;19:1175–1178.

11. Garcia E, Van Train K, Maddahi J, et al. Quantification of rotational thallium-201 myocardial tomography. *J Nucl Med.* 1985;26:17–26.

12. Eisner RL, Tamas MJ, Clononger K, et al. Normal SPECT thallium-201 bull's-eye display: Gender differences. *J Nucl Med.* 1988;29:1901–1909.

13. Van Train KF, Berman DS, Garcia EV, et al. Quantitative analysis of stress thallium-201 myocardial scintigrams: A multicenter trial. *J Nucl Med.* 1986;27(1):17–25.

14. Maddahi J, Kiat H, Van Train KF, et al. Myocardial perfusion imaging with technetium-99m sestamibi SPECT in the evaluation of coronary artery disease. *Am J Cardiol.* 1990;66(13):55E–62E.

15. DePasquale EE, Nody AC, DePuey EG, et al. Quantitative rotational thallium-201 tomography for identifying and localizing coronary artery disease. *Circulation.* 1988;77:316–327.

16. Klein J, Garcia E, DePuey E, et al. Reversibility bull's-eye: A new polar bull's-eye map to quantify reversibility of stress induced SPECT thallium-201 myocardial perfusion defects. *J Nucl Med.* 1990;31:1240–1246.

17. Cauvin JC, Boire JY, Maublant JC, Bonny JM, Zanca M, Veyre A. Automatic detection of the left ventricular myocardium long axis and center in thallium-201 single photon emission computed tomography. *Eur J Nucl Med.* 1992;19(12):1032–1037.

18. Germano G, Kavanagh PB, Su HT, et al. Automatic reorientation of three-dimensional, transaxial myocardial perfusion SPECT images [see comment]. *J Nucl Med.* 1995;36(6):1107–1114.

19. Ficaro EP, Lee BC, Kritzman JN, Corbett JR. Automatic realignment and centering of gated perfusion SPECT: Effect on quantitative reproducibility. *J Nucl Med.* 2003;44:198P (abstract).

20. Diamond GA, Forrester JS. Analysis of probability as an aid in the clinical diagnosis of coronary artery disease. *N Engl J Med.* 1979;300:1350–1358.

21. Van Train KF, Areeda J, Garcia EV, et al. Quantitative same-day rest-stress technetium-99m-sestamibi SPECT: Definition and validation of stress normal limits and criteria for abnormality. *J Nucl Med.* 1993;34(9): 1494–1502.

22. Van Train KF, Garcia EV, Maddahi J, et al. Multicenter trial validation for quantitative analysis of same-day rest-stress technetium-99m-sestamibi myocardial tomograms [see comment]. *J Nucl Med.* 1994;35(4): 609–618.

23. Van Train KF, Garcia EV, Maddahi J, et al. Multicenter trial validation for quantitative analysis of same-day rest-stress technetium-99m-sestamibi myocardial tomograms. *J Nucl Med.* 1994;35(4):609–618.

24. Ficaro EP, Fessler JA, Shreve PD, Kritzman JN, Rose PA, Corbett JR. Simultaneous transmission/emission myocardial perfusion tomography. Diagnostic accuracy of attenuation-corrected 99mTc-sestamibi single-photon emission computed tomography. *Circulation.* 1996; 93(3):463–473.

25. Grossman GB, Garcia EV, Bateman TM, et al. Quantitative Tc-99m sestamibi attenuation-corrected SPECT: Development and multicenter trial validation of myocardial perfusion stress gender-independent normal database in an obese population. *J Nucl Cardiol.* 2004; 11(3):263–272.

26. Links JM, Becker LC, Rigo P, et al. Combined corrections for attenuation, depth-dependent blur, and motion in cardiac SPECT: A multicenter trial. *J Nucl. Cardiol.* 2000;7(5):414–425.

27. Cooke CD, Garcia EV, Cullom SJ, Faber TL, Pettigrew RI. Determining the accuracy of calculating systolic wall thickening using a fast Fourier transform approximation: A simulation study based on canine and patient data. *J Nucl Med.* 1994;35(7):1185–1192.

28. Nichols K, DePuey EG, Friedman MI, Rozanski A. Do patient data ever exceed the partial volume limit in gated SPECT studies? *J Nucl Cardiol.* 1998;5(5):484–490.

29. Nichols K, Yao SS, Kamran M, Faber TL, Cooke CD, DePuey EG. Clinical impact of arrhythmias on gated SPECT cardiac myocardial perfusion and function assessment. *J Nucl Cardiol.* 2001;8(1):19–30.

30. Germano G, Kiat H, Kavanagh PB, et al. Automatic quantification of ejection fraction from gated myocardial perfusion SPECT. *J Nucl Med.* 1995;36(11):2138–2147.

31. He ZX, Cwajg E, Preslar JS, Mahmarian JJ, Verani MS. Accuracy of left ventricular ejection fraction determined by gated myocardial perfusion SPECT with Tl-201 and Tc-99m sestamibi: Comparison with first-pass radionuclide angiography. *J Nucl Cardiol.* 1999;6(4): 412–417.

32. Vallejo E, Dione DP, Bruni WL, et al. Reproducibility and accuracy of gated SPECT for determination of left ventricular volumes and ejection fraction: Experimental validation using MRI. *J Nucl Med.* 2000;41(5):874–882; discussion 883–886.

33. Chua T, Yin LC, Thiang TH, Choo TB, Ping DZ, Leng LY. Accuracy of the automated assessment of left ventricular function with gated perfusion SPECT in the presence of perfusion defects and left ventricular dysfunction: Correlation with equilibrium radionuclide ventriculography and echocardiography. *J Nucl Cardiol.* 2000;7(4):301–311.

34. Kumita S, Cho K, Nakajo H, et al. Assessment of left ventricular diastolic function with electrocardiography-gated myocardial perfusion SPECT: Comparison with multigated equilibrium radionuclide angiography. *J Nucl Cardiol.* 2001;8(5):568–574.

35. Manrique A, Faraggi M, Vera P, et al. 201Tl and 99mTc-MIBI gated SPECT in patients with large perfusion defects and left ventricular dysfunction:

Comparison with equilibrium radionuclide angiography [see comment]. *J Nucl Med.* 1999;40(5):805–809.

36. Kondo C, Fukushima K, Kusakabe K. Measurement of left ventricular volumes and ejection fraction by quantitative gated SPET, contrast ventriculography and magnetic resonance imaging: A meta-analysis. *Eur J Nucl Med Mol Imaging.* 2003;30(6):851–858.

37. Yoshioka J, Hasegawa S, Yamaguchi H, et al. Left ventricular volumes and ejection fraction calculated from quantitative electrocardiographic-gated 99mTc-tetrofosmin myocardial SPECT. *J Nucl Med.* 1999;40(10):693–698.

38. Bacher-Stier C, Muller S, Pachinger O, et al. Thallium-201 gated single-photon emission tomography for the assessment of left ventricular ejection fraction and regional wall motion abnormalities in comparison with two-dimensional echocardiography. *Eur J Nucl Med.* 1999;26(12):1533–1540.

39. Chua T, Kiat H, Germano G, et al. Gated technetium-99m sestamibi for simultaneous assessment of stress myocardial perfusion, postexercise regional ventricular function and myocardial viability. Correlation with echocardiography and rest thallium-201 scintigraphy. *J Am Coll Cardiol.* 1994;23(5):1107–1114.

40. Cwajg E, Cwajg J, He ZX, et al. Gated myocardial perfusion tomography for the assessment of left ventricular function and volumes: Comparison with echocardiography. *J Nucl Med.* 1999;40(11):1857–1865.

41. Bax JJ, Lamb H, Dibbets P, et al. Comparison of gated single-photon emission computed tomography with magnetic resonance imaging for evaluation of left ventricular function in ischemic cardiomyopathy. *Am J Cardiol.* 2000;86(12):1299–1305.

42. Faber TL, Vansant JP, Pettigrew RI, et al. Evaluation of left ventricular endocardial volumes and ejection fractions computed from gated perfusion SPECT with magnetic resonance imaging: Comparison of two methods. *J Nucl Cardiol.* 2001;8(6):645–651.

43. Ioannidis JPA, Trikalinos TA, Danias PG. Electrocardiogram-gated single-photon emission computed tomography versus cardiac magnetic resonance imaging for the assessment of left ventricular volumes and ejection fraction: A meta-analysis. *J Am Coll Cardiol.* 2002;39(12):2059–2068.

44. Lipke CSA, Kuhl HP, Nowak B, et al. Validation of 4D-MSPECT and QGS for quantification of left ventricular volumes and ejection fraction from gated 99mTc-MIBI SPET: Comparison with cardiac magnetic resonance imaging. *Eur J Nucl Med Mol Imaging.* 2004;31(4):482–490.

45. Schaefer WM, Lipke CSA, Standke D, et al. Quantification of left ventricular volumes and ejection fraction from gated 99mTc-MIBI SPECT: MRI validation and comparison of the Emory Cardiac Tool Box with QGS and 4D-MSPECT. *J Nucl Med.* 2005;46(8):1256–1263.

46. Berman D, Germano G, Lewin H, et al. Comparison of post-stress ejection fraction and relative left ventricular volumes by automatic analysis of gated myocardial perfusion single-photon emission computed tomography acquired in the supine and prone positions. *J Nucl Cardiol.* 1998;5(1):40–47.

47. Hyun IY, Kwan J, Park KS, Lee WH. Reproducibility of Tl-201 and Tc-99m sestamibi gated myocardial perfusion SPECT measurement of myocardial function. *J Nucl Cardiol.* 2001;8(2):182–187.

48. Hickey KT, Sciacca RR, Bokhari S, et al. Assessment of cardiac wall motion and ejection fraction with gated PET using N-13 ammonia. *Clin Nucl Med.* 2004;29(4):243–248.

49. Nanasato M, Ando A, Isobe S, et al. Evaluation of left ventricular function using electrocardiographically gated myocardial SPECT with (123)I-labeled fatty acid analog. *J Nucl Med.* 2001;42(12):1747–1756.

50. Schaefer WM, Lipke CSA, Nowak B, et al. Validation of an evaluation routine for left ventricular volumes, ejection fraction and wall motion from gated cardiac FDG PET: A comparison with cardiac magnetic resonance imaging. *Eur J Nucl Med Mol Imaging.* 2003;30(4):545–553.

51. Nakajima K, Higuchi T, Taki J, Kawano M, Tonami N. Accuracy of ventricular volume and ejection fraction measured by gated myocardial SPECT: Comparison of 4 software programs. *J Nucl Med.* 2001;42(10):1571–1578.

52. Schaefer WM, Lipke CSA, Nowak B, et al. Validation of QGS and 4D-MSPECT for quantification of left ventricular volumes and ejection fraction from gated 18F-FDG PET: Comparison with cardiac MRI. *J Nucl Med.* 2004;45(1):74–79.

53. Nichols K, Santana CA, Folks R, et al. Comparison between ECTb and QGS for assessment of left ventricular function from gated myocardial perfusion SPECT. *J Nucl Cardiol.* 2002;9(3):285–293.

54. Kaul S, Wismer GL, Brady TJ, et al. Measurement of normal left heart dimensions using optimally oriented MR images. *AJR Am J Roentgenol.* 1986;146(1):75–79.

55. Gerstenblith G, Frederiksen J, Yin FC, Fortuin NJ, Lakatta EG, Weisfeldt ML. Echocardiographic assessment of a normal adult aging population. *Circulation.* 1977;56(2):273–278.

56. Kennedy JW, Baxley WA, Figley MM, Dodge HT, Blackmon JR. Quantitative angiocardiography. I. The normal left ventricle in man. *Circulation.* 1966;34(2):272–278.

57. Ford PV, Chatziioannou SN, Moore WH, Dhekne RD. Overestimation of the LVEF by quantitative gated SPECT in simulated left ventricles. *J Nucl Med.* 2001;42(3):454–459.

58. Hambye A-S, Vervaet A, Dobbeleir A. Variability of left ventricular ejection fraction and volumes with quantitative gated SPECT: Influence of algorithm, pixel size and reconstruction parameters in small and normal-sized hearts. *Eur J Nucl Med Mol Imaging.* 2004;31(12):1606–1613.

59. King MA, Long DT, Bill AB. SPECT volume quantitation: Influence of spatial resolution, source size and shape, and voxel size. *Med Phys.* 1991;18:1016–1024.

60. Nakajima K, Taki J, Higuchi T, et al. Gated SPET quantification of small hearts: mathematical simulation and clinical application [erratum appears in *Eur J Nucl Med* 2000 Dec;27(12):1869]. *Eur J Nucl Med.* 2000;27(9):1372–1379.

61. Vera P, Manrique A, Pontvianne V, Hitzel A, Koning R, Cribier A. Thallium-gated SPECT in patients with major myocardial infarction: Effect of filtering and zooming in comparison with equilibrium radionuclide imaging and left ventriculography. *J Nucl Med.* 1999;40(4):513–521.

62. Moore CC, Lugo-Olivieri CH, McVeigh ER, Zerhouni EA. Three-dimensional systolic strain patterns in the normal human left ventricle: Characterization with tagged MR imaging. *Radiology.* 2000;214(2):453–466.

63. Malm S, Sagberg E, Larsson H, Skjaerpe T. Choosing apical long-axis instead of two-chamber view gives more accurate biplane echocardiographic measurements of left ventricular ejection fraction: A comparison with magnetic resonance imaging. *J Am Soc Echocardiogr.* 2005;18(10):1044–1050.

64. Maceira A, Prasad S, Khan M, Pennell D. Normalized left ventricular systolic and diastolic function by steady state free precession cardiovascular magnetic resonance. *J Cardiovasc Magn Reson.* 2006;8:417–426.

65. Bland JM, Altman DG. Statistical methods for assessing agreement between two methods of clinical measurement. *Lancet.* 1986;1(8476):307–310.

66. Ficaro EP, Kritzman JN, Corbett JR. Effect of valve plane constraint on LV ejection fractions from gated perfusion SPECT. *J Nucl Cardiol.* 2003;10(4):S23 (abstract).

67. Manrique A, Koning R, Cribier A, Vera P. Effect of temporal sampling on evaluation of left ventricular ejection fraction by means of thallium-201 gated SPET: Comparison of 16- and 8-interval gating, with reference to equilibrium radionuclide angiography. *Eur J Nucl Med.* 2000;27(6):694–699.

68. Navare SM, Wackers FJT, Liu Y-H. Comparison of 16-frame and 8-frame gated SPET imaging for determination of left ventricular volumes and ejection fraction. *Eur J Nucl Med Mol Imaging.* 2003;30(10):1330–1337.

69. Gremillet E, Champailler A, Soler C. Fourier temporal interpolation improves electrocardiograph-gated myocardial perfusion SPECT. *J Nucl Med.* 2005;46(11):1769–1774.

70. DePuey EG, Garcia EV. Updated imaging guidelines for nuclear cardiology procedures, Part 1. *J Nucl Cardiol.* 2001;8:G1–58.

CHAPTER 12

Artifacts and Quality Control for Myocardial Perfusion SPECT Including Attenuation Correction

S. James Cullom

INTRODUCTION

Myocardial perfusion single-photon emission computed tomography (SPECT) is widely implemented for the diagnosis and management of coronary artery disease. This technology requires appreciation of both technical and patient-related factors, in order to limit the likelihood of errors and to develop an appropriate response when they occur. SPECT technology has evolved at a highly accelerated rate in recent years. Todays systems options include that are highly specialized for dedicated cardiac imaging using large and small field-of-view (FOV) detectors. Hybrid SPECT computed tomography (CT) systems have gained acceptance, as well as solid-state-based detector systems. Attenuation correction options include radionuclide transmission and CT-based systems. At the same time, new "nonrotating" SPECT systems are in the clinical validation phase with the promise of new advances in clinical efficiency. A common need for all systems and applications is a laboratory quality assurance "umbrella," including equipment quality control for optimal utility. There are increasing regulatory implications for imaging guideline and quality control conformance for laboratory accreditation now related to reimbursement. In this chapter, we review the origins of image artifacts in cardiac SPECT, their impact on image quality and related resources for developing a quality control program.

Cardiac SPECT Equipment

SPECT systems characterized by single- or multi-detector sodium-iodide (NaI)-based detectors and Anger electronics[1,2] with parallel-hole collimation perform the majority of cardiac SPECT studies today. Advances in hardware design and software applications for myocardial perfusion SPECT in the last few years have been directed at improving the efficiency of SPECT studies.[3,4] Patients are conventionally imaged in the supine position but may be imaged prone[5], reclined or upright on newer systems. New solid-state detector materials such as cadmium–zinc telluride (CdZnTe)[4] are available on clinical systems. Dedicated cardiac SPECT systems have been recognized in the literature and consist of multiple (usually two) detectors in a 90-degree fixed or variable configuration to optimize efficiency for 180-degree RAO-LPO acquisition.[6] These systems may have small FOV or conventional large FOV detectors. At the time of this writing, SPECT systems that acquire data for more than 180 degrees simultaneously or near simultaneously with a combination of multiple smaller detector designs are in clinical validation studies and poised to become a part of the SPECT-installed base.[3] These systems are a departure from the conventional "step-and-shoot" approach used today and have many features comparable to positron emission tomography (PET) in their approach. The configurations of current SPECT systems are illustrated in Figure 12-1.

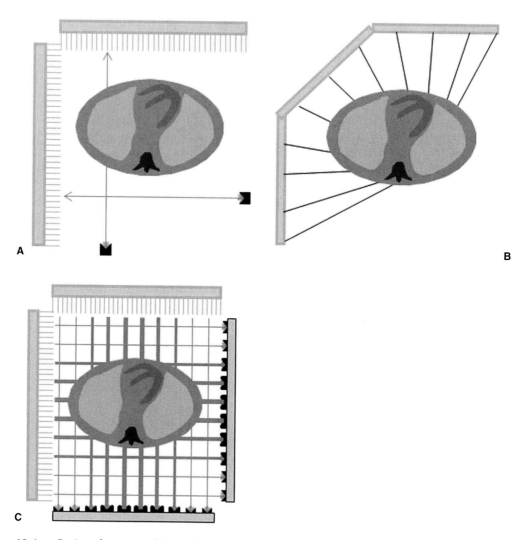

Figure 12-1. Options for myocardial perfusion SPECT imaging. A. Scanning Gd-153 line sources on a dual source 90 degree geometry system, B. Representative multi-detector geometry for 'near' 180 degree acquisition and C. Source-array approach using Gd-153 on a dual 90 degree geometry.

SPECT Equipment Quality Control

Image artifacts can result in false-positive interpretation, underestimation of the severity and extent of disease, and limit laboratory standardization and efficiency. Artifacts are best avoided through active implementation of a quality control program including both proactive and responsive components. The approach to quality control is based, in large part, on the idea that errors in the planar images should be minimized to avoid propagation into the tomographic images. Additionally, planar images are more efficient for performing quality control measurements and thus are focused on planar imaging. However, tomographic measurements are recommended periodically for a more complete assessment.

Resources for Equipment Performance and Quality Control

Multiple resources are available outlining requirements and recommendations for SPECT quality control. Nuclear and radiological imaging societies provide written guidelines. The American Society of Nuclear Cardiology (ASNC) has published imaging guidelines including protocols for quality control program details.[6] Other common sources include the Society of Nuclear Medicine (SNM)[7] and the American College of Radiology (ACR).[8] The European Society of Nuclear Medicine also provides recommendations on this topic.[9] Guidelines are used as a basis for laboratory accreditation by such groups as the Intersocietal Commission for the Accreditation of Nuclear Laboratories (ICANL)[10] and the ACR.[11] Fundamental measurements using standardized acquisition and processing protocols form a basis for the equipment quality control are published by the National Electrical Manufacturer's Association (NEMA).[12] The NEMA standards are weighted toward acceptance and performance testing but are still recognized as the standard for these measurements. As SPECT systems have become more sophisticated, many of the NEMA measurements cannot be readily performed because of geometry or other limitations, or must be performed only by service personnel. Therefore, quality control may require combined planning between clinical and manufacturer service personnel.

Myocardial perfusion SPECT studies are performed today using Tc-99m sestamibi, Tc-99m tetrofosmin, or thallium-201 chloride in single- or dual-isotope protocols.[1,2] Tc-99m undergoes gamma decay at 140 keV and thallium-201 decays by electron capture with X-ray emissions from 69 to 81 keV and by gamma decay at 167 and 135 keV. Quality control measurements must be specific to the tracer energy, or an appropriate surrogate energy source with internal correction software must be used. Attenuation correction for SPECT with external radionuclide sources uses gadolinium-153, having emissions at 100 keV, or X-ray-based CT on hybrid SPECT/CT systems.[2,13] The following sections describe the most common SPECT quality control equipment measurements.

Quality Control Measurements

Flood Field Uniformity Flood field uniformity measurements detect local and global variations in the detector's response to uniform incident radiation.[1,6] An external solid sheet source of cobalt-57 (Co-57) or a "fillable" flood source with Tc-99m is most commonly used for this measurement. Care is required with the latter to assure uniform activity concentration and to avoid warping or bubbles that may cause regional differences. The images should appear "uniform" except for statistical noise variations. Figure 12-2 shows examples of poor uniformity with visualization of the photomultiplier tubes. The standard quantity reported is the "integral" and "differential" uniformity. Integral uniformity is calculated as $100\% \times (Max - Min)/(Max + Min)$ over all pixels in the respective area.[14] Differential uniformity is calculated as $100\% \times$ the largest deviation of $(Max - Min)/(Max + Min)$ over 5×1 pixel regions in the X and Y directions.[14] Measurements are made over the central field of view (CFOV) and useful field of view (UFOV), generally defined as the central 50% to 60% of the detector surface.[14] *Extrinsic* uniformity refers to measurements with the collimator in place and *intrinsic* refers to no

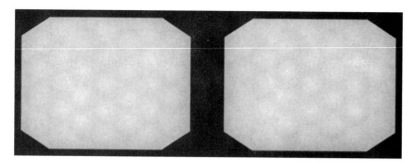

Figure 12-2. Poor flood field uniformity resulting from mismatch of the incident photon energy and the internal correction maps. The images are from the two respective detectors of a 90-degree fixed SPECT system.

collimator (exposed crystal only). All measurements are highly collimator specific.[14] The total counts to be acquired depend on the size of the FOV and number of pixels. In general, values should be in the 3% to 5% range for all measurements and checked each day when the system is used clinically. Some manufacturers recommend that testing should be less frequently. Intrinsic uniformity should be checked periodically, and have the same range for reportable quantities. This measurement is performed using a point source with a small amount of activity (0.5 mCi) placed at a distance greater than five times the central detector FOV and centered on the detector.[12] Uniformity calculations are used to correct SPECT projections for errors from the electronics prior to reconstruction. Poor uniformity (>5%) can cause structural artifacts in the transverse images with loss of contrast and spatial resolution potentially affecting diagnostic accuracy. These artifacts are not readily detected in the oblique reoriented images used for cardiac SPECT interpretation. In extreme cases, poor uniformity can result in visible artifacts resembling a "ring" pattern in the transverse plane which depends on the type of orbit.[14] Periodic high-count images (e.g., 100M) are recommended to identify any damage to the collimator that cannot be seen on lower-count measurements. Differential and integral uniformity values for CFOV and UFOV should be recorded daily and kept as part of the laboratory record. Specific methods and criteria for some emerging systems are not yet standardized. Uniformity values for Tc-99m are the reported standard. These values are typically assumed to be appropriate for imaging thallium-201 and other isotope energies. This assumption should be tested by performing a thallium-201 uniformity measurement (intrinsic or extrinsic) under the supervision of a field service engineer or medical physicist to assure optimal performance with thallium-201 or other radionuclides.

Center of Rotation Center of rotation (COR) is a quantity that measures the alignment between the electronic and mechanical axes of rotation of the detectors.[2] Significant COR errors can result in image artifacts from misalignment of the true source location and placement of counts by the reconstruction algorithm. COR measurement requires independent checking for each detector. It is measured by placement of a small Tc-99m point source "off-axis" on the imaging table. A 360-degree SPECT acquisition is performed. The source location is tracked in the projections, and the difference from the expected position is calculated and used to correct for errors at each angle. A "sinogram" reflecting the sinusoidal variation in position with respect to the system axes is produced for visual evaluation. COR measurements are highly collimator dependent.[15] For 180-degree orbital acquisitions, a fixed COR error will result in a so-called "tuning fork" artifact in the transverse plane, while a complete

360-degree acquisition will result in a circular artifact whose radius reflects the magnitude of the misalignment. However, because errors are rarely "fixed" and may be minor or nonexistent for some angles, COR errors may cause a "blurring" that is not readily identifiable as an "artifact" but may impact image accuracy. COR measurements are required to be performed each day the system is used prior to the studies, but less frequent measurements have been suggested for some systems. Software that allows quantitative assessment of the degree of misalignment and daily tracking of the COR measurements is standard on commercial systems.

System Sensitivity A less mentioned but very important QC measurement is the system sensitivity, expressed as counts per minute per microCurie of Tc-99m per NEMA standards.[6,12] System sensitivity is uniquely important for multidetector systems as significant sensitivity differences between detectors can result in image reconstruction artifacts. For example, on a dual 90-degree detector system, the contributions from one detector for more than 90 degrees would appear scaled and "smeared" across the complimentary projections from the other detector in the transverse plane. These artifacts would not be easily detected in reoriented cardiac SPECT images. Proper system sensitivity also assures the most efficient use of the injected radiation. Poor system sensitivity can yield low-count studies or require extended acquisitions to achieve desired counts. System sensitivity should be measured at installation and periodically compared to the manufacturer's specifications. This quantity is also collimator specific. NEMA specifications describe its measurement and related protocols. System sensitivity is energy dependent also and therefore should be measured for each radioisotope energy and detector with a specific energy window. Most guidelines recommend checking sensitivity at least semiannually or after servicing. It is relevant to NaI and solid-state detector systems of all geometries. The relative sensitivity of the detector can also be checked informally and tracked by calculation of

the total measured counts in the uniformity flood measurements, knowing the decay-corrected activity of the source. However, this is not a substitute for standard measurements.

Spatial Resolution and Linearity Spatial resolution reflects how well individual point sources of activity can be differentiated after the effect of blurring from the imaging system and processing. It is commonly expressed as the full width at half maximum (FWHM), usually in mm, units of from the profile of a point or line source image under specific conditions[14] (Figure 12-3). The poorer the spatial resolution (larger the FWHM), the broader the profiles and the further apart the sources must be to distinguish them as separate sources. Spatial resolution can also be measured tomographically after image reconstruction.[16] A standard method for measuring acceptable spatial resolution is the use of a multiquadrant bar or "resolution" phantom.[14] The phantom contains arrays of lead "strips" of increasing width extending below and above the systems' expected spatial resolution range. Spatial resolution can be determined semiquantitatively by identifying the

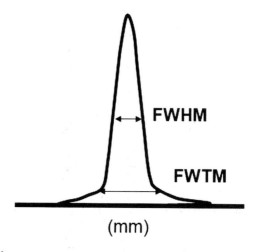

Figure 12-3. Representation of the full-width-at-half-maximum (FWHM) and full-width-at-tenth-maximum (FWTM) quantities used for evaluating spatial and energy resolutions.

smallest bars that are visually distinct. The planar measurement is performed intrinsically, using a point source of activity (per NEMA) placed greater than five times the CFOV dimension. Typical intrinsic values range from 3 to 7 mm for most SPECT systems.[6] Resolution measurements can also be performed extrinsically but should be done with caution because of sampling artifacts (Moiré patterns) from the collimator, which might result in misrepresentation of the resolution.[17] Multiple measurements can be made by rotating the phantom to evaluate resolution and linearity for different quadrants of the detector. The intrinsic spatial resolution of the system can be (roughly) estimated using a rule of thumb that the FWHM resolution (in mm) = 1.7 times smallest visible bar size.

Linearity, a measure of how accurately the imaging system spatially registers detected counts, can also be determined using the linearity or bar phantom.[6,12] This quantity is usually only visually evaluated but may be quantified. In all planar measurements, the assumption is made that the detector response does not change with angle of acquisition. This assumption can also be tested by rotating the detectors and repeating the measurement after securely attaching the bar phantom to the detector surface and repeating the measurements at different angles.

Energy Resolution

Energy Resolution   Energy resolution (ER) is a quantity representing the ability of the system to correctly identify the energy of detected photons.[1,2] Like spatial resolution, ER is expressed as the FWHM of the photopeak energy profile obtained from the energy spectrum, divided by the photopeak energy, expressed as a percentage.[12] It is measured under conditions specified by NEMA. Most NaI systems have an ER in the range of 8% to 12%,[1] while solid-state systems have reported superior ER values.[4] Superior ER is consistent with a "more narrow" photopeak profile and a reduced proportion of scatter that can affect image contrast resolution from the "blur" from scattered photons. Improved ER can allow a smaller energy window to be used, but this should be checked carefully for consistency with standards, imaging protocols, and quantitative programs. ER is specified by the manufacturer and should be checked periodically.

Quality Control on New SPECT Systems and Detector Technologies

The emergence of new cardiac SPECT technologies will certainly be reflected in quality control standards over the next few years. It is recommended that protocols be recognized by QC published imaging guidelines. Current standards are under review and will likely require updating in future publications. It is unclear to what extent emerging systems will require new measurements as part of their imaging protocols.

Patient-Related Factors and Artifacts

Patient-Related Factors and Artifacts   Quality control requires attention to patient preparation and reproducibility of acquisition methods. SPECT studies today use multiple tracers, stressing procedures, patient positioning, and other preparation steps. The guidelines cited above are highly recommended for more detailed reading on clinical and technical imaging procedures,[6,7–9] as well as aspects of review articles. A search of the nuclear medicine literature will yield an abundance of publications on these topics.

Patient and Orbital Positioning

Patient and Orbital Positioning   Patient monitoring tools and visual information should be routinely used to assure proper placement of the detectors about the patient. If the projection of the heart falls outside of the FOV for even a single projection, artifacts may result in the transverse images that cannot be corrected by any existing postprocessing algorithms. Zoom and panning factors often used in myocardial perfusion SPECT studies affect the position of the heart in the FOV, and, as the detectors move about the patient, this may cause the heart to move outside of the FOV.

When possible, identical positioning and orbital information should be applied to both rest and stress imaging unless prevented by unusual circumstances such as difficulty in raising an arm for extended periods of time. Specific considerations to assure proper positioning should be thoroughly reviewed in the manufacturer's manual. Electrocardiographic (ECG) leads and other objects should be positioned to avoid interference with the orbiting detectors causing erroneous gating signals—a source of artifacts as described below. This should be checked for all possible orbital angles when possible.

Energy Window Placement   The photon energy spectrum provides an abundance of information for assuring high-quality imaging. The photopeak consists of primary photons (those not scattered) and those that have undergone one or more energy-decreasing scatter interactions. Proper positioning of the energy window relative to the photopeak ensures efficient acquisition and is required to match the electronic correction mappings stored in the computer. Automated energy-peaking algorithms should always be visually confirmed. Energy windows are described by the center window value, which should be centered on the photopeak, and a "width" expressed as a percentage of the photopeak energy. For example, a 140-keV, 20% energy window refers to a total width that is 20% of 140 keV, or 10% on each side (i.e., 126–154 keV). A *symmetric* energy window refers to one that is centered on the photopeak with equal percentage on both sides. An *asymmetric* energy window refers to one where the center energy is not identical with the photopeak. While asymmetric energy windows have been proposed from time to time, symmetric energy windows are most commonly recommended and the standard. A significant shift (>5 keV) in energy window centerline may cause visible artifacts in the image. In extreme cases, energy window misalignment may appear in the background of the projection images as the silhouette of the photomultiplier tubes resulting from the mismatch of internal calibra-tion and energy window placement. Mispositioning can also decrease counts that could be acquired using the appropriate window or result in incorrect imaging using a disproportionate amount of lower-energy scattered photons below the photopeak.

ECG Gating Artifacts

Electrocardiographic (ECG) gating of myocardial perfusion SPECT studies is standard and well studied for assessing left ventricular cardiac function in relation to perfusion values.[18] Gating can also assist in the differentiation of fixed attenuation artifacts in patients without prior infarction.[19] Detailed technical and practical aspects of ECG gating and potential artifacts have been described in detail in other publications.[20] An important source for gating related artifacts is cardiac rhythm irregularities.[21] These cause improper placement of counts into the individual temporal bins over the cardiac cycle and inconsistent image reconstructions for each temporal frame. Errors in the ECG-gated images can be propagated into the perfusion images when the temporal frames are summed to generate the perfusion images. Both 8 and 16 frames per cardiac cycle are used clinically.[6] By reconstructing each temporal frame, time-dependent changes in position of the myocardial wall can be evaluated and quantified at stress and at rest. Left ventricular ejection fraction (LVEF), end-systolic and end-diastolic volumes, wall motion, wall thickening, and phase analysis can be extracted from the gated images using quantitative programs and visually. To minimize the potential for artifacts, ECG-gated studies can be acquired with an acceptance window defining allowable variation between R-R peaks of the cardiac cycle. Expressed as a percentage of the mean R-R time, beats that fall outside are rejected along with the counts detected during that time. However, rejecting too many beats, as can happen with significant arrhythmias, can significantly reduce image quality. Each gated frame has one-eighth (or 1/16th) the total counts of the perfusion image. While some comparative studies have been performed between 8 and 16 frames, artifacts and limitations for 16-frame acquisitions have not been described as thoroughly. Excessive rejection of beats may prevent sufficient "averaging" of the position of the heart over the cardiac cycle. A limitation for ECG-gating artifacts can occur when the end-systolic left ventricular volume becomes "small" relative to the spatial resolution of the system.[2] System blurring and noise filtering may cause the cavity size to be underestimated compared to the true size, and the amount of error is inversely related to the cavity volume. This has been reported more frequently in women, where cavity size is smaller than men on average, but small volumes may also occur in men.[22] Several processing solutions have been proposed, but a standard approach has not evolved.

In order to avoid the impact of gating irregularities on the perfusion images, modern SPECT systems allow acquisition of perfusion images without applying beat rejection to be collected, in addition to those with the beat acceptance and rejection criteria applied. In this way, the summed perfusion images are not affected by beat rejection.

Patient Motion and Related Artifacts

As conventional SPECT protocols are lengthy (12–20 minutes), patients have an increased likelihood of moving during the acquisition. Because most SPECT systems do not acquire projection data from all projections simultaneously, motion can result in severe misalignment of projection information and result in significant artifacts[23,24] (Figure 12-4). Reconstruction algorithms cannot compensate for patient motion without independent evaluation and correction prior to reconstruction. Motion artifacts have been described for all tracers and protocols of myocardial perfusion SPECT. The presence of significant patient motion is assessed by reviewing the SPECT projection images in a cine format.[25] While the potential for motion artifacts should always be

minimized through patient education and preparation, it may still occur, and automated motion detection and correction algorithms on most modern processing environments are well validated for detecting and correcting the most common types of motion. There are specific features associated with severe motion-related artifacts in the tomographic images that can sometimes be visually detected. The appearance of a "dislocation" of the walls in the long-axis slices is one described characteristic.[26] Misalignment from patient motion can also result in streaking artifacts if uncorrected, which pass through the images as counts are not properly positioned by the reconstruction algorithm.

Attenuation Processes, Artifacts, and Their Management

Attenuation of photons by the patient's body is described by a complex set of energy and material-dependent interactions.[1] Attenuation is well recognized as the problematic physical factor most affecting interpretive and quantitative accuracy of myocardial perfusion SPECT.[27] Attenuation is an exponential process described by the linear attenuation coefficient (μ) in units of cm^{-1} and represents the probability per unit path length that interactions will occur.[1] μ depends on the proportion of scatter in the measurement. In CT, μ is expressed in Hounsfield units that relate μ values to that of water.[28] The half-value layer (HVL) represents the length or thickness of tissue that reduces the beam intensity by 50%.[1] For SPECT energies, HVL is approximately 4 to 6 cm in soft tissue. As will be discussed in later sections, measurement of the attenuation distribution is required for patient-specific attenuation correction. Figure 12-5 illustrates common examples of breast and diaphragmatic attenuation artifacts in perfusion SPECT. Attenuation artifacts can also distort the left ventricular shape in severe cases.[29] The presence of attenuation artifacts may be evaluated by reviewing a cine display of the projection images.[30] Regions that are significantly attenuated relative to

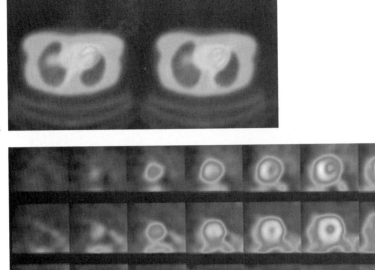

A

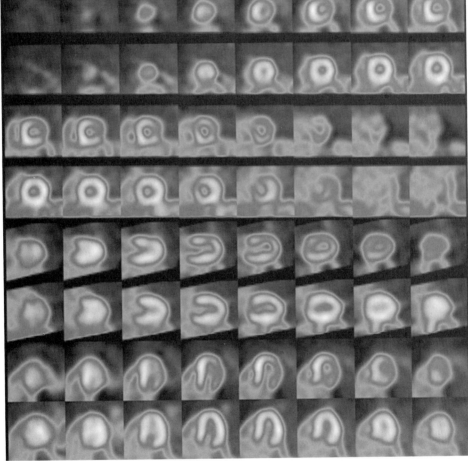

B

Figure 12-4.   Artifact resulting from the mismatch between the positioning of the attenuation map and the emission images resulting in significant artifacts. (See color insert.) A. Superposition of Rb-82 emission image onto attenuation map. Left image shows misalignment with lateral wall shifted partially into the lung region. The resulting artifact is shown in the top row of oblique images in B. The aligned images, represented by the image on the right in A, is associated with the 2nd row in B. (See color insert.)

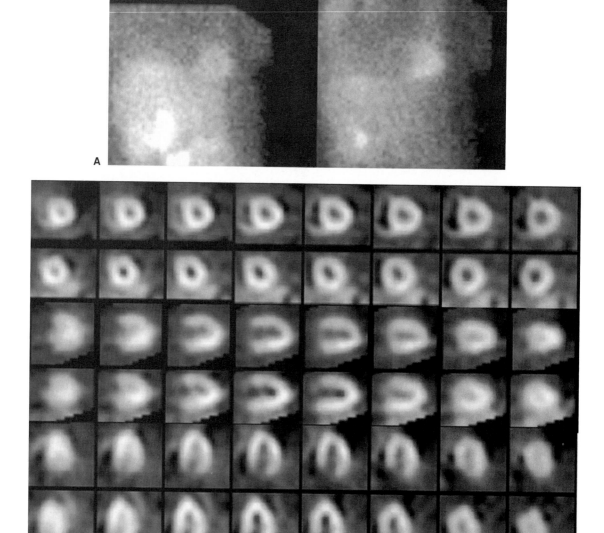

Figure 12-5. Breast attenuation artifact in the projection (left) and tomographic images (right). The lower row illustrates a diaphragmatic attenuation artifact in the projection images (left) and the artifact in the tomographic images (right).

surrounding regions, often associated with breast tissue in women overlapping the anterior wall of the heart or diaphragmatic attenuation of the inferior wall in men, are common clinical findings. While perfusion defects in the tomographic images can be recognized using review of the rotating projection images, perfusion defects can be superimposed on attenuation shadows.

Several techniques have evolved to clinically manage attenuation artifacts. A steep lateral planar image can be useful in separating the inferior wall of the heart from the effects of an overlapping hemidiaphragm.[30] In women, the left breast can be lifted up and out of the FOV or held in place by taping, or the lower border of the breast can be delineated with a lead marker, which appears as a shadow on the planar image. The marker serves as a quality control tool to help assure that the breast is positioned identically at stress and at rest imaging. With thallium-201 imaging, the early post-stress images can also be useful for visualizing and quantifying lung uptake of thallium-201.

Supine Plus Prone Imaging   Acquisition of an additional SPECT image with the patient lying prone, following supine imaging, has been shown in some patients to overcome inferior wall attenuation artifacts.[5] Its impact on diagnostic accuracy has limited validation, but a recent publication has shown that the event rate following supine-only, or supine plus prone imaging if the supine image shows an inferior wall abnormality, was similar.[26] This approach can limit laboratory throughput and efficiency and can create anterior wall defects.

SPECT Processing Artifacts

Processing and reorientation of the transverse images using standard conventions are highly important to reducing the likelihood of artifacts. Stress and rest images should be identically aligned as much as possible, using similar landmarks and criteria for each.[2,31] Most commercial processing environments provide automated or semiautomated methods directed at improving efficiency and standardization of reorientation for visual and quantitative interpretation. Stress–rest misalignment results in erroneous comparison of segments and territories where differences may be associated with the presence of cardiovascular disease or other abnormalities. ECG-gated images can also be similarly affected and can also benefit from processing standardization. It is important to be able to con-

fidently compare changes in wall motion between stress and rest associated with the same segment or territory. The use of quantitative normal databases for assisting in the detection of perfusion defects also requires standardization of processing, including filtering and reconstruction protocols. Deviation from a standardized approach can result in erroneous comparison of regions and subsequent error in calculation of quantitative parameters. The various environments available for processing have differences that are important for interpreting results and have recently been compared.[31] Another frequent finding on SPECT perfusion images is the appearance of decreased perfusion in the apical region, known as "apical thinning." This is most easily visualized in the long-axis views. The origins of this finding may be true perfusion deficit, the result of undersampling and spatial resolution, and the partial volume effect of SPECT. However, the apical region is physically thinner, with significant tissue differences between patients and the surrounding myocardium and may also move differently over the cardiac cycle.[32] Thus, this is a complicated region for perfusion interpretation.

Noise Filtering   Noise filtering of scintillation image data is required to remove the effects of statistical variations on the quality of SPECT images. Perfusion and ECG-gated images have traditionally been reconstructed using the filtered back-projection (FBP) algorithm, with different filters and parameters optimized individually for both perfusion and gated images caused by the noise differences. The impact of filtering on the detection of disease, and how improper filtering can result in artifacts, has been well described extensively in several previous technical publications.[2,33]

A balance must be achieved so that noise variations are minimized without removing important image information defining features such as defect size and shape, extent of disease, LV cavity size, and wall thickness. Noise variations can overlap the image components describing these features. Image contrast is a key image measure most degraded by overfiltering. Stress and resting images may be filtered differently but should be consistent from patient to patient for a given tracer and acquisition protocol. Deviations from standardized processing protocols should be avoided except when absolutely required. ECG-gated images have inherently fewer counts (proportionately higher noise) than the summed perfusion images. Therefore, filtering that further smoothes the images is often applied to gated images but should also be standardized for both visual assessment and quantitative processing. Filtering can be applied to the projections prior to reconstruction, during image reconstruction, or to the reconstructed images. Noise filtering should not be confused with "ramp" filtering used with the FBP reconstruction algorithm, which is a geometric requirement relating the projection measurements to the transverse plane. However, ramp and noise filters may be combined mathematically for efficient computation and are often displayed this way for the operator.

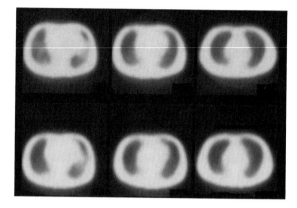

Figure 12-6.   Illustration of a high-quality attenuation map acquired using Gd-153 line sources. High-quality maps are characterized by uniformity in regions of similar tissues, well-defined boundaries between regions of significantly different attenuation coefficients, and quantitatively accurate representations of all tissue regions.

Transmission-Based SPECT Attenuation Correction

Equipment Overview   Over the last decade, SPECT systems have evolved which incorporate equipment for imaging the patient's anatomy to provide a quantitative measure of the attenuation. The principles and technical aspects are given in recent reviews.[34,35] It is well accepted that the quality of the resulting attenuation map affects the accuracy of attenuation-corrected images (Figure 12-6). Thus, improper application or technical errors in applying the attenuation map can be a source of artifacts. Commercialized SPECT attenuation correction systems measure the nonhomogeneous attenuation distribution using external collimated radionuclide sources,[36] source-array approaches,[37] or hybrid SPECT CT systems.[38] The options are shown in Figure 12-1. Essentially all commercial systems today with radionuclide sources use Gd-153 in scanning line or array-based configurations. X-ray CT systems are designed to allow lower-dose acquisition protocols that provide sufficient information for attenuation correction without high radiation dose. However, these protocols are not sufficient for detailed radiological examination of the thorax and surrounding regions. The latter uses conventional diagnostic X-ray sources with lower-dose protocols and detector arrays in serial alignment with the SPECT scanner. Both approaches have unique technical requirements as well as implications for laboratory efficiency and are part of the quality control program.[39]

Scanning Line Source Methods   The quality of a scanning line source data relies, in large part, on the quality control measurements for conventional SPECT emission imaging. A few additional steps specific to the transmission scanning are required. Important to both approaches to attenuation correction is the alignment of the emission and the transmission data.[34] Significant misalignment of these two images can result in severe artifacts that can degrade the accuracy of SPECT attenuation correction imaging. The type and degree of misalignment are specific to the system and acquisition protocol. Stone et al.[40] showed that, for transverse and axial shifts of 2.9 cm, the normalized myocardial SPECT activity was decreased in certain regions of the heart by 20% to 35%. For a 12-degree rotational shift, the error was on the order of 10% to 20%, compared to a normalized variation of 20% to 25% in the image with no attenuation correction. The results indicate that registration errors of 2 to 3 cm can seriously affect image quality in both the phantom and the human images.

Simultaneous acquisition using scanning line sources acquires the emission and transmission images without movement of the patient position. Because of the relatively low flux and limited spatial resolution of this approach compared to X-ray methods, the heart is imaged over multiple cardiac cycles and minimizes misalignment errors.[41] X-ray CT methods, by definition, are necessarily acquired sequentially and, therefore, require repositioning of the patient in the CT scanner with a greater chance of misalignment. X-ray CT images are acquired in a few seconds and have a very high degree of spatial resolution compared with scanning line source images.[41] An important consideration of this very high spatial resolution acquired in such short time, essentially capturing the heart at a fixed position for some protocols, is that an almost a 10-fold difference existing in the attenuation coefficients makes alignment critical.[42] Some SPECT systems require sequential emission/transmission imaging. The ASNC has published, in their imaging guidelines, recommendations for quality control of attenuation correction systems.[6]

QUALITY CONTROL SPECIFIC TO ATTENUATION CORRECTION

A high-quality attenuation map applied appropriately is essential for accurate attenuation correction.[34] However, early studies with attenuation correction reported little on quality control methods. Quality control of the attenuation maps

is an indicator of the overall quality of the study. High-quality attenuation maps are characterized by high-count density, minimal or no truncation of the transmission projections, high-quality reference scans, and alignment of emission and transmission.

With radionuclide source systems, equipment errors can negatively impact attenuation map quality. Mechanical misalignment or malfunction of the source housing has been shown to create artifacts in the attenuation map, which can be propagated into the corrected emission images. Physically decayed transmission sources or insufficient imaging acquisition time is also a limitation causing artifacts and becomes more significant in patients with large body habitus or excessive attenuating tissue regions. Some systems provide software to estimate optimal acquisition time requirements for sufficient counts and quality attenuation maps, using a short prescan with the transmission sources.[43] With X-ray CT transmission, the abundant photon flux from these systems provides adequate counts for accurate reconstruction of the attenuation maps, provided proper calibration is maintained.

Image Truncation and Truncation Compensation

Truncation of the transmission scan occurs when a portion of the patient's body moves outside of the FOV for a finite number of angles and must be minimized or prevented.[44,45] The measured attenuation distribution can have significant error and may produce attenuation correction artifacts, as correction algorithms attempt to produce images consistent with the errors. The location of the artifact is critical and depends on the angular range affected. Chen et al. have recently demonstrated the impact of truncation artifacts on attenuation-corrected images for small FOV studies based on simulated truncation from large FOV systems.[45] Case et al. developed a conjugate symmetry reconstruction method to compensate for transmission truncation on small FOV systems.[46] Iterative reconstruction algorithms are less sensitive to the missing information.[47,48] However, specialconsideration should be given to the orbital setup of the study to avoid or minimize truncation. Interestingly, early landmark studies showing the value of attenuation correction used iterative reconstruction algorithms that compensated intrinsically for truncation, and attenuation maps were not a direct part of the process. However, these systems[49] were not commercialized.

The likelihood of truncation increases with increasing body size and decreasing detector FOV.[45] A current trend in gamma camera design is toward the use of small FOV detectors which increases truncation likelihood based on their smaller dimensions. Figure 12-7 illustrates a patient attenuation map reconstructed without truncation and with severe truncation on a small FOV system, and the results of the truncation compensation algorithms.

The Reference ("Blank") Scan

Attenuation correction requires independent measures of the response of the detectors to the incident flux in the absence of attenuating media (table, gantry components, etc.). Figure 12-8 shows examples of acceptable and unacceptable reference scans for Gd-153 transmission scanning. For radionuclide and X-ray CT systems, "reference scans" provide this information. The reference scans are assumed to remain stable over time, as a single scan acquired each day may be applied to multiple transmission studies. The reference scan appearance is determined by the geometry of the source–detector combination and the shape of the incident photon beam. Evans and Hutton have described potential artifacts in the reference scan and described the impact on these errors in the attenuation maps and images for Gd-153 scanning line source geometry.[50] Some systems use multiple measures of the reference scans at various angles to compute an average response in order to minimize variation. X-ray CT systems use a similar approach to reference scan mea-

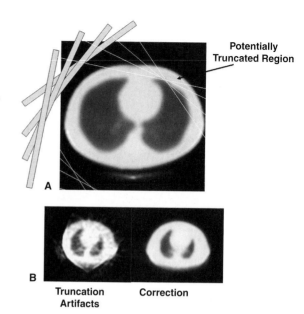

Figure 12-7.   (**A**) Truncation of the attenuation map illustrated for radionuclide-based transmission scanning, showing portions of the body outside the field of view for larger patients or for smaller field-of-view systems. For 180-degree myocardial perfusion SPECT acquisitions, the location of the truncation is important. Left-sided truncation is more significant, as these artifacts tend to be directly within the path of the emission projections when performing attenuation correction. Right-sided truncation is less likely to be in the path of the projections, or weighting regions that are relatively low in counts compared to the heart and other higher-uptake structures. In the second image (**B**), a single transverse slice is shown with truncation artifacts on both sides (left), and after correction (right). (See color insert.)

surement, or they may use an indirect approach whereby the attenuation coefficients are calibrated against a phantom (Figure 12-9).

Downscatter Artifacts in the Attenuation Map

Figure 12-10 illustrates the impact of Tc-99m-tracer photons detected in the Gd-153 transmission energy window and the characteristic

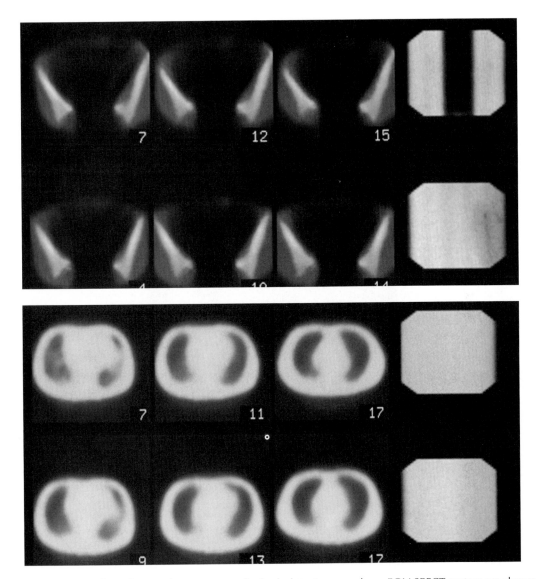

Figure 12-8. Top). The Gd-153 references scans for both detectors on a large FOV SPECT system are shown on the right side of this illustration. A dark band can be seen in the top image where the table was not removed for acquisition. The image below this shows the reference scan for the other detector acquired simultaneously, and the pillow can be seen as a darker area on the right side of this image. The 6 images on the left of these two are representative transverse slices processed with these reference scans. Bottom). The corrupted reference scans at the top were required and are shown on the right side. The properly reconstructed transverse attenuation maps are shown in this image to their left.

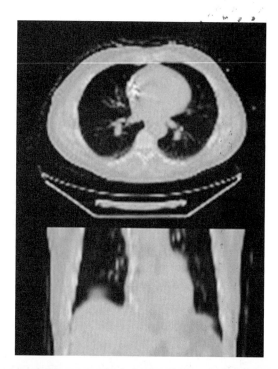

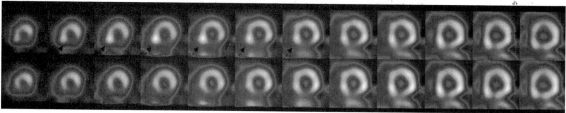

Figure 12-9. Top) Example of transverse and coronal plane images of an attenuation map obtained using an x-ray CT acquisition, illustrating artifacts that can result from X-ray imaging of implantable objects such as an ICD (shown here), which are highly opaque to X-rays. Bottom) The resulting artifact in the emission images is shown for a myocardial perfusion stress study (top row). The artifact appears as a hot spot in the inferior septal region of the short-axis images at the mid-heart level. Immediately below are the corresponding images after application of a correction algorithm (case reference). (See color insert.)

underestimation of attenuation coefficients.[51] The appearance of these artifacts indicates a compromised attenuation correction study. Thallium-201 SPECT studies require special consideration for downscatter in a different sense. In this case, Gd-153 at 100 keV can scatter and be detected in the thallium-201 emission energy window (70–80 keV) and can be substantial as a result of the relatively low count rates of thallium-201. X-ray-based system studies are performed sequentially,

and the very high flux dominates the count rates from Tc-99m and Thallium-201 crossover and essentially negates any crossover artifacts.

Iterative Reconstruction Protocols

Attenuation correction, in large part, introduced a new class of reconstruction algorithms referred to collectively as iterative algorithms. Iterative algorithms provide a broad mathematical

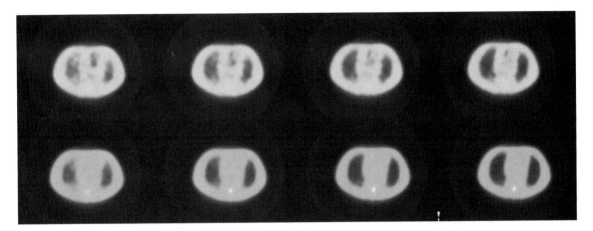

Figure 12-10. Severe error in attenuation map estimates (top row) in a phantom study resulting from downscatter of Tc-99m photons detected in the Gd-153 energy window. The same images are shown in the bottom row in the absence of downscatter.

framework permitting modeling of physical processes and image noise characteristics. These algorithms are applied to reconstruct attenuation maps and for reconstruction of the attenuation-corrected images. Attenuation correction reconstruction is most commonly accomplished using algorithms related to the maximum-likelihood expectation-maximization (MLEM) algorithm,[47] or the ordered subset expectation maximization (OSEM).[48] OSEM accelerates reconstruction by using subsets of the projection data in a specified order. While mathematically different, they are similar in their clinical performance. Starting with an estimate of the image on each transverse plane, estimated projections are calculated using a forward projection process through the attenuation map. Differences between these estimates and the measured projections are used to "update" the transverse image estimate to a more accurate image. Successive application of this process increases the likelihood that the estimated transverse image is the source of the measured projections until this likelihood is maximized—hence the name maximum likelihood. While theoretical descriptions exist for the number of iterations to terminate the reconstruction, most practical applications are based largely on empirical study of the various tasks. The reconstruction model may also include other

factors such as distance-dependent spatial resolution of the collimated detector.[52] Figure 12-11 illustrates iterative reconstruction of an attenuation map, using a Bayesian approach applied to the transmission projection data acquired from Gd-153 scanning line sources and the reconstruction of the transverse emission images corrected using the calculated attenuation map. SPECT/CT systems for attenuation correction have also incorporated iterative methods for attenuation map reconstruction. However, given the abundant flux of these systems, CT reconstruction uses FBP for estimating the attenuation map. Iteratively reconstructed images have a unique appearance compared with FBP images, especially as the number of counts decreases. Incomplete reconstruction and poor image contrast resolution can result from improper parameters for iterative reconstruction. Insufficient iterations can fail to extract the optimal contrast resolution in the image and can result in a blur of the images and missed features critical to interpretation and quantitation. Applying an excessive number of iterations can result in increased noise in the images and degradation of image quality. As with other protocols, it is best to adhere to the standardized parameters optimized for each type of study.

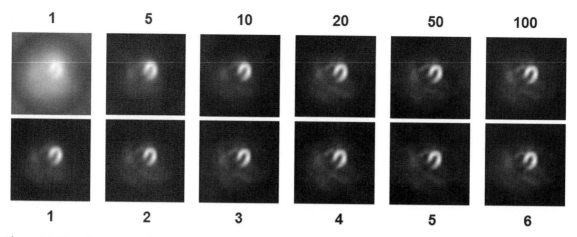

Figure 12-11.   Top: successive iterations from MLEM reconstruction of a representative Tc-99m perfusion transverse images, showing corresponding improvements in the image detail (spatial and contrast resolutions). Bottom: the same images reconstructed using the accelerated OSEM algorithm (eight subsets).

Attenuation Correction and Extracardiac Activity

In the non-attenuation-corrected SPECT scan, attenuation of counts by subdiaphragmatic tissues greatly suppresses the appearance of activity in this region, which may be greater with pharmacological stress or at rest.[53] When attenuation correction is applied, the effect is "unmasked" and the activity may be superimposed on the inferior parts of the heart[34] (Figure 12-12). Visualization of uptake in this region may be compromised. Improper scaling of other regions of the myocardium causing the appearance of reduced perfusion in the more anterior regions of the heart may occur. This ef-

fect can occur with both radionuclide and X-ray CT-based systems. Patients should present after 4 to 8 hours of fasting, and imaging may need to be delayed up to 45 minutes after resting or posthyperemic pharmacologic stress. If necessary, the study should be repeated after appropriate steps are taken to clear the activity, including ingestion of fatty or other substances.[54]

Quantitation

Quantitative analysis of myocardial perfusion compares a patient's relative distribution of tracer at stress and at rest against a database of patients with a low likelihood of disease and a set of abnormality

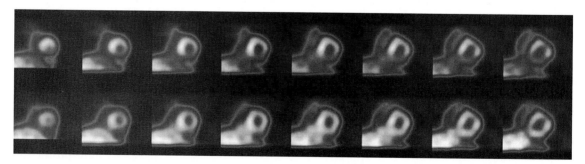

Figure 12-12.   Example of how attenuation correction can unintentionally enhance the appearance of extracardiac activity compared with conventional uncorrected images. Noncorrected images (top row). Attenuation-corrected images (bottom row). (See color insert.)

criteria validated prospectively to determine regional thresholds for the likelihood of true coronary artery disease.[55] Quantitative methods on non-attenuation-corrected studies factor in the effects of attenuation on the regional appearance of uptake. Different criteria may result for abnormalities in women and men and broader limits of acceptance of normality for the anterior wall in women and the inferior wall in men. Normal databases for tracer uptake have been developed and validated for attenuation-corrected scans.[56] As with non-attenuation-corrected scans, processing errors, registration errors, and the factors that affect noncorrected scans can also lead to artifacts when employing normal databases. These methods rely critically on standardization of protocols and parameter selection to assure optimal results.

SUMMARY

In summary, image artifacts represent errors in the images from a multitude of sources, both technical and patient related. The major concern with artifacts is their potential impact on interpretive and quantitative accuracy, and limitations in laboratory efficiency. Artifacts may be subtle and, therefore, not easily recognizable as structural inconsistencies in the images, which do not correlate with expected anatomy, or the clear presence of unsubstantiated variations in apparent activity. The best approach to avoiding artifacts includes a comprehensive quality control program, where testing is performed independently from the patient studies that meet specific performance criteria, and continued education on how to respond when problems occur. Additionally, the future will require increased scrutiny on quality control as part of accreditation and regulatory requirements, and these requirements are expected to evolve as new types of systems and detectors become more widespread.

REFERENCES

1. Cherry SR, Sorenson JA, Phelps ME. *Physics in Nuclear Medicine*. 3rd ed. Philadelphia, PA: Saunders; 2003.
2. Garcia EV, Galt JR, Faber TL, Chen J. Principles of nuclear cardiology imaging. In: Dilsizian V, Narula J, eds. *Atlas of Nuclear Cardiology*. Philadelphia, PA: Current Medicine, LLC; 1995.
3. Patton JA, Slomka PJ, Germano G, Berman DS. Recent technologic advances in nuclear cardiology. *J Nucl Cardiol*. 2007;14(4):501–513.
4. O'Connor MK, Kemp BJ. Single-photon emission computed tomography/computed tomography: Basic instrumentation and innovations. *Semin Nucl Med*. 2006;36(4):258–266.
5. Segall GM, Davis MJ. Prone versus supine thallium myocardial SPECT: A method to decrease artifactual inferior wall defects. *J Nucl Med*. 1989;30:548–555.
6. American Society of Nuclear Cardiology. Imaging guidelines for nuclear cardiology. *J Nucl Cardiol*. 2006;13:e25–e41.
7. Society of Nuclear Medicine. *Procedure Guideline for General Imaging*. Version 3.0. Reston, VA: Society of Nuclear Medicine; 2004 May 30:10.
8. ACR Technical Standard for Medical Nuclear Physics Performance Monitoring of Nuclear Medicine Imaging Equipment, 2003.
9. Hesse B, Tagil K, Cuocolo A, et al. EANM/ESC procedural guidelines for myocardial perfusion imaging in nuclear imaging. *Eur J Nucl Med Mol Imaging*. 2005;32(7):855–897.
10. Intersocietal Commission for the Accreditation of Nuclear Medicine Laboratories. http://icactl.org/icactl/apply/standards.htm.
11. American College of Radiology. http://www.acr.org/accreditation/nuclear/nuc_med_reqs.aspx.
12. National Electrical Manufacturers Association (NEMA). Performance measurements of gamma cameras, NU 1-2007;35:1117–1123.
13. McQuaid SJ, Hutton BF. Sources of attenuation-correction artefacts in cardiac PET/CT and SPECT/CT. *Eur J Nucl Med Mol Imaging*. 2008.
14. Nichols KJ, Galt JR. Quality control for SPECT imaging. In: DePuey EG, Berman DS, Garcia EV, eds. *Cardiac SPECT imaging*. 2nd ed. Philadelphia: Lippincott Williams & Wilkins; 2001:17–40.
15. Cerqueira MD, Matsuoka D, Ritchie JL, Harp GD. The influence of collimators of SPECT center of rotation measurements: Artifact generation and acceptance testing. *J Nucl Med*. 1988;29:1393–1397.
16. Hines H, Kayayan R, Colsher J, et al. National Electrical Manufacturers Association recommendation for implementing SPECT instrumentation quality control. *J Nucl Med*. 2000;41:383–389.
17. Graham LS. Quality control for SPECT systems. *Radiographics*. 1995;15(6):1471–1481.
18. Abidov A, Germano G, Hachamovitch R, Berman DS. Gated SPECT in assessment of regional and global left ventricular function: Major tool of modern nuclear imaging. *J Nucl Cardiol*. 2006;13(2):261–279.

19. DePuey EG, Rozanski A. Using gated technetium-99m-sestamibi SPECT to characterize fixed myocardial defects as infarct or artifact. *J Nucl Med*. 1995;36(6):952–955.

20. Germano G, Nichols KJ, Cullom SJ, Faber TL, Cooke CD. Gated perfusion SPECT: Technical considerations. In: DePuey EG, Berman DS, Garcia EV, eds. *Cardiac SPECT Imaging*. 2nd ed. Philadelphia: Lippincott Williams & Wilkins; 2001:103–115.

21. Nichols K, Yao SS, Kamran M, Faber TL, Cooke CD, DePuey EG. Clinical impact of arrhythmias on gated SPECT cardiac myocardial perfusion and function assessment. *J Nucl Cardiol*. 2001;8:19–30.

22. Kakhki VR, Sadeghi R. Gated myocardial perfusion SPECT in patients with a small heart: Effect of zooming and filtering. *Clin Nucl Med*. 2007;32(5):404–406.

23. Wheat JM, Currie GM. Impact of patient motion on myocardial perfusion SPECT diagnostic integrity: Part 2. *J Nucl Med Technol*. 2004;32(3):158–163.

24. Wheat JM, Currie GM. Incidence and characterization of patient motion in myocardial perfusion SPECT: Part 1. *J Nucl Med Technol*. 2004;32(2):60–65.

25. Hendel RC, Gibbons RJ, Bateman TM. Use of rotating (cine) planar projection images in the interpretation of a tomographic myocardial perfusion study. *J Nucl Cardiol*. 1999;6(2):234–240.

26. Hayes SW, DeLorenzo A, Hachamovitch R, et al. Prognostic implications of combined prone and supine acquisitions in patients with equivocal or abnormal supine myocardial perfusion SPECT. *J Nucl Med*. 2003; 44:1633–1640.

27. King MA, Tsui BM, Pan TS. Attenuation compensation for cardiac single-photon emission computed tomographic imaging: Part 1. Impact of attenuation and methods of estimating attenuation maps. *J Nucl Cardiol*. 1995;2(6):513–524.

28. Schoenhagen P, Stillman AE, Halliburton SS, White RD. CT of the heart: Principles, advances, clinical uses. *Cleve Clin J Med*. 2005;72(2):127–138.

29. Hansen CL, Kramer M. Attenuation smear: A 'paradoxical' increase in counts due to attenuation artifact. *Int J Card Imaging*. 2000;16(6):455–460.

30. DePuey EG, Garcia EV. Optimal specificity of thallium-201 SPECT through recognition of imaging artifacts. J Nucl Med. 1989;30(4):441–449.

31. Burrell S, Macdonald A. Artifacts and Pitfalls in myocardial perfusion imaging. *J Nucl Med Technol*. 2006;34:193–211.

32. Links JM, Becker LC, Anstett F. Clinical significance of apical thinning after attenuation correction. *J Nucl Cardiol*. 2004;11:26–31.

33. Zubal IG, Wisniewski G. Understanding Fourier space and filter selection. *J Nucl Cardiol*. 1997;4(3):234–243.

34. Bateman TM, Cullom SJ. Attenuation correction single-photon emission computed tomography

35. Bailey DL. Transmission scanning in emission tomography. *Eur J Nucl Med*. 1998;25(7): 774–787.

36. Tan P, Bailey DL, Meikle SR, Eberl S, Fulton RR, Hutton BF. A scanning line source for simultaneous emission and transmission measurements in SPECT. *J Nucl Med*. 1993;34(10):1752–1760.

37. Cellar A, Sitek A. Transmission SPECT scans using multiple collimated line sources. In: Proc IEEE Medical Imaging Conference, Anaheim; 1995:1121–1125.

38. Bailey DL. Transmission scanning in emission tomography. *Eur J Nucl Med*. 1998;25(7):774–787.

39. ICACTL Standards for Computed Tomography (CT) Laboratory Operations. www.icactl.org/icactl/apply/standards.htm.

40. Stone CD, McCormick JW, Gilland DR, Greer KL, Coleman RE, Jaszczak RJ. Effect of registration errors between transmission and emission scans on a SPECT system using sequential scanning. *J Nucl Med*. 1998; 39(2):365–373.

41. Bacharach SL. PET/CT attenuation correction: breathing lessons. *J Nucl Med*. 2007;48(5):677–679.

42. Harris CC, Greer KL, Jaszczak RJ, Floyd CE Jr, Fearnow EC, Coleman RE. Tc-99m attenuation coefficients in water-filled phantoms determined with gamma cameras. Med Phys. 1984;11(5):681–685.

43. Zhao Z, Ye J, Durbin M, Coles D, and Shao L. Estimation of the optimum transmission scan time by using the subjects weight, height and the transmission source strength. *J Nucl Med*. 2001;42(5):195P.

44. Kadrmas DJ, Jaszczak RJ, McCormick JW, Coleman RE, Lim CB. Truncation artifact reduction in transmission CT for improved SPECT attenuation compensation. *Phys Med Biol*. 1995;40(6):1085–1104.

45. Chen J, Galt JR, Durbin MK, Ye J, Case JA, Cullom SJ, Shao L, Garcia EV. Significance of transmission scan truncation in attenuation corrected myocardial perfusion SPECT images [abstract]. *J Nucl Cardiol*., to be published.

46. Case JA, Hsu BL, Cullom SJ, Bateman TM, Galt JR, Garcia EV. Correcting for transmission truncation artifacts using conjugate sonogram data as a posteriori information for transmission reconstruction in cardiac SPECT. *IEEE Trans Nucl Sci*. 2003.

47. Tsui BM, Gullberg GT, Edgerton ER, et al. Correction of nonuniform attenuation in cardiac SPECT imaging. *J Nucl Med*. 1989;30(4):497–507.

48. Hudsonn HM, Larkin RS. Accelerated image reconstruction using ordered subsets of projection data. *IEEE Trans Med Imaging*. 1994;13:601–609.

49. Ficaro EA, Fessler JA, Shreve PD, et al. Simultaneous transmission/emission myocardial perfusion tomography: Diagnostic accuracy of attenuation myocardial perfusion imaging. *Semin Nucl Med*. 2005; 35(1):37–51.

corrected Tc-99m sestamibi single-photon emission computed tomography. *Circulation*. 1996;93: 463–473.

50. Evans SG, Hutton BF. Variation in scanning line source sensitivity: A significant source of error in simultaneous emission-transmission tomography. *Eur J Nucl Med Mol Imaging*. 2004;31:703–709.

51. Almquist H, Arheden H, Arvidsson AH, Pahlm O, Palmer J. Clinical implication of down-scatter in attenuation-corrected myocardial SPECT. *J Nucl Cardiol*. 1999;6(4):406–411.

52. Hutton BF. Cardiac single-photon emission tomography: Is attenuation correction enough? *Eur J Nucl Med*.

53. Heller EN, DeMan P, Yi-Hwa L, et al. Extracardiac activity complicates quantitative cardiac SPECT imaging using a simultaneous transmission-emission approach. *J Nucl Med*. 1997;38:1882–1890.

54. Thompson RC, et al. The problem of radiotracer abdominal activity in myocardial perfusion imaging studies. *J Nucl Cardiol*., to be published.

55. Van Train KF, Garcia EV, Maddahi J, et al. Multicenter trial validation for quantitative analysis of same-day rest–stress technetium-99m-sestamibi myocardial tomograms. *J Nucl Med*. 1994;35:609–618.

56. Grossman GB, Garcia EV, Bateman TM, et al. Quantitative technetium-99m sestamibi attenuation corrected SPECT: Development and multicenter trial validation of myocardial perfusion stress gender-independent normal database in an obese population. *J Nucl Cardiol*. 2004;11:263–272.

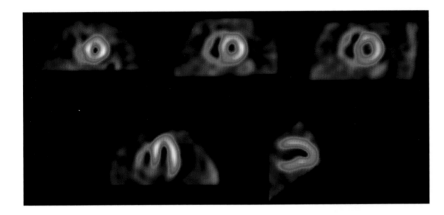

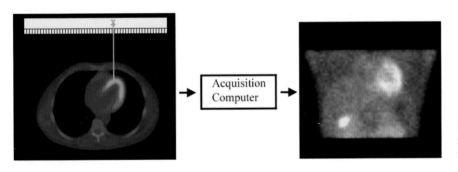

Figure 1-1. Representative slices of a myocardial perfusion SPECT examination.

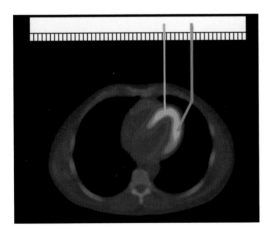

Figure 1-2. Simplified schematic of image formation.

Figure 1-3. An ideal photon detection is indicated by the green path in the cross section of a collimator and crystal. The red path represents a "scattered" photon whose path has been altered by bone.

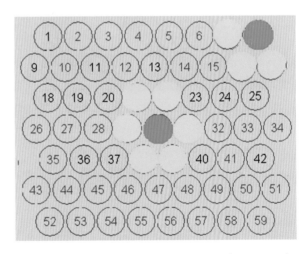

Figure 1-5. Red PMT's represent primary locations of scintillation. Adjacent tubes (yellow) also observe the event.

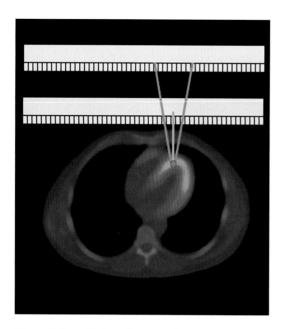

Figure 1-9. Photon dispersion increases as a function of distance.

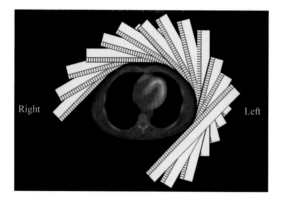

Figure 1-10. Acquisition projection range for myocardial perfusion SPECTimaging.

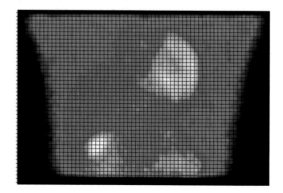

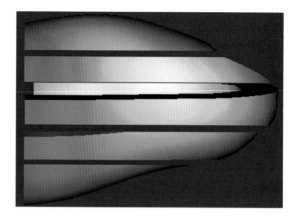

Figure 1-13. Example of 3D rendered stacked trans-axial images of the left ventricle.

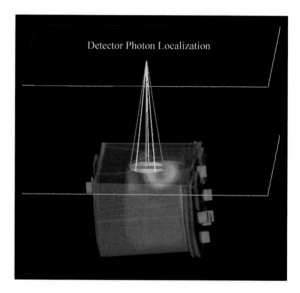

Figure 1-19. Representation of FBP (green), 2D (blue) and 3D (yellow) beam modeling techniques illustrating theoretical photon origination distributions.

Figure 1-11. A standard projection image displayed in a 64 x 64 matrix.

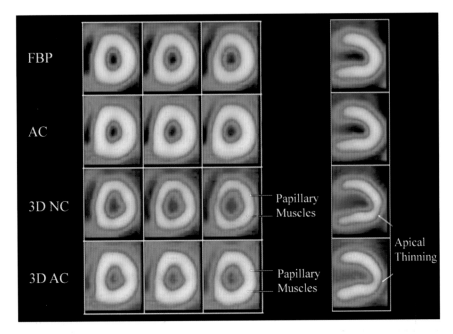

Figure 1-20. 3D beam modeled reconstructions illustrate more "anatomic" cardiac images including papillary musculature and anatomic apical thinning not apparent using standard reconstruction techniques.

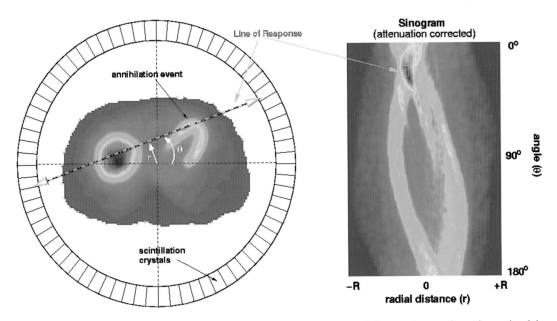

Figure 2-5. Binning the PET signal. The two detection points of the annihilation photons form the ends of the line-of-response (LOR). The LOR is characterized by its axial position (z), the radial distance from the center of the scanner (r), and the angle that the LOR makes with the x-axis (θ). LOR data can be binned into a sinogram with each point in the sinogram corresponding to the number of events detected along the LOR at (r,θ).

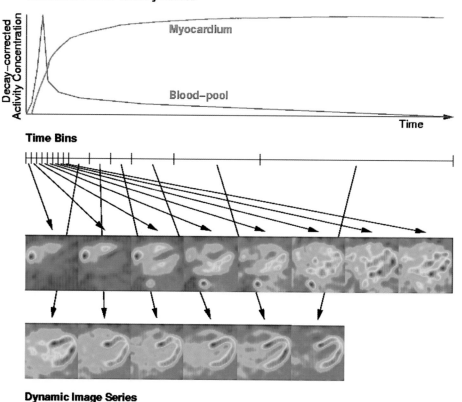

Radiotracer Time–Activity Curves

Myocardium

Blood–pool

Time

Time Bins

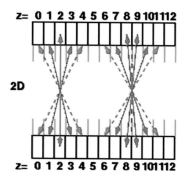
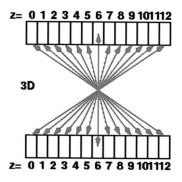

Dynamic Image Series

Figure 2-7. Dynamic Acquisition. PET data can be acquired in a series of images with variable duration in order to capture the changing temporal behavior of the tracer. Dynamic imaging is important because it allows absolute quantitative measurement of physiological parameters such as blood flow and receptor density. In these Rb-perfusion images, the injected tracer is seen first in the right chambers of the heart, followed by the left chambers of the heart and the descending aorta, and finally accumulates in the myocardium and clears from the bloodpool.

z= 0 1 2 3 4 5 6 7 8 9 10 11 12

2D

z= 0 1 2 3 4 5 6 7 8 9 10 11 12

z= 0 1 2 3 4 5 6 7 8 9 10 11 12

3D

z= 0 1 2 3 4 5 6 7 8 9 10 11 12

Figure 2-9. 2D vs 3D acquisition. In 2D acquisition, septa made of an absorbing material like tungsten are placed between the crystal elements of the detectors (shown in green). This restricts the axial span of the LOR to those along which the photons do not intersect the septa (blue) and removes those that do intersect septa (red). In 3D acquisition mode, the septa are removed and much larger axial angles are still accepted.

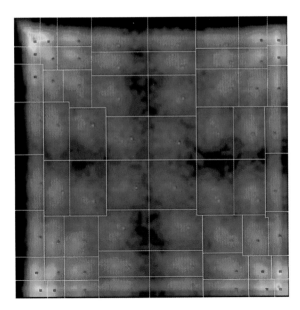

Figure 2-10. Block uniformity map. The uniformity map is segmented into areas corresponding to each crystal element in the block (indicated by the white lines). Red dots mark the computer's identification of each crystal element. The grid pattern is distorted due to the differences in sensitivity and amplification between the edge and the center of the PMTs.

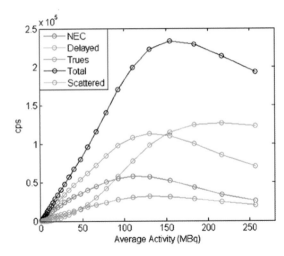

Figure 2-13. Noise-equivalent count rate. This example shows the contributions to the total number of prompts (black) detected in a PET scanner as the amount of activity in the scanner increases. The true (red) and scattered (purple) event rates initially increase in proportion to the singles rate (activity), but the randoms or delayed rate (green), increases with the square of the singles rate. Deadtime in processing events leads to a peak in the measured count rate (here at 130 MBq for the true rate, and 150 MBq for the total rate). The noise-equivalent count rate (blue) peaks even earlier at about 110 MBq.

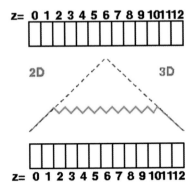

Figure 2-11. Axial sensitivity profiles for 2D (green) and 3D (blue) acquisitions.

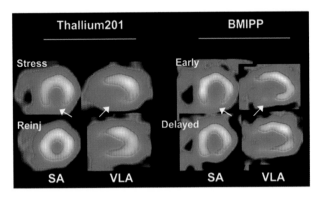

Figure 5-4. BMIPP detection of ischemic memory after demand ischemia. Left, Thallium-201 stress and reinjection (Reinj) images after treadmill exercise in the short-axis (SA) and vertical long-axis (VLA) SPECT tomograms (left). Thallium images demonstrate a severe reversible inferior defect (arrows), consistent with exercise stress-induced ischemia. Right, A similar defect is seen on the early BMIPP images in the same tomographic cuts (arrows), with BMIPP injected 22 hours after the stress-induced ischemia. The defect on the delayed BMIPP image is less prominent than on the early image. These image data suggest that BMIPP detects prolonged postischemic suppression of fatty acid metabolism for up to 22 hours after stress-induced ischemia. (Adapted from Dilsizian V, Bateman TM, Bergmann SR, et al. Metabolic imaging with ß-methyl-*p*-[^{123}I]-iodophenyl-pentadecanoic acid identifies ischemic memory after demand ischemia. *Circulation* 2005;112:2169–2174.)

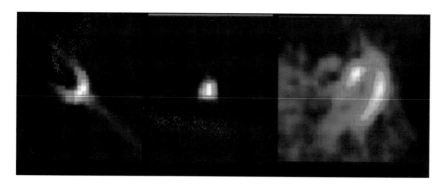

Figure 9-6. (A) Tuning Fork artifact (B) Normal COR image (C) Apical artifact a result of COR deviation (From Mann A. Quality control for myocardial perfusion imaging. In: Heller GV & Hendel RC, eds. *Nuclear Cardiology: Practical Applications.* New York, NY: McGraw Hill Companies Inc; 2004.)

Figure 10-7. The same transaxial image slice, with six different variations of a Butterworh filter applied. In the left column, the power is constant at 5, and critical frequencies vary: 0.22 (A), 0.52 (B) and 0.82 (C). In the right column, the critical frequency is constant at 0.52, and the power varies: 20 (D), 5 (E) and 2.5 (F). The critical frequency makes more difference in the appearance of the image. A and C are quite different in image texture, though the critical frequency is different by less than a factor of 4. D and F are similar even though the power differs by a factor of 8. The expected difference in effect of two filters can be approximated by noting the difference in the area under the two filter curve definitions.

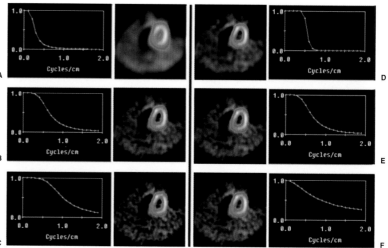

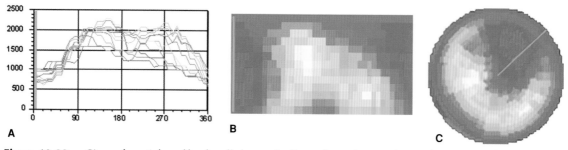

Figure 10-22. Circumferential profiles for all short axis slices of a patient study are shown in A. The green line represents the starting point of sampling, which is 45 degrees right-anterior-oblique. When the counts from these profiles are converted into colors, and stacked, they form the array shown in B. The top row is the apex, the bottom row is the base. Here the ventricular counts are plotted in rectangular coordinates, giving equal area to each slice. This creates distortion in the shape of the ventricle being represented, especially at the apex, which is over represented, being stretched out across the top of the array. The counts in the array can also be plotted in polar coordinates (C), to form the familiar polar map, or bull's-eye map, roughly equivalent to looking at the heart from the apical end, while still seeing the entire ventricle. Here there is a different kind of distortion. The apex is given less area than it should be, and the base is given more area than it should be.

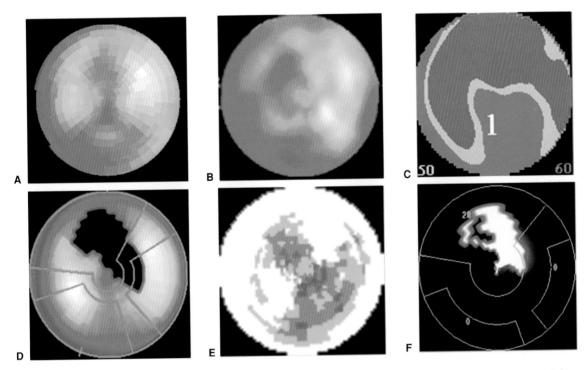

Figure 10-23. Different types of polar map displays of myocardial perfusion, taken from various commercial programs. These plots, from six different patients, show raw perfusion (A), raw smoothed perfusion (B), quantized perfusion, in which counts have been grouped by value (C), raw perfusion with defect extent indicated in black and coronary territories overlaid (D), defect severity indicated by the number of standard deviations below mean normal (E), and thresholded reversibility, shown in white, with overlaid coronary territories (F).

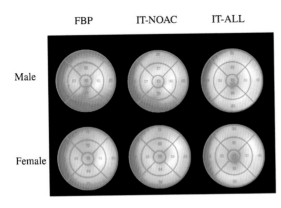

Figure 11-5. Comparison of male and female normals database distributions for different reconstruction algorithms. The filtered backprojection (FBP) databases are significantly different for males and females and are also significantly different from distributions derived from iterative algorithms. The middle column databases (IT-NOAC) generated using an iterative algorithm that modeled scatter and collimator response but not photon absorption are different from FBP databases. The maps for IT-ALL were reconstructed with an iterative algorithm that corrected for photon absorption as well as scatter and collimator response. These distributions are statistically equivalent in males and females. The differences between databases generated using different reconstruction algorithms demonstrate the importance of matching clinical patient data and the appropriate normals database similarly processed.

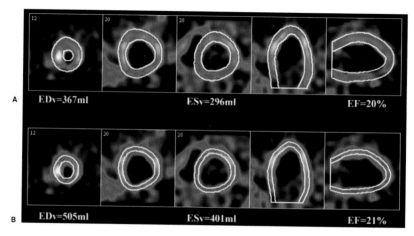

Figure 11-6. Resolution effects on wall thickness estimates. The surfaces in row (A) are determined from an edge detection gradient operator and reflect the poor resolution of SPECT images, resulting in an average myocardial wall thickness of 22 mm for the end diastolic frame. In row (B), the wall thickness estimates are scaled to provide a mean myocardial thickness of 10 mm. Scaling the surface locations significantly affects the end-diastolic volume (EDv) and end-systolic volume (ESv), but the ejection fraction (EF) is essentially unaffected as the errors in EDv and ESv cancel.

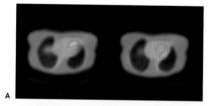

A

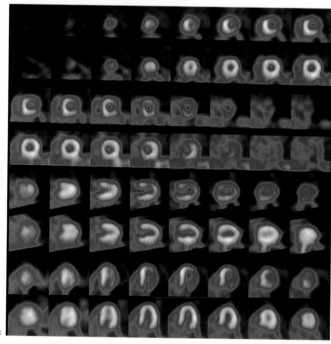

B

Figure 12-4. Artifact resulting from the mismatch between the positioning of the attenuation map and the emission images. This example is the result of a severe lateral shift causing the lateral wall to extend into the lung area where the attenuation coefficients are significantly less than soft tissue values. The result is severe under correction for attenuation. The shift can be seen in the representative transverse plane (A) of overlaid images of the emission and attenuation map (left, misregistered; right, properly registered). In B, the corresponding short, vertical and horizontal long axis images are shown where the appearance of a severe defect is seen in the lateral and anterior walls (top), and the corresponding correct values for each image directly below for each.

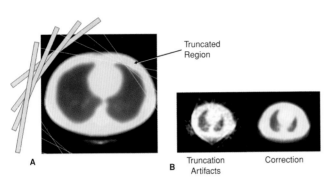

Truncated Region

A

B Truncation Artifacts   Correction

Figure 12-7. (**A**) Truncation of the attenuation map illustrated for radionuclide-based transmission scanning, showing portions of the body outside the field of view for larger patients or for smaller field-of-view systems. For 180-degree myocardial perfusion SPECT acquisitions, the location of the truncation is important. Left-sided truncation is more significant, as these artifacts tend to be directly within the path of the emission projections when performing attenuation correction. Right-sided truncation is less likely to be in the path of the projections, or weighting regions that are relatively low in counts compared to the heart and other higher-uptake structures. In the second image (**B**), a single transverse slice is shown with truncation artifacts on both sides (left), and after correction (right).

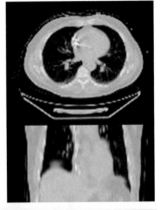

Figure 12-9. Top) Example of transverse and coronal plane images of an attenuation map obtained using an x-ray CT acquisition, illustrating artifacts that can result from X-ray imaging of implantable objects such as an ICD (shown here), which are highly opaque to X-rays. Bottom) The resulting artifact in the emission images is shown for a myocardial perfusion stress study (top row). The artifact appears as a hot spot in the inferior septal region of the short-axis images at the mid-heart level. Immediately below are the corresponding images after application of a correction algorithm (case reference).

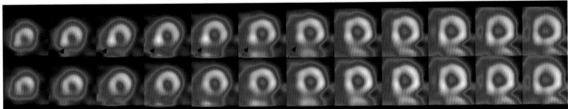

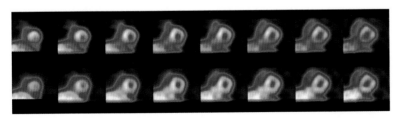

Figure 12-12. Example of how attenuation correction can unintentionally enhance the appearance of extracardiac activity compared with conventional uncorrected images. Noncorrected images (top row). Attenuation-corrected images (bottom row).

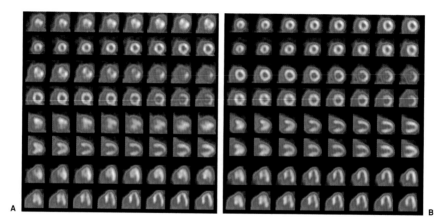

A   B

Figure 13-5. The stress images (top rows) show an extensive abnormality (A), not present at rest. The technologists noted patient movements during the stress but not the rest acquisition. With repeat stress imaging, the scan is normal (B).

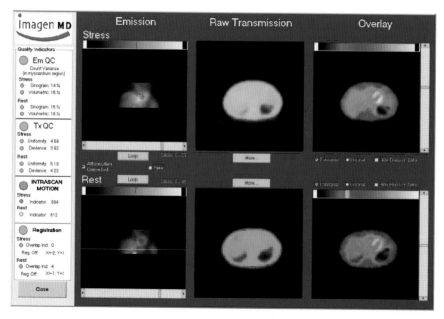

Figure 13-7. Example of a software program (ImagenMD®) that indicates technical violations that could result in image artifacts. Note the red light next to the motion quality control indicator for the stress images. This indicator was for the study shown in Figure 13-5.

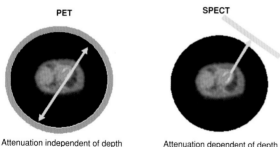

PET   SPECT

Attenuation independent of depth   Attenuation dependent of depth

Figure 15-2. Detection of coincidence pair results in depth-independent attenuation in PET as opposed to SPECT with depth-dependent attenuation.

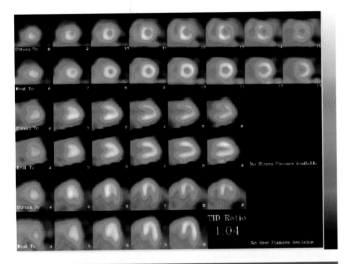

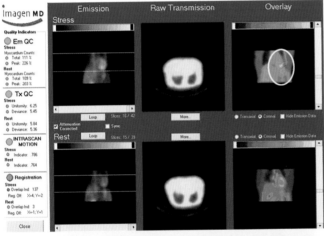

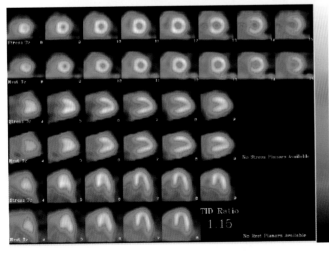

Figure 15-3. An example of transmission/emission misregistration in cardiac PET. Part of the myocardium in the lung fields creates perfusion defects in lateral and high-lateral segments (top row). With proper realignment in both lateral and axial directions, the images show normal perfusion in those segments (bottom row).

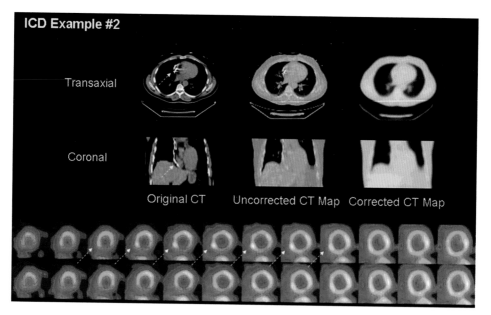

Figure 15-7. An example of patient who wears intravascular cardiodefibrillator (ICD) whose tip locates next to the septal wall. The metal object in CT maps produces focal tracer artifacts in Rb-82 images. The artifact can be removed with corrected CT maps.

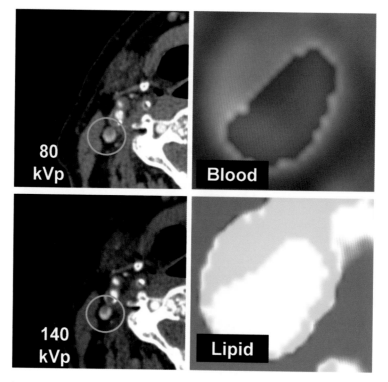

Figure 16-16. Dual-energy CT image opens up the possibility of charcterizing plaques based on the intrinsic signature different material make on the different kVp images. In this image the iodine in the blood can be segmented to locate lumen and the lipid in the plaque can also be identified.

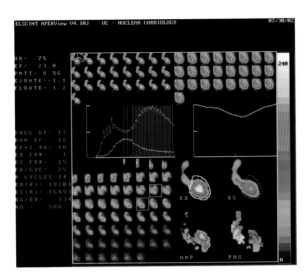

Figure 17-1. FPRNA (anterior projection) images are shown, with the serial images at the lower left, demonstrating tracer transit from the superior vena cava, to right atrium, to right ventricle to the pulmonary phase, left heart phase, and systemic circulation. Using regions of interest (ROIs) drawn over the LV and left lung (far upper left image, also blue and green), histograms are obtained (shown above serial images, in blue and green respectively), which show overlapping RV counts with systoles (curve valleys) and diastoles (curve peaks) from which the cardiac cycles (CYC) are derived which comprise the representative cycle. Each cardiac cycle is marked (red for diastole, green for systole). The pulmonary curve is used to compute the pulmonary mean transit time (PMTT). The length of the representative cycle in frames (FR) is used to derive the heart rate (HR). The images of the raw representative cycle are shown at upper right. This is subjected to the frame method of background subtraction (i.e., using the background to end-diastolic image ratio (BG/ED) and the washout factor (WO) needed to set the pulmonary area to zero counts), in order to derive the corrected representative cycle (upper left images) from which single ROI ejection fraction (SNGL EF), which is higher than the raw EF, but lower than the dual ROI derived EF, which is used to account for valve plane motion. The Fourier amplitude (AMP) and phase (PHS) images at the lower right demonstrate reduced inferior wall amplitude and delayed contraction of the inferior wall and apex, respectively.

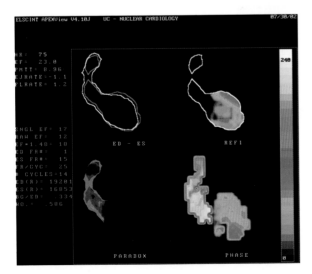

Figure 17-2. FPRNA (anterior projection) functional images are shown, with end-diastolic and end-systolic perimeter image at the upper left (ED-ES), a paradox image (lower left), regional ejection fraction index (REFI, upper right), and Fourier phase images (lower right) shown. The Fourier phase image demonstrates delayed contraction of the inferior wall and apex. These functional images allow assessment of regional function without the use of visual interpretation of cine images.

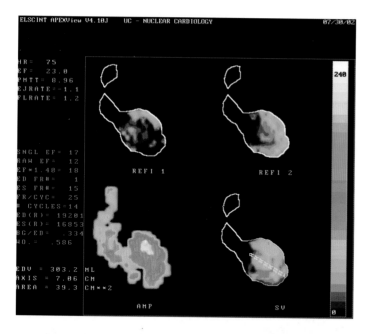

HR = 75
EF = 23.0
PMTT = 8.96
EJRATE = -1.1
FLRATE = 1.2

SNGL EF = 17
RAW EF = 12
EF*1.48 = 18
ED FR# = 1
ES FR# = 15
FR/CYC = 25
CYCLES = 14
ED(R) = 19201
ES(R) = 16853
BG/ED = .334
NO. = .586

EDV = 303.2 ML
AXIS = 7.06 CM
AREA = 39.3 CM**2

REFI 1   REFI 2

AMP   SV

Figure 17-3. Additional FPRNA (anterior projection) functional images are shown, with regional ejection fraction index for the first and second halves of systole (REFI1 and REFI2, upper frames), an alternative method of determining the presence of delayed contraction. Note that the inferior and apical regions have more ejection fraction in the latter half of systole, compared with the anterolateral wall. Fourier amplitude (AMP, lower left) and stroke volume (SV, ED minus ES, lower right) images are shown. The graphic extending from the valve plane to the apex on the SV image is used to compute the LV volume using the Sandler and Dodge equation for the anterior projection.

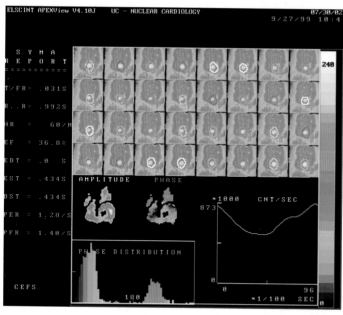

S Y M A
R E P O R T
=============

T/FR = .031S

R..R = .992S

HR = 60/M

EF = 36.8%

EDT = .0 S

EST = .434S

DST = .434S

PER = 1.28/S

PFR = 1.40/S

CEFS

AMPLITUDE   PHASE

PHASE DISTRIBUTION

180

*1000   CNT/SEC
873

0   96
0   *1/100   SEC

Figure 17-6. GERNA analysis is shown for images obtained in the left anterior oblique 45 degrees projection. The 32 ECG-gated frames are analyzed using a guiding region of interest (ROI, in cyan, frame 1) obtained either manually or using Fourier phase and amplitude images to automatically locate and outline the LV. Automated LV edge detection is performed using a combination of first and second derivatives of count profiles inside the guiding or master ROI. Background correction is performed based on the counts per pixel within a small periventricular ROI (in cyan, frame 16) drawn carefully to avoid the ventricle or the spleen. The counts within the 32 ROIs are shown after background correction in the lower right histogram. The first derivative of this ventricular volume curve is used to compute the peak filling and emptying rates (PFR and PER). The Fourier phase and amplitude functional images demonstrate inferoapical and septal hypokinesis with late contraction, when compared with the RV and the basal lateral portion of the LV.

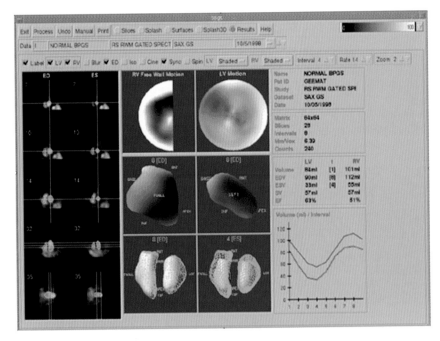

Figure 17-8. Gated SPECT blood pool images are shown analyzed with the commercially available QBS program (Cedars-Sinai) used for display and automated calculation of RV and LV ejection fraction and volume. Changes in volume are tracked from ED to ES, for calculation of wall motion and regional thickening, displayed in polar map format. Three-dimensional diagrams (above) and actual SPECT slices with fitted edges (below) are also shown. (Images courtesy of Dr. Guido Germano.)

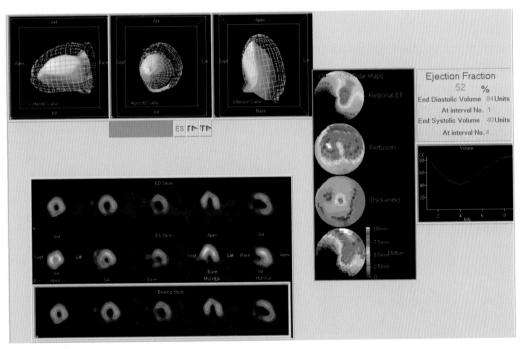

Figure 17-9. Gated SPECT myocardial perfusion images are shown analyzed with the commercially available QGS program (Cedars-Sinai), as in Figure 8, but obtained with Tc-99-tetrofosmin. The images demonstrate hypoperfusion and hypokinesis with reduced thickening in the inferior wall. The apparent septal hypokinesis on the 3D, regional EF, and motion maps is an artifact due to previous median sternotomy with coronary artery bypass surgery and can be distinguished from ischemic dysfunction by the presence of normal systolic thickening of the septal myocardium.

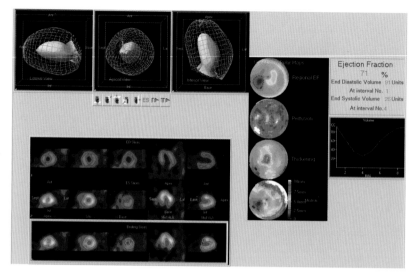

Figure 17-10. Gated SPECT myocardial perfusion images are shown analyzed with the commercially available QGS program (Cedars-Sinai) used for display and automated calculation of ejection fraction and volume. Changes in volume are tracked from ED to ES, for calculation of wall motion and regional thickening, displayed in polar map format. Three-dimensional diagrams (above) and actual SPECT slices with fitted edges (below) are also shown. These images were obtained with thallium-201 in a normal patient.

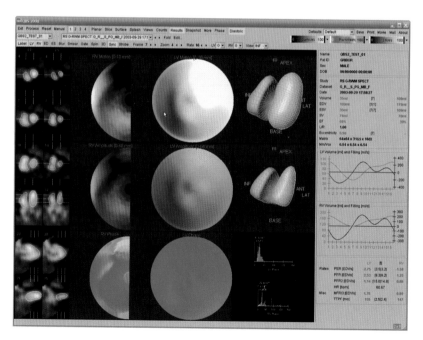

Figure 19-2. Example of a gated blood pool SPECT study. This screen capture from a commercially available program (QBS, Cedars-Sinai) shows representative tomographic views on the left side of the figure, and volumetric, 3D reconstructions on the right side of the figure (left ventricle in red, right ventricle in blue). Left and right ventricular volume curves and calculated ejection fractions are shown at the far right. (Courtesy of G. Germano, PhD)

SECTION 5

MYOCARDIAL PERFUSION IMAGING PET TECHNIQUES

Positron Emission Tomographic Techniques and Procedures: Myocardial Perfusion Imaging

Timothy M. Bateman

Technical aspects of myocardial perfusion imaging using positron emission tomography (PET) differ from the more frequently employed single-photon tracers in a number of respects. As discussed in prior chapters, the tracers and the equipment are much different from those used in SPECT perfusion imaging, which impacts on space requirements, room design, patient education, and preparation for imaging, quality control routines, stress-testing protocols, inspection of data for artifacts, and transmission and emission scan interpretive steps. This chapter will be devoted to highlight the unique technical requisites of PET perfusion imaging, often comparing and contrasting these with the more familiar SPECT perfusion imaging.

SPACE DESIGN

PET scanners are much larger and heavier than current-generation SPECT devices. Typical scanning rooms are often four times larger, in the range of 400 ft^2, compared to those commonly allocated for a SPECT scanner. A control room of at least 100 ft^2 is also needed. Furthermore, the 511 keV photons were used for PET mandate lead-shielding in walls, floors, and ceilings. Different than for SPECT, nuclear technologists and physicians who may be in attendance during active PET scanning will be out of the scanning room and in the control room, monitoring the patient through a leaded glass partition. If the PET scanner is a PET/CT device, the CT component may require a separate room for a chiller. For stress testing using the very short-lived tracer Rb-82, there needs to be sufficient space in the scanning room for the ECG-monitoring module, an intravenous pole, a crash cart, and the Rb-82 infusion pump. All of these imply much greater space requirements and higher initial construction costs. Figure 13-1 shows a typical PET scan room design for Rb-82 myocardial perfusion PET imaging.

The need for lead shielding arises because of the high energy of the 511 keV photons. More

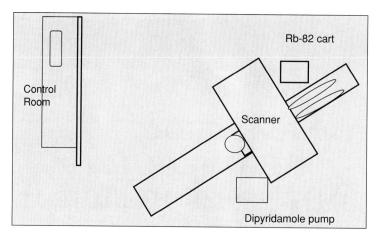

Figure 13-1.   Typical layout of a PET or PET/CT cardiac imaging suite.

than 13 mm of lead would be required to attenuate 90% of the energy of these photons. Since this is impracticable, room design for perfusion PET relies on a combination of lead shielding between the patient and the attending personnel (or others who may be in the vicinity of the scanning room), distance between others and the patient, and maintaining distance from the patient for several minutes after tracer infusion. Distance is a potent attenuator of 511 keV photons: a distance of 2.5 m is roughly equivalent to 1 cm of lead! Time is also important because of the short half-life of Rb-82 and NH3-ammonia. By example, after 5 minutes a 60 mCi dosage of Rb-82 will have decayed to <0.2 mCi.

Because staff is not in the room with the patient during scanning, there needs to be provision for remote monitoring of the patient's vital signs, heart rhythm, and well-being. This can be done by using an automated blood pressure apparatus and by displaying at least one ECG lead on a visible LCD monitor. Verbal communication is typically maintained via a speaker system that needs either to be left on throughout the scanning period or to be voice-activated by the patient.

Staff need to be particularly attentive to patients while they are being scanned, because of the fact that they are not actually in the patient's im-

mediate presence. Motion or deep breathing or sighing or coughing, just as with SPECT, can result in artifacts that can make interpretation difficult or impossible and can lead to scan interpretive errors. If the patient is positioned in the scanner feet-first, it may be difficult for the staff to visualize whether the patient is moving his or her body; a television camera/monitoring system is inexpensive and can be useful. If staff notice patient motion during the scan, the options are to repeat imaging immediately, keep the patient in the premises until the data are processed and the physician interpreter makes a judgment as to adequacy of the scans, or determine that the patient simply cannot lie still for the duration of the acquisition and choose a different imaging modality. Motion *recognition* algorithms are now commercially available for PET; motion *correction* algorithms are not available as of yet.

PATIENT PREPARATION FOR PET PERFUSION ASSESSMENT

Unlike the majority of SPECT scanners, dedicated and hybrid PET scanners are solid gantry devices with a table that slides the patient into the device. Especially when the scanner positioning is such that the patient goes in head-first, there may be an issue of claustrophobia for some patients. Intravenous sedation such as versed may be useful in such cases. By law, conscious-sedation records must be maintained, appropriate consents obtained, and patients need to be counseled about not driving or performing tasks that require a high level of attention or physical stability for several hours afterward. Sedatives should not be administered without ensuring that there is a transportation option besides the patient driving.

Except for a small percent of patients who are not candidates for vasodilator stress, most will be tested with adenosine or dipyridamole. They, therefore, need to be informed about no caffeine for 12 to 24 hours, no dipyridamole-containing medications (such as oral dipyridamole or aggrenox) for 24 hours, no nitrates for 6 to 24 hours, no calcium-channel blockers for 24 hours, and no β-blocking agents for 24 hours beforehand.[1-4] In selected instances, it may be important that patients be tested on β-blockers or calcium-channel blockers; this needs to be determined ahead of time and the interpreting physician should be made aware as to whether a given patient was tested on or off medications.

If the PET perfusion study will be done with stand-alone PET, the only immediate pretest patient education needed is to emphasize the importance of not moving, breathing normally, and avoiding talking or sighing or sleeping or coughing during the transmission and emission scan acquisitions. To improve the chances of adherence, patients should be made aware of the symptoms that commonly accompany the chosen pharmacologic stress agent, and staff should stay in the room at the patient's side until the time of Rb-82 infusion.

When the acquisition will be performed with a PET/CT hybrid, the patient needs breathing instructions to ensure a high-quality CT transmission scan. The options are free breathing, end-inspiration breath hold, or light end-expiration breath hold. The choice will, to some extent, depend on the number of CT detector rows and patient capability to hold breath.

STRESS TESTING PROTOCOLS FOR PET

Exercise

NH3-ammonia studies can be performed with either pharmacologic or exercise stress, as the 10-minute half-life is logistically amenable to permitting time delays between injection of the tracer at peak stress and the start of imaging. Because of the short 75-second half-life of Rb-82, almost all clinical studies are done using pharmacologic stress, with the patient lying in the camera. One study[5] has demonstrated the technical feasibility and comparable diagnostic accuracy of performing Rb-82 stress imaging with exercise, but the authors emphasized the logistic challenges of moving the patient from a treadmill to the camera, attaining correct positioning, and completing imaging while there are still sufficient myocardial counts for a high-quality scan. In addition, such protocols carry a potential for higher radiation exposure to staff.

Dipyridamole

Intravenous dipyridamole is an excellent vasodilator for stress Rb-82 and for NH3-ammonia perfusion PET; it induces a long effective hyperemia, permitting adequate time to acquire both emission and transmission scans during hyperemia. The standard infusion is 6 mg/kg for more than 4 minutes, with the transmission scan being acquired 2 to 4 minutes later, followed by the ECG-gated emission acquisition.

There are some differences in typical protocols with Rb-82 vs. NH3-ammonia. Because NH3-ammonia is injected as a bolus, and, because the tracer has a longer half-life, it is acceptable if necessary to reverse the effects of dipyridamole with 75 to 150 mg of intravenous aminophylline before beginning imaging. With Rb-82, the dipyridamole side effects cannot be reversed with aminophylline until completion of imaging. The acquisition of images under the effects of hyperemia carries the bonus of being able to quantitate the function correlates of vasodilation, which may include augmentation of contraction and LVEF in normals and a loss of regional contraction and a drop in LVEF in those with severe CAD. Staff stay in the room with the patient during the infusion and leave the scanning room with the start of the Rb-82 infusion or the NH3-ammonia injection. Staff need to educate the patient about frequent side effects, and yet the importance of lying still during imaging.

Monitoring of the ECG for ischemic changes and for arrhythmias is important, as some patients with severe CAD can develop a "steal" syndrome in which intense myocardial ischemia can occur. One group has reported that transient ST depression with dipyridamole is less specific for ischemia than has been reported for SPECT vasodilator stress[6]; in this study, patients with transient ST depression but a normal PET scan had a very low incidence of CAD at follow-up coronary angiography and remained free of coronary events.

Adenosine

Adenosine is commonly used with NH3-ammonia, as the tracer can be injected during the adenosine infusion and the patient is then imaged several minutes later. The images reflect the initial uptake of the tracer, which does not redistribute. Imaging during the adenosine infusion has not been reported for NH3-ammonia; imaging after the infusion, if discontinued, loses peak hyperemia function information.

We have been using a modified adenosine protocol with PET/CT, as a comparison study with dipyridamole showed a strong trend toward larger perfusion defects with adenosine.[7–9] After completion of rest imaging, we infuse adenosine at 140 μg/kg/min for 7 minutes. After 2 minutes we begin the Rb-82 infusion, and 120 seconds later we start a 3.5-minute peak hyperemia ECG-gated emission acquisition. The CT transmission scan is acquired immediately thereafter. This provides the superior hyperemia afforded by adenosine, with higher sensitivity and specificity for perfusion defects. We have not attempted this with radioactive-source attenuation correction—

presumably the only issue would be that the longer transmission scan acquisition would mean that much of this would be done when coronary flows and adenosine side effects were abated. It would be necessary to validate use of the poststress transmission scan for attenuation correction of the peak stress emission scan.

The protocol introduces a potential logistic concern, as staff should not be in the room when Rb-82 is being infused and yet the patient is still receiving the adenosine infusion. In this protocol, staff stay at the patients' sides during the first 2 full minutes of adenosine infusion. Most instances of heart block occur before this time, if they are going to occur. Staff then leave the room and the Rb-82 infusion is begun. To prevent "pushing" the adenosine and perhaps causing transient heart block, we use intravenous tubing and needles that have two channels (one for Rb-82 and one for adenosine). We also position the infusion cart and generator behind the camera gantry (see Figure 13-1), so that if staff needed to come into the room during the Rb-82 infusion or immediately after it, they would be shielded by the metal in the PET/CT gantry. Thus far, we have had no instances where staff members have needed to enter the room during infusion or during the first few moments of scanning.

Dobutamine

Pharmacologic stress testing using dobutamine will follow the same protocols as with SPECT, when the PET tracer used is NH3-ammonia. This agent is administered as a bolus when the patient has achieved a diagnostic level heart rate, and imaging takes place several minutes later. It is a more difficult and challenging protocol when the PET tracer is Rb-82. This is because the short half-life of Rb-82 mandates that the tracer be infused during the dobutamine infusion and that imaging is also completed during the infusion. This introduces two logistic challenges. The first is that the patient needs to be maintained at the peak infusion rate of dobutamine for up to 10 minutes, sufficient time to complete the Rb-82 infusion (usually 20–30 seconds), leave approximately 120 seconds for blood pool clearance, and then allow sufficient time to acquire the emission images (3.5–5 minutes). The dobutamine infusion can then be discontinued, and the stress transmission scan can be acquired at that time (if it was not acquired earlier during the infusion). Some patients may be intensely uncomfortable during the last several minutes, especially if there is a marked tachycardia or stress-induced angina. The second concern is that, just as with adenosine, the staff will not be in the room during and for a few moments after the Rb-82 has been infused, the time when the dobutamine is at its peak rate and patients likely to be most uncomfortable. Needless to say, vasodilator stress is much preferred.

ACQUISITION PROTOCOLS

The American Society of Nuclear Cardiology has published imaging protocol guidelines for myocardial perfusion PET.[10] The specific protocol that will optimize the imaging characteristics of the many different types of PET and PET/CT scanners in operation today is beyond the scope of this chapter. However, some general protocols in wide use can serve to exemplify the basics of how PET perfusion imaging is performed.

NH3-Ammonia

NH3-ammonia is not very frequently used in a rest/stress protocol to identify myocardial ischemia, mainly because it requires an on-site cyclotron and its throughput efficiency is low compared to Rb-82. However, there is substantive literature documenting its accuracy, which is generally believed to be higher than that of SPECT perfusion imaging. The typical imaging protocol is fairly simple, entailing a transmission scan, a resting bolus injection of NH3-ammonia, followed by emission imaging several minutes later for approximately 5 to 10 minutes. After a time interval of approximately 1 hour, to permit decay of background activity, the stress component is repeated exactly the same. One nuance is the timing of start of acquisition, which can vary by patient and by scan (rest or poststress). During the first minute or 2 after injection, there can be rapidly changing myocardial uptake, as significant blood activity persists for 2 or 3 minutes, so a variable several-minute time delay postinjection before starting imaging is needed.

Rb-82

A typical acquisition protocol for rest/stress Rb-82 perfusion PET is shown in Figure 13-2. On most scanners, the gantry is quite narrow so that correct positioning of the heart within the field of view can be an issue. Risk to "missing" a portion of the heart can be minimized by using a small test bolus of Rb-82 and then marking the patient's chest in relation to laser beams on the scanner. We have found that this step is not essential however. Acquisition of the transmission scan is an easier and faster way to perform this step. The transmission scan itself can then be used for small adjustments in positioning for the emission scan. In the unlikely event that the transmission scan is too malpositioned, it can simply be repeated.

The transmission scan itself is often as short as 1 or 2 minutes, using the BITGA algorithm for its reconstruction[11–13] (see next chapter). The emission image is then acquired for 3.5 to 5 minutes, with ECG gating. The gating is usually eight frames, although technically this could be acquired

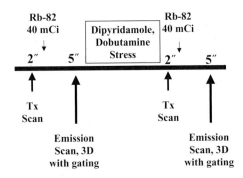

Figure 13-2. Typical acquisition protocol for Rb-82 rest/stress perfusion PET.

with many more frames; each frame needs to be attenuation corrected, and the work-flow as well as the storage requirements increase exponentially. With the patient still on the table, the pharmacologic stress agent is infused, and then the same sequence of transmission and emission scan acquisitions is performed under the effects of the stress agent. This permits a full ECG-gated rest perfusion/function study paired to a peak stress perfusion/function study, all within approximately 35 minutes total time.

Hybrid PET/CT

The typical acquisition protocol for a perfusion study on a hybrid device is similar, except that the much faster CT acquisition permits the opportunity to use adenosine as the stress pharmaceutical. The adenosine protocol, described above, can shorten the entire study to the range of less than 20 minutes (Figure 13-3). Most hybrid devices do not have an option for acquiring the transmission scan other than by CT.

Several issues need to be considered when performing PET perfusion studies on a hybrid device. These include how best to acquire the transmission scan, whether or not to acquire a calcium score, and whether or not to incorporate CT coronary angiography into the study. There are not sufficient published data, especially from perspective of clinical results in day-to-day practice, to make definitive conclusions about any of these alternatives.

Options for transmission scan acquisition include a relatively long free-breathing acquisition, scanning at end-inspiration breath hold, or scanning at end-inspiration breath hold. To some extent, the choice will depend on the specific equipment being used. For example, a four-slice CT scanner may preclude a breath-hold acquisition, because of how long it takes to acquire the scan. On 16-slice scanners and above, breath holds of just a few seconds will suffice. Because of the large amount of attenuation inherent in PET scanning, free breathing can result in portions of the heart not being assigned correct attenuation coefficients; this can result in false-positive scans. Our protocol is to instruct patients that we want them to breathe normally and, when instructed, to simply quit breathing at end expiration. After a few practice sessions, most patients find this easy to understand and are able to do this comfortably.

A related issue is what the optimal CT scanner settings for optimizing information content are. The CT attenuation coefficients (Hounsfield units) are converted to radionuclide units (mu's), such that for the purposes of attenuation correction, a low-quality or noisy CT scan is adequate for the purpose. Figure 13-4 shows the difference in CT-scan appearances between a short, low-mA, nongated, relatively thick slices scan at one level, compared to a longer, higher-mA, ECG-gated, thin slices scan at the same level. The latter approach will permit recognition of numerous noncardiovascular findings and will also enable calculation of a coronary calcium score. However,

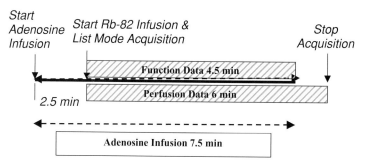

Figure 13-3.   Rapid acquisition adenosine PET/CT imaging protocol.

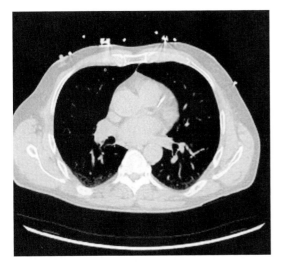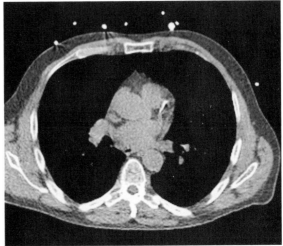

Figure 13-4. Examples of CT scans acquired for attenuation correction. The scan on the left was acquired at 250-mA, 3-mm-thick slices, and ECG gating. The scan on the right was acquired with 9-mA, 5-mm-thick slices, and no ECG gating.

the radiation exposure to the patient will be much higher than is necessary to perform the requested test—an assessment of myocardial perfusion at rest and at stress. For example, the acquisition parameters on the right-hand image in Figure 13-4 subjected the patient to only 0.26 mSv, compared to 5.5 mSv using those parameters that provided the high-quality CT scan on the left panel.

In some cases, it may be requested by the referring physician that a coronary calcium score be reported along with the perfusion findings. One option is to perform the transmission scan with thin slices, high mA, ECG gating, dose modulation, and breath hold. Another is to acquire the transmission scan with low mA and thick slices without gating and then acquire the calcium scan as a separate acquisition. Interestingly, the latter approach actually reduces radiation exposure to most patients, as the transmission scan needs to cover a much greater amount of thorax than is necessary for the calcium scoring.

In selected instances, a combined perfusion and coronary CT angiographic study may be clinically indicated.[14] More often this might be done as part of a research study. While there are sev-

eral steps to the protocol, the entire procedure including calcium scoring, rest and stress perfusion and function, and coronary CTA can be completed in less than 1 hour. There are several challenges that include appropriate patient identification, appropriate patient preparation, and processing and interpreting each component as completed to be sure that there is indication, and also no contraindication, to proceed to the next phase. Patient preparation is important because the perfusion study will optimally be performed off β-blockers and the vasodilator used for stress will likely increase heart rate. Then intravenous β-blockers need to be administered to bring heart rate down, in order to obtain a quality CT angiogram. The administered radiation dose can be quite high for such protocols.

IMAGE QUALITY CONTROL/ ARTIFACT RECOGNITION

Prior to image interpretation, the physician needs to be sure that what is going to be visualized on the scan represents physiology and not artifact. Just as with SPECT, there are a number of common technical problems that can result in artifacts in the images. The most common of these are discussed here.

Scanner malfunction: Inspection of raw data prior to and after attenuation correction is important, as with SPECT. Dark lines across the field of view, or dark blobs within the field of view, can be indications that counts are not being registered in those areas.

Poor counts/noisy images: Imaging too early after the Rb-82 infusion can result in a poor signal-to-noise ratio, with excess counts in the blood pool and low counts in the myocardium. Imaging too late can result in poor myocardial count statistics. Standardized times of beginning imaging 90 to 120 seconds after completion of the Rb-82 infusion will work satisfactorily in most patients, but those with congestive heart failure, right ventricular dysfunction, or pulmonary hypertension may have much slower circulation times, and younger patients and those with renal failure may have much faster circulation times. Optimally, the scanner will acquire its data in list mode, permitting optimization of the reconstruction interval to that of lowest noise/best myocardial uptake.

Patient motion during the acquisition: Patients need to be instructed about the importance of lying very still during the rest and peak stress acquisitions. They also need to know that deep breathing, sighing, talking, chewing, or falling asleep can cause the heart to be in a different position at different time intervals during the acquisition. This can result in misalignment of the counts within the heart, with varying degrees of impact on the final images. In extreme cases, when motion occurs during the stress acquisition but not during the rest scan, the study may suggest multivessel distribution ischemia (Figure 13-5A). Note that the repeated stress scan (Figure 13-5B) is normal. In less extreme cases, there may be a blurring or smearing of the myocardium to suggest that motion has occurred (Figure 13-6). We use a software program (ImagenMD®) (Figure 13-7) to help us

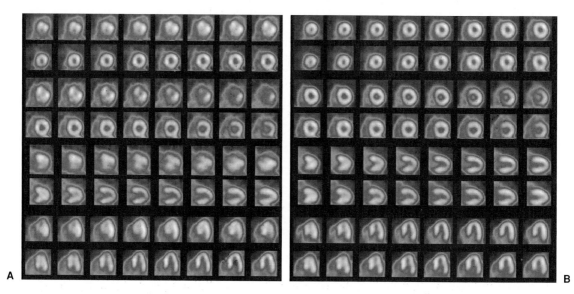

Figure 13-5.   The stress images (top rows) show an extensive abnormality (**A**), not present at rest. The technologists noted patient movements during the stress but not the rest acquisition. With repeat stress imaging, the scan is normal (**B**). (See color insert.)

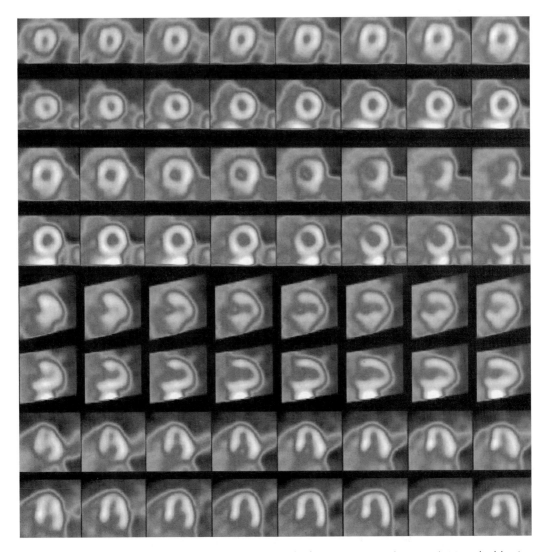

Figure 13-6.   Example of less extreme motion, affecting only the stress images (top rows). Note the blurring or smudging of detail of the inferior wall.

identify when sufficient motion has occurred to cause scan artifacts. The best option then is to repeat the scan, as motion correction software currently does not exist for PET.

Misregistration of transmission and emission scans. This problem must be recognized before interpreting the study, because even small portions of myocardium that are not assigned proper attenuation coefficients will make the scans ap-

pear nonuniform, potentially resulting in a misdiagnosis. The most extreme errors occur when the lateral border of the heart is assigned lung coefficients, with less "correction" being applied, resulting in an apparent large perfusion defect of the anterior and lateral walls. This can mimic left main distribution ischemia. A quality control program is essential both for recognizing and for correcting misregistration. The

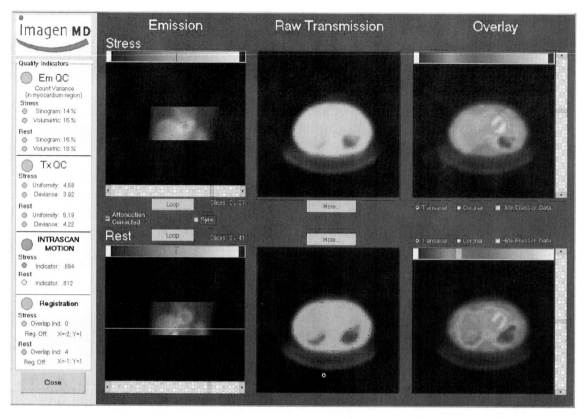

Figure 13-7.   Example of a software program (ImagenMD®) that indicates technical violations that could result in image artifacts. Note the red light next to the motion quality control indicator for the stress images. This indicator was for the study shown in Figure 13-5. (See color insert.)

frequency with which sufficient misregistration to cause an erroneous interpretation varies is probably in the range of 20%.[15] The important point is to recognize that this has occurred and then to correct the problem before interpreting the images, as even small amounts of misregistration in PET scans can cause artifacts.[16]

NORMAL AND ABNORMAL SCAN APPEARANCES

Transmission Scans

The transmission scans should always be inspected, both for quality and for recognition of unexpected but clinically relevant findings. Several investigators have reported that 20% to 50% of CT scans acquired for attenuation correction contain incidental findings of potential clinical importance.[17–19] These include calcifications in coronaries, the aorta, valves and valve annulus, and the pericardium; hiatal hernias; pleural and pericardial effusions; various types of cysts; thoracic aorta aneurysms; mediastinal adenopathy; lung nodules; parenchymal lung diseases; anatomic anomalies; and breast tumors. Figure 13-8 shows an example of a CT transmission scan with a pleural effusion noted incidentally. Many of these findings will also be evident when the CT scan is performed at low-mA settings. One important point to emphasize

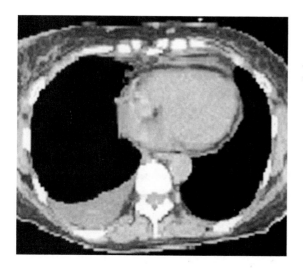

Figure 13-8.   CT scan acquired for attenuation correction, showing a right pleural effusion and a thickened pericardium.

is that if the CT scan is acquired without ECG gating, coronary calcium may be seen and can be commented on, but if not seen cannot be inferred not to be present, as the coronary arteries move during the cardiac cycle and a calcified region may simply not be in any field of view.

It is also important to inspect the transmission scans when they have been acquired using radioactive sources. Many of the same incidental findings will be easily recognized, including pleural effusions (Figure 13-9), parenchymal lung disease, and even larger lung tumors (Figure 13-10).

Emission Scans

PET perfusion emission images are consistently of higher quality than are SPECT images and afford higher diagnostic accuracy.[20,21] Scans that are normal have the following characteristics: uniform distribution of myocardial counts at stress and at rest independent of gender, and a cavity at stress that is generally equal to or smaller than the cavity

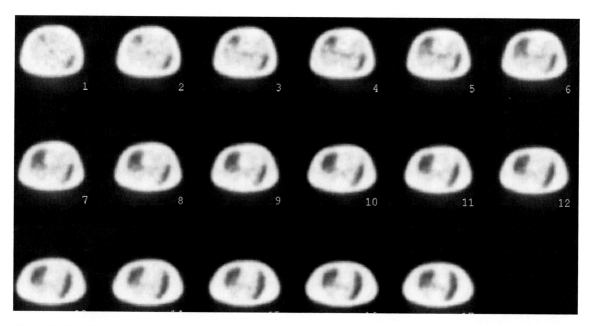

Figure 13-9.   The transmission scans obtained with radioactive sources can also be used to identify unexpected pathology. This scan shows a small right-sided pleural effusion.

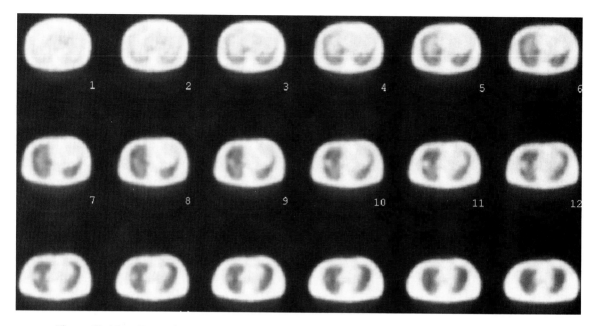

Figure 13-10. Transmission scan acquired with radioactive sources showing a right lung tumor.

at rest.[22] Ejection fraction will be higher at stress than at rest, and end-systolic volume will be lower.[23] In abnormals, there will be perfusion defects whose severity will approximate the relative degree of regional flow reduction. This is because of the superior tracer uptake characteristics in relation to coronary flows than is attainable with current SPECT tracers. The cavity is often larger at stress than at rest,[22] and, in the case of severe CAD, there may be a reduction in LVEF and an increase in end-systolic volume comparing the stress and rest images.

REFERENCES

1. Shehata AR, Gillam LD, Herman SD, et al. Impact of acute propanolol administration on dobutamine-induced myocardial ischemia as evaluated by myocardial perfusion imaging and echocardiography. *Am J Cardiol.* 1997; 80:268–272.
2. Sharir T, Rabinowitz B, Livschitz S, et al. Underestimation of extent and severity of coronary artery disease by dipyridamole stress thallium-201 single photon emission computed tomographic myocardial perfusion imaging in patients taking antianginal drugs. *J Am Coll Cardiol.* 1998;31:1540–1546.
3. Bottcher M, Refsgaard J, Madsen MM, et al. Effect of antianginal medication on resting myocardial perfusion and pharmacologically induced hyperemia. *J Nucl Cardiol.* 2003;10:345–352.
4. Taillefer R, Ahlberg AW, Masood Y, et al. Acute beta-blockade reduces the extent and severity of myocardial perfusion defects with dipyridamole Tc-99m sestamibi SPECT imaging. *J Am Coll Cardiol.* 2003;42: 1475–1483.
5. Chow BJW, Ananthasubramaniam K, deKemp RA, et al. Comparison of treadmill exercise versus dipyridamole stress with myocardial perfusion imaging using rubidium-82 positron emission tomography. *J Am Coll Cardiol.* 2005;45:1227–1234.
6. Chow BJ, Wong JW, Yoshinaga K, et al. Prognostic significance of dipyridamole induced ST depression in patients with normal Rb-82 myocardial perfusion PET imaging. *J Nucl Med.* 2005;7:1095–1101.
7. Bateman TM. Cardiac positron emission tomography and the role of adenosine pharmacologic stress. *Am J Cardiol.* 2004;94(Suppl):19D–25D.
8. Moser KW, Cullom SJ, Case JA, Hertenstein GK, Volker LL, Bateman TM. An evaluation of adenosine peak-stress myocardial perfusion imaging with ECG-gated rubidium-82 PET. *JNC.* 2005;12:S119.

9. McGhie AI, Bateman TM, Volker L, Case JA, Cullom SJ. Adenosine peak stress Rb-82 PET imaging: Feasibility and comparison with dipyridamole stress. *J Nucl Cardiol.* 2006;13:S6 (abstract).

10. Machac J, Bacharach SL, Bateman TM, et al. Positron emission tomography myocardial perfusion and glucose metabolism imaging. *J Nucl Cardiol.* 2006;13: e121–e151.

11. Moser KW, Hsu BL, Cullom SJ, Bateman TM, Case JA. Count-based attenuation maps reconstructed with a Bayesian algorithm for more efficient cardiac PET imaging. *J Nucl Med.* 2005;46:262P.

12. Hsu BL, Moser KW, Cullom JS, Bateman TM, Heller GV, Case JA. A novel Bayesian reconstruction method to correct CT image artifacts in cardiac PET/CT. *JNC.* 2005;12:S57.

13. Hsu BL, Moser KW, Bateman TM, Stoner C, Case JA. Validation of a rapid transmission scan and Bayesian reconstruction algorithm in dedicated PET imaging. *JNC.* 2005;12:S116.

14. Di Carli MF, Dorbala S, Hachamovitch R. Integrated cardiac PET-CT for the diagnosis and management of CAD. *J Nucl Cardiol.* 2006;13:139–144.

15. Loghin C, Sdringola S, Gould KL. Common artifacts in PET myocardial perfusion images due to attenuation–emission misregistration: Clinical significance, causes, and solutions. *J Nucl Med.* 2004;45:1029–1039.

16. Case JA, Heller GV, Cullom SJ, et al. Sensitivity of myocardial perfusion PET/CT imaging scan appearance on accurate transmission/emission registration. *J Nucl Cardiol.* 2005;12:S117 (abstract).

17. Thompson RC, Bateman TM, McGhie AI, O'Keefe JH, Bybee KA, Hsu BL. CT for attenuation correction in myocardial perfusion PET. *Int J Card Imaging.* 2006;822:8.

18. Goetze S, Pannu HK, Wahl RL. Clinically significant abnormal findings on the "nondiagnostic" CT portion of low-amperage-CT attenuation-corrected myocardial perfusion SPECT/CT studies. *J Nucl Med.* 2006;47: 1312–1318.

19. Osman MM, Cohade C, Fishman EK, Wahl RL. Clinically significant incidental findings on the unenhanced CT portion of PET/CT studies. *J Nucl Med.* 2005;46:1352–1357.

20. Conaway DG, Bateman TM, Moutray KL, et al. Impact of myocardial perfusion PET following non-diagnostic SPECT: Follow-up procedures and patient outcomes. *J Nucl Med.* 2005;46:58P (abstract).

21. Bateman TM, Heller GV, McGhie AI, et al. Diagnostic accuracy of rest/stress ECG-gated rubidium-82 myocardial perfusion PET: Comparison with ECG-gated Tc-99m sestamibi SPECT. *J Nucl Cardiol.* 2006;13: 24–33.

22. Bateman TM, McGhie AI, Heller GV, et al. Significance of changes in left ventricular cavity size in dipyridamole stress rubidium-82 myocardial perfusion PET. *J Am Coll Cardiol.* 2005;45:306A (abstract).

23. Goeke JA, Bateman TM, Cullom SJ, Case JA, McGhie AI. Normal limits for stress-induced changes in left ventricular function for ECG-gated dipyridamole Rb-82 PET imaging in women. *J Nucl Cardiol.* 2006;13:S9 (abstract).

CHAPTER 14

PET for Assessing Myocardial Viability

Marcelo F. Di Carli

Left ventricular (LV) function is a well-established and powerful predictor of outcome after myocardial infarction (MI).[1] Indeed, the occurrence of severe LV systolic dysfunction (i.e., LV ejection fraction <35%) post MI, especially when combined with heart failure, is associated with very poor survival if treated with medical therapy alone.[2] In selected patients, high-risk surgical revascularization appears to afford long-term survival benefit.[3] However, selection of patients with severe LV dysfunction for high-risk revascularization remains controversial.

In some patients with CAD, LV dysfunction results from MI with attendant necrosis and scar formation. However, it is now clear that in many patients such myocardial dysfunction may be reversible with revascularization; this is otherwise referred to as hibernating[4] and/or stunned[5] myocardium. Consequently, the distinction of LV dysfunction caused by fibrosis from that arising from viable but dysfunctional myocardium is a diagnostic issue with important implications for patients with low ejection fraction. In these patients, severe heart failure may be attributed to severe, widespread hibernation (or stunning or both) rather than to necrosis of a critical mass of myocardium.[6] Failure to identify patients with these potentially reversible causes of heart failure may lead to progressive cellular damage, heart failure, and death.

This chapter will review the principles of positron emission tomography (PET) viability imaging, fundamentals of patient preparation, and imaging protocols.

METHODOLOGY FOR ASSESSING MYOCARDIAL VIABILITY WITH PET

Many protocols have been proposed to evaluate myocardial viability using PET. By far, the combined assessment of regional myocardial perfusion and glucose use is the most widely used protocol in routine clinical practice. With this protocol, regional myocardial perfusion is first evaluated with PET, following the administration of ^{13}N-ammonia, [82]rubidium, or ^{15}O-water, or using SPECT with ^{99m}Tc tracers. Regional glucose use is then assessed with ^{18}F-deoxyglucose (FDG) and PET, providing an index of myocardial metabolism and, thus, cell viability.

[18F]Fluorodeoxyglucose

Normal myocardium uses a variety of energy-producing substrates to fulfill its energy requirements.[7] In the fasting state, free fatty acids (FFA) are mobilized in relatively large quantities from tryglicerides stored in adipose tissue. Thus, the increased availability of FFA in plasma makes them the preferred energy-producing fuel in the myocardium.[7] In the fed state, however, the increase in plasma glucose and the subsequent rise in insulin levels significantly reduce FFA release from adipose tissue and, consequently, its availability in plasma. In addition, the increased insulin levels mobilize glucose transporters (especially GLUT 4) onto the cell membrane, resulting in an increased transport and use of exogenous glucose by the myocardium.[8]

FFA metabolism via beta-oxidation in the mitochondria is highly dependent on oxygen availability, and, thus, it declines sharply during myocardial ischemia.[9,10] Under this condition, studies in animal experiments[9] and in humans[11] have shown that the uptake and subsequent metabolism of glucose by the ischemic myocardium are markedly increased. This shift to preferential glucose uptake plays a critical role in the survival of functionally compromised myocytes (i.e., stunned and hibernating), as glycolytically derived high-energy phosphates are thought to be critical for maintaining basic cellular functions. Consequently, noninvasive approaches that can assess the magnitude of exogenous glucose use play an important role in the evaluation of tissue viability in patients with myocardial dysfunction because of CAD. For these metabolic adaptations to occur, sufficient nutrient perfusion is required to

supply energy-rich substrates (e.g., glucose) and oxygen, and for removal of the by-products of glycolysis (e.g., lactate and hydrogen ion). A prolonged and severe reduction of myocardial blood flow rapidly precipitates depletion of high-energy phosphate, cell membrane disruption, and cellular death. Therefore, assessment of regional blood flow also provides important information regarding the presence of tissue viability within dysfunctional myocardial regions.

Imaging Protocols

Because dysfunctional myocardium that improves functionally after revascularization must retain sufficient blood flow and metabolic activity to sustain myocyte viability, the combined assessment of regional myocardial perfusion and glucose metabolism appears most attractive for delineating myocardial viability (Figure 14-1). With this approach, regional myocardial perfusion is first evaluated. Since information regarding the magnitude of stress-induced ischemia and resting viability are both important for management decisions, the ideal approach should include both rest and stress perfusion imaging. However, the selection of the approach (i.e., rest vs. stress/rest) should be tailored to the clinical question being addressed in an individual patient.

Regional glucose uptake is then assessed with FDG (a marker of exogenous glucose uptake), providing an index of myocardial metabolism and, thus, cell viability. After intravenous administration, FDG traces the initial transport of glucose across the myocyte membrane and its subsequent hexokinase-mediated phosphorylation to FDG-6-phosphate.[12] Since the latter is a poor substrate for further metabolism and is rather impermeable to the cell membrane, it becomes virtually trapped in the myocardium (Figure 14-2).

Patient Preparation for FDG Imaging

As mentioned above, use of energy-producing substrates by the heart muscle is largely a function

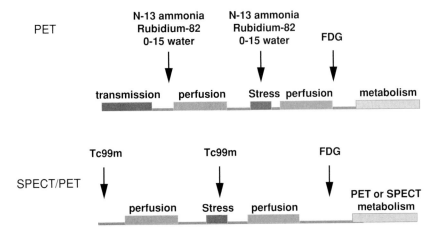

Figure 14-1.   Myocardial viability protocols using PET and the hybrid SPECT/PET approach.

of their concentration in plasma and hormone levels (especially plasma insulin, insulin/glucagon ratio, growth hormone, and catecholamines) and of oxygen availability for oxidative metabolism. For a detailed step-by-step description of the available methods for FDG imaging, the reader should review the *Guidelines for PET Imaging* published by the American Society of Nuclear Cardiology and the Society of Nuclear Medicine.[13]

These approaches for FDG imaging include the following:

1. *Fasting*: This is the simplest method because it does not require any substrate manipulation. With this approach, ischemic but viable tissue is shown as a "hot spot" because of the preferential FFA use by normal (nonischemic) myocardium.

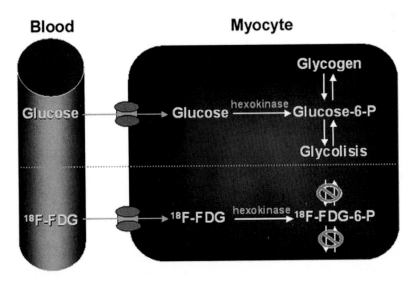

Figure 14-2.   Schematic of uptake and trapping mechanisms for FDG.

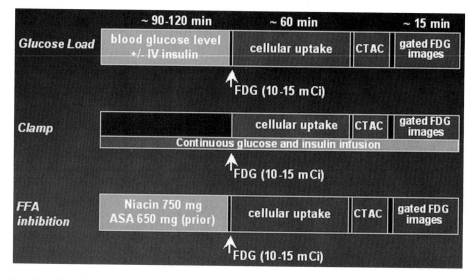

Figure 14-3.   Timeline of protocols for patient preparation before FDG imaging.

While imaging interpretation would seem straightforward, the lack of tracer uptake in normal (reference) myocardium may occasionally lead to an overestimation of the amount of residual viability within a dysfunctional territory. Indeed, the predictive accuracy of this approach is lower[14] than with the glucose-loaded approach.[15]

2. *Oral or intravenous glucose loading*: This is the most commonly used approach to FDG imaging (Figure 14-3). The goal of glucose loading is to stimulate the release of endogenous insulin in order to decrease the plasma levels of FFA and to facilitate the transport and use of FDG. Patients are usually fasted for at least 6 hours and then receive an oral or intravenous glucose load. Most patients require the administration of IV insulin to maximize myocardial FDG uptake. With this approach, image quality is generally of diagnostic quality and the reported diagnostic accuracy very good.[15]

3. *Hyperinsulinemic-euglycemic clamp*: This approach is technically demanding and time consuming (Figure 14-3). However, it provides the highest and most consistent image quality.[16] Based on the reported predictive accuracies, however, this does not necessarily translate in improved predictions of functional outcome.[17] Because it is technically demanding, most laboratories reserve this approach for challenging conditions (e.g., diabetes and severe congestive heart failure).

4. *Free-fatty acid inhibition*: Acipimox (not available in the United States) and Niacin are both nicotinic acid derivatives that inhibit peripheral lipolysis, thereby reducing plasma FFA levels and, indirectly, forcing a switch to preferential myocardial glucose use. These drugs are usually given 60 to 90 minutes prior to FDG administration (Figure 14-3). The approach is practical and provides consistent image quality.[16,18] However, Acipimox is not available for clinical use in the United States.

Myocardial Perfusion and Glucose-Loaded FDG Patterns

Using the sequential perfusion–FDG approach, four distinct perfusion–metabolism patterns can be observed in dysfunctional myocardium:

1. Normal perfusion associated with normal FDG uptake

2. Reduced perfusion associated with preserved or enhanced FDG uptake (the so-called *perfusion–metabolism mismatch*), which reflects myocardial viability (Figure 14-4)

3. Proportional reduction in perfusion and FDG uptake (the so-called *perfusion–metabolism match*), which reflects nonviable myocardium (Figure 14-4)

4. Normal or near-normal perfusion with reduced FDG uptake (the so-called *reversed perfusion–metabolism mismatch*) (Figure 14-5)[19,20]

The patterns of normal perfusion and metabolism or of a PET mismatch identify potentially reversible myocardial dysfunction; the PET match pattern identifies irreversible myocardial dysfunction. The reversed perfusion–FDG mismatch has been described in the context of repetitive myocardial stunning[19] and in patients with left bundle branch block.[20] Quantitation of regional myocardial perfusion and FDG tracer uptake and their difference can be helpful to objectively assess the magnitude of viability.

Combining SPECT Perfusion and FDG PET Imaging

In current clinical practice, FDG PET images are often performed and interpreted in combination

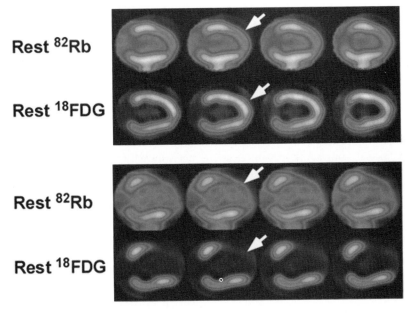

Figure 14-4.   Top panel: Mid-ventricular long-axis slices of myocardial perfusion (obtained with [82]Rb) and FDG uptake demonstrating decreased perfusion in the anterior LV wall (arrow) with preserved FDG uptake, consistent with viable myocardium (the so-called perfusion–metabolic mismatch). Bottom panel: Mid-ventricular long-axis slices of myocardial perfusion (obtained with [82]Rb) and FDG uptake demonstrating concordant reduction in perfusion and FDG uptake in the anterior LV wall (arrow), consistent with nonviable myocardium (the so-called perfusion–metabolic match).

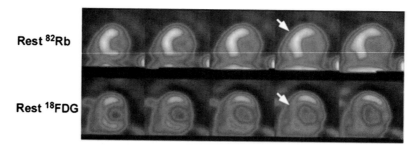

Figure 14-5.   Mid-ventricular short-axis slices of myocardial perfusion (obtained with [82]Rb) and FDG uptake demonstrating preserved perfusion to the anterior and septal walls (arrow) with reduced FDG uptake (the so-called perfusion–metabolic reversed mismatch). This pattern has been associated with myocardial stunning[19] and with LBBB.[20]

with SPECT myocardial perfusion images (Figure 14-1). The interpretation of the specific viability patterns shown in Figures 14-4 and 14-5 should be performed carefully, especially when comparing non-attenuation-corrected SPECT myocardial perfusion images with attenuation-corrected FDG PET images. Myocardial regions showing an excessive reduction in tracer concentration as a result of attenuation artifacts on the perfusion images, such as the inferior wall or the anterior wall in females, may result in falsely positive perfusion–FDG mismatches. Two approaches have proved useful for overcoming this limitation. First, because assessment of viability is relevant only in myocardium with regional contractile dysfunction, gated SPECT or gated PET images offer a means for determining whether apparent perfusion defects are associated with abnormal regional wall motion. Second, quantitative analysis of regional myocardial perfusion using polar map displays that are compared to tracer- and (for SPECT images) gender-specific databases may be a useful aid to the visual interpretation.

Gated Imaging to Assess LV Volumes and Function

FDG PET provides excellent gated images, and the parameters of global and regional LV function derived from these images correlate closely with those obtained with MRI.[21] As mentioned above, gated images are particularly useful when FDG PET patterns are interpreted in relation to non-attenuation-corrected SPECT perfusion images. In addition, measures of global LV function and remodeling (i.e., LVEF and volumes) are also useful for predicting improvement in LV function after revascularization.[22] Indeed, increased LV volumes and cavity size are predictors of poor outcome in patients with ischemic cardiomyopathy who are undergoing CABG. For example, a preoperative LV end-diastolic dimension 70 mm, as assessed by echocardiography, has been shown to be a marker of poor outcome after revascularization.[23] Similarly, others have shown that a preoperative LV end-systolic volume index (LVESVI) >100 mL/m^2, as assessed by contrast left ventriculography, was a predictor of mortality and postoperative heart failure.[24] Patients with LVESVI >100 mL/m^2 failed to improve regional and global LV function after CABG, resulting in lower survival and a higher probability of postoperative heart failure. Significantly, these poor results in patients with severe LV dilation were observed even in the patients with severe anginal symptoms, suggesting that progressive LV remodeling after MI may limit the benefits of revascularization on ventricular function and survival, even if there is evidence of viable (ischemic) myocardium.

CONCLUSIONS

PET imaging is an accurate and reproducible technique for the noninvasive evaluation of myocardial ischemia and viability. The FDG approach can be technically challenging, especially in patients with diabetes and congestive heart failure, and aggressive patient preparation is mandatory to optimize diagnostic accuracy. The available evidence suggests that this approach can provide accurate predictions of functional, symptomatic, and prognostic improvement after revascularization and, thus, improve management decisions in patients with poor cardiac function.

REFERENCES

1. Risk stratification and survival after myocardial infarction. *N Engl J Med.* 1983;309:331–336.
2. Emond M, Mock, MB, Davis, KB, et al. Long-term survival of medically treated patients in the Coronary Artery Surgery Study (CASS) Registry. *Circulation.* 1994;90:2645–2657.
3. Baker D, Jones R, Hodges J, Massie BM, Konstam MA, Rose EA. Management of heart failure. III. The role of revascularization in the treatment of patients with moderate or severe left ventricular systolic dysfunction. *JAMA.* 1994;272:1528–1534.
4. Rahimtoola SH. The hibernating myocardium. *Am Heart J.* 1989;117:211–221.
5. Braunwald E, Kloner RA. The stunned myocardium: Prolonged, postischemic ventricular dysfunction. *Circulation.* 1982;66:1146–1149.
6. Di Carli MF, Asgarzadie F, Schelbert HR, et al. Quantitative relation between myocardial viability and improvement in heart failure symptoms after revascularization in patients with ischemic cardiomyopathy. *Circulation.* 1995;92:3436–3444.
7. Opie LH. *The Heart. Physiology and Metabolism.* 2nd ed. New York: Raven Press; 1991.
8. Young LH, Coven DL, Russell RR III. Cellular and molecular regulation of cardiac glucose transport. *J Nucl Cardiol.* 2000;7:267–276.
9. Opie LH. Effects of regional ischemia on metabolism of glucose and fatty acids. *Circ Res.* 1976;38:152–174.
10. Liedtke AJ. Alterations of carbohydrate and lipid metabolism in the acutely ischemic heart. *Progr Cardiovasc Dis.* 1981;23:321–336.
11. Camici P, Araujo LI, Spinks T, et al. Increase uptake of 18F-fluorodeoxyglucose in postischemic myocardium of patients with exercise-induced angina. *Circulation.* 1986;74:81–88.
12. Phelps ME, Hoffman EJ, Selin C, et al. Investigation of [18F]2-fluoro-2-deoxyglucose for the measure of myocardial glucose metabolism. *J Nucl Med.* 1978;19:1311–1319.
13. Bacharach SL, Bax JJ, Case J, et al. PET myocardial glucose metabolism and perfusion imaging with 18FDG, 13NH3 and 82Rb. Part 1—Guidelines for data acquisition and patient preparation. *J Nucl Cardiol.* 2003;10:545–556.
14. Tamaki N, Yonekura Y, Yamashita K, et al. Positron emission tomography using fluorine-18 deoxyglucose in evaluation of coronary artery bypass grafting. *Am J Cardiol.* 1989;64:860–865.
15. Schoder H, Campisi R, Ohtake T, et al. Blood flow-metabolism imaging with positron emission tomography in patients with diabetes mellitus for the assessment of reversible left ventricular contractile dysfunction. *J Am Coll Cardiol.* 1999;33:1328–1337.
16. Bax JJ, Veening MA, Visser FC, et al. Optimal metabolic conditions during fluorine-18 fluorodeoxyglucose imaging; a comparative study using different protocols. *Eur J Nucl Med.* 1997;24:35–41.
17. Pagano D, Bonser RS, Townend JN, Ordoubadi F, Lorenzoni R, Camici PG. Predictive value of dobutamine echocardiography and positron emission tomography in identifying hibernating myocardium in patients with postischaemic heart failure. *Heart.* 1998;79:281–288.
18. Vitale GD, deKemp RA, Ruddy TD, Williams K, Beanlands RS. Myocardial glucose utilization and optimization of (18)F-FDG PET imaging in patients with non-insulin-dependent diabetes mellitus, coronary artery disease, and left ventricular dysfunction. *J Nucl Med.* 2001;42:1730–1736.
19. Di Carli MF, Prcevski P, Singh TP, et al. Myocardial blood flow, function, and metabolism in repetitive stunning. *J Nucl Med.* 2000;41:1227–1234.
20. Nowak B, Sinha AM, Schaefer WM, et al. Cardiac resynchronization therapy homogenizes myocardial glucose metabolism and perfusion in dilated cardiomyopathy and left bundle branch block. *J Am Coll Cardiol.* 2003;41:1523–1528.
21. Schaefer WM, Lipke CS, Nowak B, et al. Validation of an evaluation routine for left ventricular volumes, ejection fraction and wall motion from gated cardiac FDG PET: A comparison with cardiac magnetic resonance imaging. *Eur J Nucl Med Mol Imaging.* 2003;30:545–553.
22. Yamaguchi A, Ino T, Adachi H, Mizuhara A, Murata S,

Kamio H. Left ventricular end-systolic volume index in patients with ischemic cardiomyopathy predicts postoperative ventricular function. *Ann Thorac Surg.* 1995;60:1059–1062.

23. Louie HW, Laks H, Milgalter E, et al. Ischemic cardiomyopathy. Criteria for coronary revascularization and cardiac transplantation. *Circulation.* 1991;84: III290–III295.

24. Yamaguchi A, Ino T, Adachi H, et al. Left ventricular volume predicts postoperative course in patients with ischemic cardiomyopathy. *Ann Thorac Surg.* 1998;65: 434–438.

CHAPTER 15

Attenuation and Scatter Correction in Cardiac PET

James A. Case

Bai-Ling Hsu

INTRODUCTION

From the past decade to recent years, cardiac positron emission tomography (PET) with Rb-82 or N-13-ammonia perfusion tracers has been recognized as a clearly superior imaging method over myocardial perfusion single-photon emission computed tomography (SPECT) for accessing a patient's coronary artery disease.[1-7] One of the major attractions of cardiac PET imaging is the relative simplicity of attenuation and scatter correction when compared to myocardial perfusion SPECT imaging. Attenuation and scatter correction for PET is both straightforward and necessary when the correction techniques have been solidly built for clinical use day by day. One of the consequences of routinely applied attenuation and scatter correction in PET is a measurable improvement in diagnostic accuracy. Since the early introduction of myocardial perfusion PET imaging, most studies directly comparing SPECT and PET demonstrate improved accuracy (mainly specificity) with

PET.[1-4] More recently, in a retrospective study of 112 matched Rb-82 PET and SPECT (same-day Tc-99m sestamibi studies), patients demonstrated an overall improvement in sensitivity of 79% (SPECT) to 89% (PET) for 70% lesions ($p = 0.03$).[6] For multivessel detection, the improvement was more dramatic: 48% (SPECT) to 71% (PET) ($p = 0.02$). In addition, overall reader confidence was substantially improved using Rb-82 myocardial perfusion PET imaging versus Tc-99m sestamibi imaging. Specificity was also improved from 73% (SPECT) to 93% (PET). Although this study did not specifically look at the incremental gain of applying attenuation and scatter correction in PET, since both corrections are required in PET, it did demonstrate significant improvements over SPECT in diagnostic accuracy in areas known to be challenging, as soft-tissue attenuation and photon scatter are largely overcome.

Photon attenuation is recognized as one of the most significant sources of diagnostic uncertainty in myocardial perfusion SPECT imaging.

Despite the recommendations to perform attenuation correction from the American College of Cardiology, American Society of Nuclear Cardiology, and the Society of Nuclear Medicine,[8,9] most myocardial perfusion SPECT studies were performed without attenuation correction. For most clinicians, there are two major reasons for not performing attenuation correction: (1) inconsistent results from different attenuation correction systems require clinicians to look at both attenuation- and non-attenuation-corrected data set for diagnosis and (2) added cost of performing attenuation correction. In contrast, virtually all myocardial perfusion PET studies are performed with attenuation correction because attenuation correction is relatively simple, accurate, and necessary. This routine use of attenuation correction is likely one of the major reasons that PET has significantly higher diagnostic specificity when compared to SPECT.

A less recognized limitation of SPECT is the presence of scattered photons in the photopeak window. These photons reduce defect contrast and render a significant number of nondiagnostic cases. Myocardial perfusion PET is routinely corrected for scatter. This may be part of the reason for observations of increased sensitivity and image quality with scatter correction.[6]

BASIC PHYSICS OF ATTENUATION IN PET

The origin of attenuation in myocardial perfusion PET imaging is identical to that in SPECT: photon scatter off of electron in the patient. The fundamental reaction can be described by two physics phenomena as Compton scatter and photoelectric effects. However, because these photons are of considerably higher energy than typical SPECT photons, they almost exclusively scatter via Compton scattering: a photon knocks out an electron using part of its energy, resulting in ionization of the atom.[10]

The Compton scattering cross section of 511-keV photons colliding with electrons is considerably less than it is for photons commonly used for SPECT imaging (72 keV, 141 keV, etc.); therefore, the amount of photons attenuated per unit length is much lower at 511 keV, as a result of a lower attenuation coefficient (0.183 cm^{-1} for Tl-201 (72 keV), 0.15 cm^{-1} for Tc-99m (140 keV), and 0.098 cm^{-1} for positron annihilation (511 keV)) (Figure 15-1). Annihilation photons scattered by the medium will lose energy as a function of the angle these are scattered into. For these photons, the Compton formula assumes a simple form:

$$E' = \frac{511\,keV}{2 - \cos(\theta)}$$

Most of the scattered photons in the patient are scattered into angles that either miss the detector or are below the acceptance energy of the PET scanner. For example, a modern PET/CT system would have an energy window of $\pm 15\%$ or a lower acceptance window of 425 keV to reject Compton-scattered photons from 511 keV.[11] This corresponds to a scattering angle of 37 degrees, compared to the 53 degree acceptance angle for Tc-99m photons in SPECT imaging (20% energy window). For this reason, the vast majority, almost 80%, of scattered photons are scattered into angles that allow them to be excluded by the energy discrimination of the camera and, thereby, are considered completely attenuated by the medium. However, that is not to say that scatter is not an important consideration, as will be discussed later.

ATTENUATION CORRECTION IN PET

In PET, it is necessary to measure both of the photons that are emitted from an annihilation event. Because of this, the amount of attenuation that is measured for a single coincidence is the sum of the attenuation along the entire line of sight (in contrast to SPECT, where the total attenuation is from the source to the detector). In a 180-degree acquisition, attenuation correction of PET is necessary because the amount of attenuating medium that the coincidence pair must penetrate is considerably

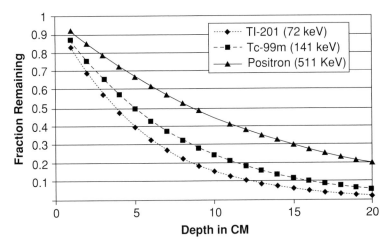

Figure 15-1.   Photon attenuation of 72 (TI-201), 141 (Tc-99m), and 511 keV (position emitter) corresponded to distance. With smaller attenuation coefficient compared to SPECT, 511-keV photons have less attenuation at the same distance.

more than in SPECT (Figure 15-2). In a typical patient study, the attenuation length can be as much as 40 cm or more. However, because of the unique property of depth-independent attenuation, applying attenuation correction is rather simple for PET attenuation. By multiplying each pixel of the attenuation correction factor, the sinogram data can be corrected for attenuation. In contrast, SPECT attenuation correction is applied iteratively during image reconstruction.

OBTAIN ATTENUATION ESTIMATE

Dedicated PET System

A dedicated PET system uses external rod or point sources to project gamma radiation through the patient. The most common external source is a system of rotating rod sources, typically loaded with Ge-68 (a positron emitter, half-life = 270 days) or point sources with Cs-137 (gamma photon emitter, 662 keV, half-life = 30.7 years). The

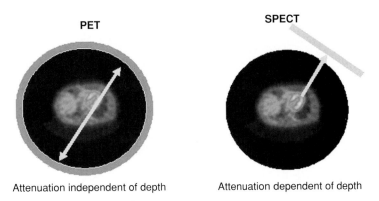

Attenuation independent of depth   Attenuation dependent of depth

Figure 15-2.   Detection of coincidence pair results in depth-independent attenuation in PET, as opposed to SPECT with depth-dependent attenuation. (See color insert.)

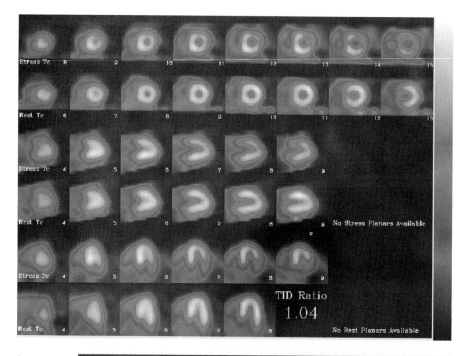

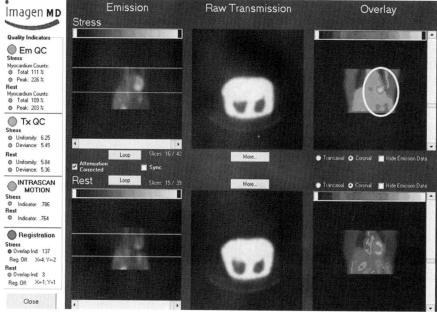

Figure 15-3. An example of transmission/emission misregistration in cardiac PET. Part of the myocardium in the lung fields creates perfusion defects in lateral and high-lateral segments (top row). With proper realignment in both lateral and axial directions, the images show normal perfusion in those segments (bottom row). (See color insert.)

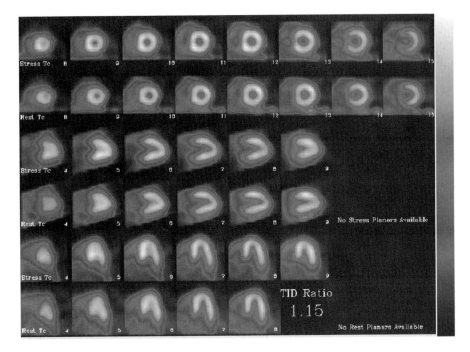

Figure 15-3. (*Continued*)

advantage of performing dedicate PET myocardial perfusion imaging is that the transmission and emission data both represent an average of diaphragm positions of multiple cardiac and breath cycles, making the technique for attenuation correction robust and accurate. The major drawback with dedicated PET imaging is that the transmission imaging times are often prolonged, in order to obtain accurate attenuation estimate. Another limitation is the common use of positron emitters as a transmission source. As the transmission and emission photons are at the same energy, simultaneous imaging is not possible. This incapability reduces the efficiency of the imaging protocol and introduces the possibility of misregistration between the transmission and emission data sets (Figure 15-3 (center)).

Recent advances in reconstruction algorithms have been introduced to significantly reduce the transmission acquisition times. Hsu et al. reported that with acquisition times as short as 70 seconds, there was little difference between high-count filtered backprojection images and their OSEM-based Bayesian reconstruction[12] (Figure 15-4). Considering the improvements that have been made in the acquisition times using the OSEM-B algorithm, the use of a dedicated PET scanner for myocardial perfusion PET imaging is robust, accurate, and efficient.

Hybrid PET/CT System

In recent years, the use of combined PET and CT (X-ray computed tomography) has become standard in the diagnosis and management of cancer. However, the utility of PET/CT for the management of cardiovascular disease is currently being developed.[13] X-ray computed tomography was first demonstrated in 1972[14] and was awarded the Noble prize in 1978 for its demonstrated value to medicine. This technique uses a rotating X-ray tube to acquire a series of transmission images around the patient. The quality of the CT image is governed by several parameters:

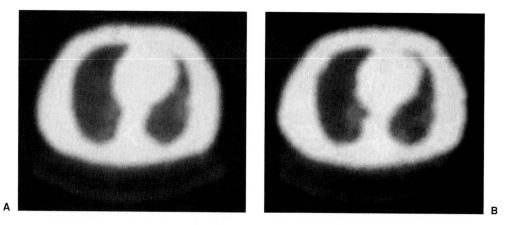

Figure 15-4.   Ge-68 maps reconstructed with OSEM-B algorithm: (**A**) acquired with 4 minutes (65 million cts) and (**B**) 70 seconds (20 million cts). The shortened TX scan does not show significant difference of map quality as compared to the longer TX scan.

1. Tube voltage (measured in kVp): The higher the tube voltage the higher the photon energy produced by the X-ray tube, typically 80 to 140 kVp.

2. Tube current (mAs): Measure of the current in the X-ray tube. The higher the current the higher the signal-to-noise ratio in the image, Typically between 10 and 250 mAs, depending on the application.

3. In-plane resolution: The resolution of a pixel within a particular tomographic slice, typically 0.5 to 1.0 mm.

4. Axial resolution (or slice thickness): Typically much large than in-plane resolution, 1.5 to 5 mm.

5. Number of slices: A measure of the number of slices that can be simultaneously acquired for each rotation of the CT scanner. The higher the number of slices, the larger the volume in each slice and the faster the scan time. The faster the scan time, the more flexibility the user will have on breathing protocols.

The primary use of the cardiac CT image in myocardial perfusion PET imaging is to create a high-quality transmission imaging for attenuation correction. X-ray computed tomography is different from radionuclide-based tomography in that the X-rays are produced with relatively low-energy, polyenergetic photons from an X-ray tube. To use an X-ray-based CT transmission image as an attenuation estimate, attenuation coefficients must be translated from Houndsfield units to the standard units of attenuation (cm^{-1}) at 511 keV. The simplest approach is to use a linear model for adapting the CT transmission data to the 511-keV attenuation coefficients.[15] This has the limitation of assigning systematically high attenuation confidents for bone and higher-density material. A more sophisticated algorithm using a two-stage model for mapping the X-ray CT transmission data has been developed and shown to provide a much more robust and accurate mapping between the CT and 511-keV attenuation coefficients.[16]

One of the challenges facing clinicians in using PET/CT for myocardial perfusion imaging is assessing the relative value of acquiring a diagnostic-quality CT imaging on a patient who is being assessed for obstructive coronary disease. Although the relative radiation risk for a patient who is being imaged with higher radiation dose is relatively small, what to do with clinical CT data remains undefined. Anecdotally, secondary findings and the presence of coronary calcium appear to be useful in the management of patients imaged with PET/CT. However, it has not been demonstrated what value clinicians should place on those secondary findings, how they should be interpreted, and what obligations and training are assumed when interpreting diagnostic-quality PET/CT images. Until these challenges are better understood, limiting patient radiation exposure is an important consideration.

CORRECTION FOR SCATTER IN PET

Physically similar to SPECT, Compton scatter in PET is a result of the interaction of emitted photons with the attenuating medium (e.g., patient). When photons scatter off the electrons in the medium, they impart some of their energy to the electrons, thereby reducing the energy of the resulting photon. In PET, most of the scatter photons can be excluded as a result of this change in energy (Compton scattering). However, scattered photons, which have a final energy high enough to be included in the final image, will degrade the image quality and potentially introduce artifacts (Figure 15-5). The major impacts of Compton scatter in cardiac PET imaging are decreased image contrast of the myocardial boundary, the reduced size, and the depth of perfusion defects and spillover from extra activity (Figure 15-6 (top row)).

The energy resolution of a PET system is directly related to the light output of the scintillator crystal used. BGO-based scanner systems employ an energy window from 350 to 720 keV. LSO scintillator-based scanners have 3.75 times the light output of BGO and can use a more narrow energy window, typically from 425 to 650 keV. Another technique for reducing scatter in PET imaging is to employ a system of lead septa to separate coincidence events in the transverse direction. When the sinogram data are acquired in two-dimensional (2D, septa extended), the scatter fraction (the ratio between the number of scatter events and the total number of coincidence events) ranges from 10% to 15%,[17] depending on the scanner geometry, the energy window, and the patient size. With septa retracted or no septa in the 3D mode, the scatter fraction can even increase to 30% to 50%,[17] depending on the maximum ring difference and span of the 3D data acquisition.[18]

For 2D PET imaging, nonstationary convolution-subtraction methods have been used to compensate for the impact of scatter on the photon-peak image. These methods utilize a model based on a point spread function dependent on locations, object size, etc.[19,20] The methods of 3D scatter correction require more robust modeling. These models primarily rely on physical models for simulating the scatter

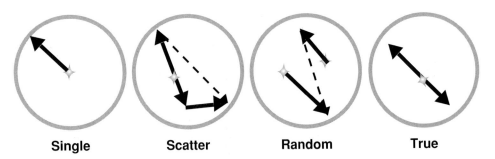

Single   **Scatter**   **Random**   **True**

Figure 15-5.   Four different types of events in PET. The LOR of scatter event is created when one or both 511-keV photons interact with the attenuating medium.

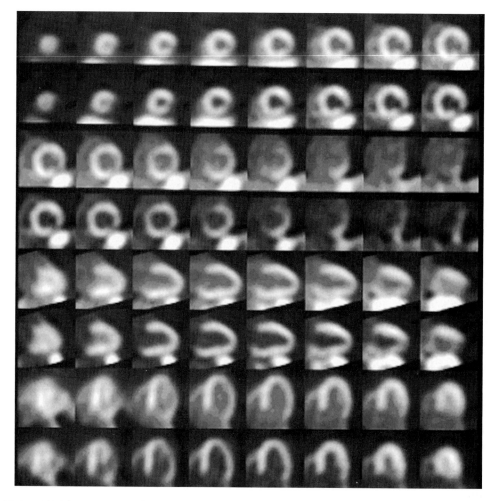

Figure 15-6.   3D Rb-82 images w/o (top row) and with scatter correction (bottom row).[17] The scatter-corrected images show improved image contrast with free of hot-spot artifact in the myocardial wall adjacent to the hot bowel.

process.[21,22–26] These models use a patient-specific attenuation map obtained from a transmission scan (either external radionuclide source or x-ray CT).

Scatter correction of myocardium perfusion PET images is essential for maintaining defect sensitivity. Although PET scatter artifacts are less spatially correlated to the source distribution than what is seen in SPECT, they do represent a significant degradation in image quality. For this reason, all PET images are routinely corrected for photon scatter, in addition to correcting for attenuation.

CHALLENGES FOR ATTENUATION AND SCATTER CORRECTION IN PET

TX/EM Misregistration

Misregistration between transmission and emission data sets has been recognized as major source image artifacts in myocardial perfusion Rb-82 PET imaging. In a study of rest myocardial perfusion images, it was observed that 21% of all resting perfusion studies have a significant amount of misregistration.[28] Although this study did not look at the prevalence of misregistration in stress studies, experience indicates that the prevalence of misregistration in stress imaging may be significantly higher.

In a recent study, it was demonstrated that misregistration of more than 7.8 mm in the left lateral direction did introduce a significant change in the septal and lateral wall ratios.[29] Furthermore, misregistration in both the positive transverse ("up") and the negative transaxial ("down") resulted in significant changes in the anterior to inferior wall ratios. In contrast, opposite translations (right lateral and negative transverse) may not introduce a significant artifact in the emission images.

Misregistration artifacts are most common in the anterior, high lateral, and lateral walls of the heart and can often be mistaken for left circumflex, diagonal, or left main disease (although misregistration artifact can introduce unusual finding in all vascular territories) (Figure 15-3 (top)). Because the artifacts arise in high-risk regions of the heart, they are difficult to overlook with substantial complimentary evidence. Misregistration artifacts are best detected by careful examination of fused transmission and emission data (Figure 15-3 (center)). Although some investigators have looked at using external marker, these have been shown to be of limited value because of cardiac and diaphragmatic motion. The careful examination of the combined (or fused) transmission and emission data sets is a required quality control step on every patient regardless of whether or not misregistration is suspected.

Compensation for misregistration is relatively intuitive and should be considered a necessary step in image processing. The most common technique for re-registering the images is using a rigid translation of the transmission data relative to the emission data. Either visually or as a process of trial and error, a set of 3D offsets is determined for the emission data. The emission sinogram is then adjusted

to represent a different center of rotation and then reconstructed.

Some authors have considered modifying the transmission images by growing attenuation coefficients to soft-tissue values in lung region where the heart is mispositioned into because of patient motion.[30] This technique may not be capable of performing accurate attenuation compensation, as the original attenuation determined by the transmission maps is no longer conserved.

Diaphragm Motion

A major challenge in cardiac PET/CT is how to merge the rapidly acquired CT data with the PET data that are integrated over several minutes. The difficulty arises in coregistering the diaphragm positions during the respiratory cycle with the average position that is present during the PET acquisition. Diaphragm motion can introduce a wide variety of artifacts ranging from regions of artificial hot and cold areas to more realistic dark artifacts resembling hypoperfusion.

Several investigators have explored the use of different breathing protocols to reduce the impact of diaphragm motion. It has been reported that a slow scan with a shallow free breath protocol has produced high-quality results.[31] More recently, others have reported success using an end-expiration breath-hold protocol.[32,33] This latter protocol is typically more practical with scanners capable of performing a chest CT in less than 10 seconds (8- and 16-slice PET/CT systems).

Another approach is to acquire sequential respiratory-gated CT used to create attenuation data similar to data acquired with multiple breathing cycles with radionuclide rod sources.[34] Although the technique may be capable of simulating free-breathing transmission by averaging multiple-phased CT images, it can introduce higher radiation exposure. Compared to routine diagnostic CT, the CT dose in such a protocol is also considerably high (23–70 mGy), particularly without the ability to provide physicians with useful clinical information from CT images, given such a high dose.

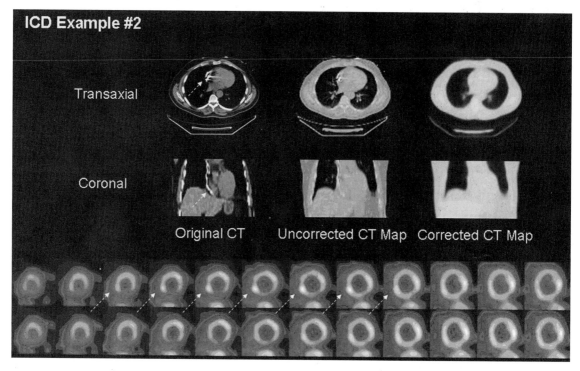

Figure 15-7. An example of a patient who wears intravascular cardiodefibrillator (ICD) whose tip locates next to the septal wall. The metal object in CT maps produces focal tracer artifacts in Rb-82 images. The artifact can be removed with corrected CT maps. (See color insert.)

Implanted Devices

Implanted devices are another major challenge for attenuation correction. DiFilippo and Brunken demonstrated that metal artifacts from implanted devices such as pacemakers, intravascular cardiodefibrillator (ICD), and surgical clips can introduce significant artifacts in the attenuation-corrected myocardial perfusion PET image[35] (Figure 15-7). At present, very few solutions exist for correcting the artifacts caused by metal artifacts. Hsu et al. developed a correction algorithm without using CT sinogram data. The method effectively removes metal objects in CT images and corrects for the streak artifact and beam-hardening effect accompanied with metal objects using OSEM-B transmission reconstruction algorithm.[36] Another method was independently developed by Hamill et al., which gives a similar performance in metal artifact reduction.[37]

3D Scatter Correction

The challenges for model-based scatter correction for fully 3D PET data are the substantially demanded computation when the simulation takes into account a large number of scattering points and multiple scatter events. Single scatter simulation (SSS) as only one of the two 511-keV photons is considered scatter, and coarse sampling of scatter sites has been used to accelerate the computation speed with preserved accuracy.[17,23] As originally developed, most algorithms do not consider scatter from outside the FOV. Some implementation took the effect of multiple scattering into

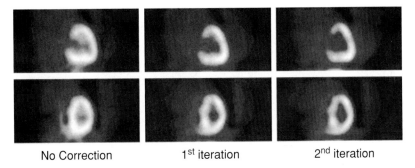

No Correction   1st iteration   2nd iteration

Figure 15-8.   Image example of fast Monte Carlo scatter correction of fully 3D PET.

account by convolving the estimated single scatter component with a Gaussian function and approximates the contribution from activity out of FOV empirically.[25] Accounted for multiple scatter and adequate normalization of activity profile were reported to be crucial for stabilizing the performance of analytical model-based methods.[17] Figure 15-6 (bottom row) shows the effect of scatter correction with an analytical method.[17]

Monte Carlo methods give an insight of scatter process in PET and potentially offer an accurate correction procedure.[26,27] Direct Monte Carlo scatter compensation approach intrinsically accounts for the contribution of multiple scatter and scatter from out of FOV. Although sophisticated simulation has been proposed to effectively eliminate scatter problem in 3D PET imaging,[26] it is recognized that a direct Monte Carlo scatter correction may not be practical for clinical routine applications with common computing facilities. The complexity and computing requirements of Monte Carlo simulation demand new development of simulation tools upon simplifying approximations to improve the speed of operation. More recent approaches use a hybrid scatter-correction method for fully 3D PET by combining Monte Carlo approach and fast statistical reconstruction. This method uses Monte Carlo simulation for only simulating single scatter events in image and incorporates with a coarse sampling approach to accelerate the speed. When the scatter is estimated from simulation, the method removes scatter from sinogram data with a statistical-type reconstruction that preserves the noise property in original data Figure 15-8.

The challenge of cardiac PET continues. The introduction of LSO-crystal PET/CT system with higher photon sensitivity and listmode acquisition of dynamic and ECG-triggered data ideally create a new imaging method of cardiac PET with more consistent image quality across a broad range of patient populations.[33,38] Recent breakthrough in electronic timing limitation moves time-of-flight PET a step forward for clinical use.[39] Optimal data processing has been proposed for time-of-flight PET based on the methods previously developed for traditional PET.[40-42] Although time-of-flight PET can perform improved signal-to-noise level with a better ability to resolve small structures,[43,44] effective corrections for attenuation, scatter, and other imaging factors would still be the turnkeys to prove whether time-of-flight PET can outperform traditional PET, hopefully moving time-of-flight PET a step closer to clinical use.

REFERENCES

1. Tamaki N, Yorekura Y, Senda M, et al. Value and limitation of stress thallium-201 single photon emission computed tomography: Comparison with nitrogen-13 ammonia positron tomography. *J Nucl Med.* 1988;29: 1181–1188.
2. Go RT, Marwick TH, MacIntyre WJ, et al. A prospective comparison of rubidium-82 PET and thallium-201 SPECT myocardial perfusion imaging utilizing a single

dipyridamole stress in the diagnosis of coronary artery disease. *J Nucl Med.* 1990;31:1899–1905.

3. Berman DS, Kiat H, Van Train KF, Friedman J, Garcia EV, Maddahi J. Comparison of SPECT using technetium-99m agents and thallium-201 and PET for the assessment of myocardial perfusion and viability. *Am J Cardiol.* 1990;66(13):72E–79E.

4. Stewart RE, Schwaiger M, Molina E, Popma J, Gacioch GM, Kalus M. Comparison of rubidium-82 PET and thallium-201 SPECT imaging for detection of coronary artery disease. *Am J Cardiol.* 1991;67: 1303–1310.

5. Lodge MA, Braess H, Mahmoud F, et al. Developments in nuclear cardiology: Transition from single photon emission computed tomography to positron emission tomography-computed tomography [review]. *J Invasive Cardiol.* 2005;17(9):491–496.

6. Bateman TM, Heller GV, McGhie AI, et al. Diagnostic accuracy of rest/stress ECG-gated Rb-82 myocardial perfusion PET: Comparison with ECG-gated Tc-99m sestamibi SPECT. *J Nucl Cardiol.* 2006;13(1): 24–33.

7. Di Carli MF, Hachamovitch R. Should PET replace SPECT for evaluating CAD? The end of the beginning. *J Nucl Cardiol.* 2006;13(1):2–7.

8. Klocke FJ, Baird MG, Lorell BH, et al.; American College of Cardiology; American Heart Association; American Society for Nuclear Cardiology. ACC/AHA/ ASNC guidelines for the clinical use of cardiac radionuclide imaging—executive summary: A report of the American College of Cardiology/American Heart Association Task Force on Practice Guidelines (ACC/AHA/ASNC Committee to Revise the 1995 Guidelines for the Clinical Use of Cardiac Radionuclide Imaging). *J Am Coll Cardiol.* 2003;42(7):1318–1333.

9. Heller GV, Links J, Bateman TM, et al. American Society of Nuclear Cardiology and Society of Nuclear Medicine joint position statement: Attenuation correction of myocardial perfusion SPECT scintigraphy. *J Nucl Cardiol.* 2004;11(2):229–230.

10. Cherry SR, Sorenson JA, Phelps ME. *Physics in Nuclear Medicine.* Chapter 6. Philadelphia, PA: Saunders/ Elsevier Science; 2003. ISBN 0-7216-8342-X.

11. Erdi YE, Nehmeh SA, Mulnix T, Humm JL, Watson CC. PET performance measurements for an LSO-based combined PET/CT scanner using the National Electrical Manufacturers Association NU 2-2001 standard. *J Nucl Med.* 2004;45(5):813–821.

12. Hsu BL, Case JA, Moser KW, Bateman TM, Cullom SJ. Reconstruction of rapidly acquired Germanium-68 transmission scans for cardiac PET attenuation correction. *J Nucl Cardiol.* 2007;14(5):706–714.

13. Di Carli MF, Dorbala S. Integrated PET/CT for cardiac imaging [review]. *Q J Nucl Med Mol Imaging.* 2006; 50(1):44–52.

14. Hounsfield GN. A method of and apparatus for examination of the body by radiation such as X or gamma radiation. British patent No. 1283915;1972.

15. Kinahan PE, Townsend DW, Beyer T, Sashin D. Attenuation correction for a combined 3D PET/CT scanner. *Med Phys.* 1998;25(10):2046–2053.

16. Carney JP, Townsend DW, Rappoport V, Bendriem B. Method for transforming CT images for attenuation correction in PET/CT imaging. *Med Phys.* 2006;33(4): 976–983.

17. Visvikis D, Griffiths D, Costa DC, Bomanji J, Ell PJ. Clinical evaluation of 2D versus 3D whole-body PET image quality using a dedicated BGO PET scanner. *Eur J Nucl Med Mol Imaging.* 2005;32(9):1050–1056.

18. Fahey FH. Data acquisition in PET imaging. *J Nucl Med Technol.* 2002;30(2):39–49.

19. Bentourkia M, Msaki P, Cadorette J, Lecomte R. Nonstationary scatter subtraction-restoration in high-resolution PET. *J Nucl Med.* 1996;37(12): 2040–2046.

20. Bentourkia M, Lecomte R. Energy dependence of nonstationary scatter subtraction—restoration in high resolution PET. *IEEE Trans Med Imaging.* 1999; 18(1):66–73.

21. Watson CC. New, faster, image-based scatter correction for 3D PET. *IEEE Trans Nucl Sci.* 2000;47:1587–1594.

22. Levin CS, Dahlbom M, Hoffman EJ. A Monte Carlo correction for the effect of Compton scattering in 3-D PET brain imaging. *IEEE Trans Nucl Sci.* 1995;42: 1181–1188.

23. Watson CC, Newport D, Casey ME, deKemp A, Beanlands RS, Schmand M. Evaluation of simulation-based scatter correction for 3-D PET cardiac imaging. *IEEE Trans Nucl Sci.* 1997;44:90–97.

24. Ollinger JM. Model-based scatter correction for fully 3D PET. *Phys Med Biol.* 1996;41:153–176.

25. Zaidi H. Statistical reconstruction-based scatter correction: A new method for 3D PET. *Proc 22nd Annu Int Conf IEEE.* 2000;1:86–89.

26. Zaidi H. Relevance of accurate Monte Carlo modeling in nuclear medical imaging. *Med Phys.* 1999;26: 574–608.

27. Attix FH. *Introduction to Radiological Physics and Radiation Dosimetry.* Chapter 7. New York: John Wiley & Sons; 1986.

28. Gould KL, Pan T, Loghin C, Johnson NP, Guha A, Sdringola S. Frequent diagnostic errors in cardiac PET/CT due to misregistration of CT attenuation and emission PET images: A definitive analysis of causes, consequences, and corrections. *J Nucl Med.* 2007;48: 1112–1121.

29. Case JA, Heller GV, Cullom SJ, et al. Sensitivity of myocardial perfusion PET/CT imaging scans appearance on accurate transmission/emission registration [abstract]. *J Nucl Cardiol.* 2005;12(4):S117.

30. Moller AM, Martinez M, Ziegler SI, Navab N, Schwaiger M, Nekolla SG. Emission driven motion correction in PET/CT cardiac imaging [abstract]. *J Nucl Med.* 2005;46:163P.

31. Brunken RC, Difilippo FP, Bybel B, Neumann DR, Kaczur T, White RD. Clinical evaluation of cardiac PET attenuation correction using "fast" and "slow" CT images. *J Nucl Med.* 2004;45:120P.

32. de Juan R, Seifert B, Berthold T, von Schulthess GK, Goerres GW. Clinical evaluation of a breathing protocol for PET/CT. *Eur Radiol.* 2004;14(6):1118–1123; Epub Dec 16, 2003.

33. Hsu BL, Case JA, Helmuth PA, Schoonover S, McGhie AIMD, Bateman TM. Initial experience of new LSO-crystal PET/CT scanner enabled simultaneous dynamic and gated listmode acquisition for myocardial Rb-82 imaging [abstract]. ASNC 2006 Scientific Conference.

34. Pan T, Mawlawi O, Nehmeh SA, et al. Attenuation correction of PET images with respiration-averaged CT images in PET/CT. *J Nucl Med.* 2005;46(9):1481–1487.

35. DiFilippo FP, Brunken RC. Do implanted pacemaker leads and ICD leads cause metal-related artifact in cardiac PET/CT? *J Nucl Med.* 2005;46(3):436–443.

36. Hsu BL, Moser KW, Cullom SJ, Bateman TM, Helmuth PA, Case JA. Correction of imaging artifacts from implanted leads in cardiac PET/CT: A phantom evaluation. *J Nucl Med.* 2005;46:174P.

37. Hamill JJ, Brunken RC, Bybel B, DiFilippo FP, Faul DD. A knowledge-based method for reducing attenuation artefacts caused by cardiac appliances in myocardial PET/CT. *Phys Med Biol.* 2006;51(11):2901–2918; Epub May 24, 2006.

38. Nekolla SG. Dynamic and gated PET: Quantitative imaging of the heart revisited [review]. *Nuklearmedizin.* 2005;44(Suppl 1):S41–S45.

39. Bercier Y, Casey M, Young J, Wheelock T. LSO PET/CT pico performance improvements with ultra Hi-Rez option. IEEE Medical Imaging Conf. Record, Rome, Italy, October 16–22, 2004.

40. Defrise M, Casey ME, Michel C, Conti M. Fourier rebinning of time-of-flight PET data. *Phys Med Biol.* 2005;50:2749–2763.

41. Vandenberghe S, Daube-Witherspoon ME, Lewitt RM, Karp JS. Fast reconstruction of 3D time-of-flight PET data by axial rebinning and transverse mashing. *Phys Med Biol.* 2006;51(6):1603–1621.

42. Watson CC. Extension of single scatter simulation to scatter correction of time-of-flight PET 2005. IEEE Medical Imaging Conf. Record, Puerto Rico, October 23–29, 2005.

43. Conti M, Bendriem B, Casey M, et al. First experimental results of time-of-flight reconstruction on an LSO PET scanner. *Phys Med Biol.* 2005;50(19):4507–4526.

44. Surti S, Karp JS, Popescu LM, Daube-Witherspoon ME, Werner M. Investigation of time-of-flight benefit for fully 3-D PET. *IEEE Trans Med Imaging.* 2006;25(5):529–538.

SECTION 6

CARDIAC COMPUTERIZED TOMOGRAPHY

CHAPTER 16

Fundamentals of Computed Tomography and Computed Tomography Angiography

James A. Case
Bai Ling Hsu
S. James Cullom

X-rays were originally discovered by Wilhelm Conrad Röentgen on November 8, 1895, while exploring the discharges from high-voltage vacuum tubes. He discovered in working with these tubes that despite his efforts to make the box containing the tube light tight. Something mysterious was going on; a faint shimmering of light from a bench more than a meter away. Two weeks later, he reproduced the experiment with the assistance of his wife, Anna Bertha, taking the world's first radiogram (see Figure 16-1). He postulated that this mysterious new form of energy (which he termed the 'X-ray') was produced as a direct result of the high-energy electrons interacting with the equipment he was using.[1] His production of the first X-ray tube and subsequent explanation of X-rays earned him the Nobel Prize in Physics in 1901.

This discovery revolutionized medicine. For the first time, physicians had the opportunity to visualize a patient's anatomy without cutting open their body. In the offering of the first Nobel prize in physics to Röentgen in 1901, the committee, summarized its amazing properties in its award, said[2]:

Let us remind ourselves of but one of the properties which have been found in Röentgen rays; that which is the basis of the extensive use of x-rays in medical practice.... The importance of this for practical surgery, and how many operations have been made possible and facilitated by it is well known to all.

This tremendous discovery was expanded into three dimensions in 1973 by Hounsfield and Cormack with the invention of X-ray computed tomography (CT). Again, the Nobel committee recognized the revolutionary impact this technology would have on the field by awarding the Nobel Prize in Medicine to the pair in 1979[3]:

An X-ray examination usually implies the passage of x-rays through an organ with a resulting image of the organ on x-ray film. The dark areas on the film vary according to the anatomy and the structure of the tissues being x-rayed.

A peculiarity of this picture is that it is two-dimensional. In the reproduction the dimension of depth is lost.... In computer-assisted tomography these problems have been ingeniously solved. When the method was introduced into medical care six years ago it quickly became apparent that it signified something revolutionarily new, with great repercussions with x-ray diagnostics and the medical disciplines that make use of it.

Those images required hours of acquisition time and days of computer-processing time to create a three-dimensional (3D) volume. Although these important advances made possible the imaging of most organs in the body, they were insufficient for imaging the cardiovascular system.

First reports of injectable contrast date back to the early 1900s with experiments using mercury and cadavers. The first case of injectable contrast

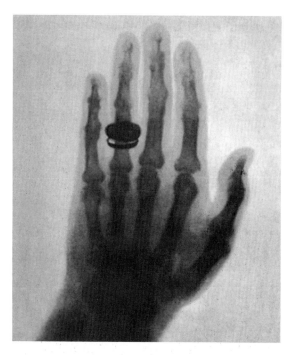

Figure 16-1. Wilhelm Conrad Röentgen's first radiograph of his wife Anna Bertha's hand revolutionized medicine, allowing for the first time the ability to noninvasively image internal structure. For this he received the first Nobel Prize awarded for Physics.

into a living subject was in 1929, when Dr. Werner Forssmann, using an incision in his arm and a urinary catheter, injected contrast media in his arm and walked up a flight of stairs to take an X-ray of his heart.[4] Although this action cost him his job at the hospital, it earned him the Nobel Prize in Medicine in 1956.[5] It was the use of contrast that allowed for the imaging of the vascular system, but this technology alone was insufficient for imaging of the coronary arteries.

CT and computed tomography angiography (CTA) were well on their way to revolutionizing medicine, but reliable techniques for imaging the heart were elusive. Imaging the coronaries represents unique challenges when compared to the rest of the vasculature. First, the vessels to be imaged are small (<3 mm); second, the lesions of the heart are of comparable density to soft tissue (fat = −40 Hounsfield units (HU), blood and muscle = 10 HU, and fibrous tissue = 70 HU); and, most of all, the heart is constantly in motion. In a typical cardiac cycle of 60 beats/min, the blood vessels will move on average 10 mm/s. To achieve 1-mm resolution over the entire cardiac cycle requires temporal resolution of 100 milliseconds. In 1983, Imatron released the first commercial electron beam-based computed tomography system (EBCT). This system, unlike traditional CT scanners, used a small linear accelerator to create a beam of electrons. Then using a system of magnets, the electron beam could be "steered" in an arc around the patient. Because this system did not require any moving parts, it could achieve extremely fast temporal resolution (~50 ms), capable of imaging the entire cardiac cycle at very high speeds.[6–9]

EBCT was used primarily in the assessment of coronary arterial calcium. Because of limitations in beam flux and spatial resolution, it was not considered a feasible technology for angiography of the coronary arteries.[10,11] In 1998, Siemens Medical Solutions introduced the first subsecond-rotation-speed, multislice mechanical CT scanner. This scanner was quickly validated for coronary calcium screening and also opened up the door to contrast-enhanced vascular studies.[12–15]

A hundred years after the invention of the X-ray tube, the achievement of true noninvasive, submillimeter, isotropic, 3D imaging of the heart is now achievable. State-of-the-art cardiovascular CT, typically performed on a 64-slice system with very high rotation speed ($>120/\text{min}$), has become the mainstay of this work.[16–20] Current uses for cardiovascular CT include

1. quantitative measurement of coronary calcium,

2. assessment of peripheral artery disease (with and without iodinated contrast), and

3. assessment of CAD and atherosclerotic burden with iodinated contrast.

The future of cardiac CT will rely on how well this imaging capability can be put into a clinically meaningful context, as has been done with traditional coronary angiography and nuclear cardiology.

PHYSICS OF CT

The X-Ray Tube

At the heart of the multislice CT scanner is the X-ray tube. In many ways, the X-ray tube can be thought of as a "light bulb" producing a stream of photons that can be projected through the patient onto a system of detectors (see Figure 16-2). The X-ray tube consists of two ends of an electric potential: the cathode and the anode (see

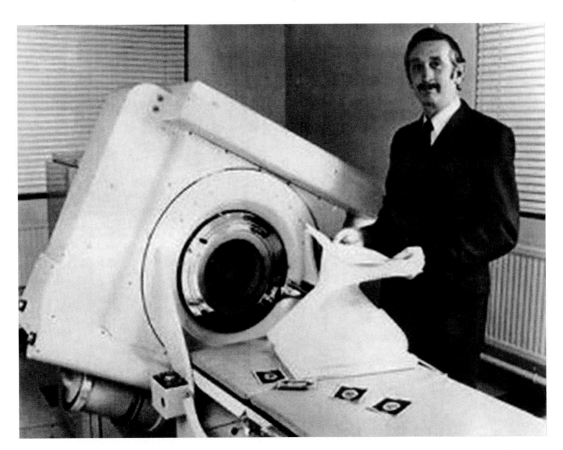

Figure 16-2. Godfrey N. Hounsfield stands next to the CT scanner that he received, together with Allan Cormack, the Nobel Prize for in Physics in 1979.

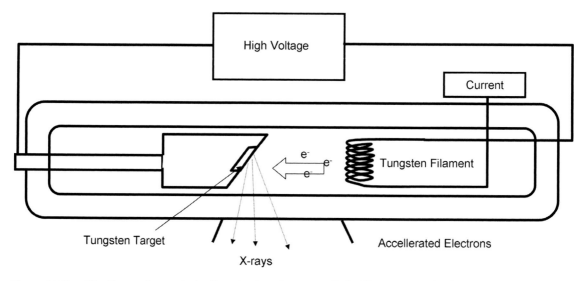

Figure 16-3. The X-ray tube works by first ejecting electrons off of a filament or cathode into a vacuum. Then those electrons are accelerated by the high voltage until they collide with the tungsten target. Those electrons give up their kinetic energy in the form of X-rays.

Figure 16-3). When high enough voltage is applied to the cathode and the anode, the electrons are stripped off of the cathode and accelerated across the electric potential, ultimately colliding with the anode. The higher the voltage, the faster the electrons will be traveling when they strike the anode.

Once they strike the anode, they immediately begin to slow down, giving up much of their energy in the form of photons (or light). This type of radiation is referred to as Bremstraulung radiation, literally meaning "breaking radiation." It is this radiation that we commonly refer to as X-rays.

The parameters that describe the performance of the X-ray tube are the following:

- kVp = kilovolt potential. This represents the accelerating electric potential across the cathode and anode. The higher the voltage, the faster the electrons and the higher-energy photons that can be produced.
- mAs = milliamp seconds. This is a measure of the total electron flux across the potential. This number will directly relate to the

signal-to-noise ratio in the final transmission image.

Gamma rays produced from radionuclide decay will produce a coherent radiation at discrete energies (Co-68 at 122 keV and Tc-99m at 141 keV). In contrast, photons produced from an X-ray tube will produce a continuous distribution of photon energy distributed from 0 keV to complete conversion of the electrons' kinetic energy to photon energy (see Figure 16-4).

Rotational CT

Tomographic imaging requires the acquisitions of multiple projections of the patient, at different angles around the patient. For X-ray CT, this is accomplished using an array of detectors and an X-ray tube mounted on a gantry that rapidly rotates around the patient. This mechanical rotation requires precision engineering to maintain alignment, center of rotation, and speed.

For most applications, the rotational speed of the scanner is not directly related to the

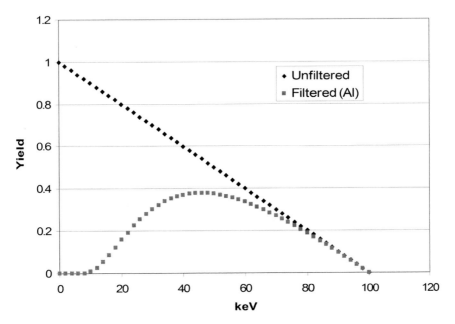

Figure 16-4.   The theoretical spectrum from an X-ray tube in a linear decrease in photon flux with increasing photon energy. This spectrum in reality is complicated by the characteristic X-rays of tungsten and "filtering" materials used to remove the lower-energy, soft X-rays.

ultimate image quality of the clinical study. However, in cardiac CT, this is crucial. The first report of using ECG gating with CT was in the late 1970s.[21,22] This technique was limited in its application until the late 1990s when manufacturers released the first subsecond, multislice CT scanners. These scanners enabled a true "freezing" of a slice of the heart within a single heart beat.

During the last decade, rotational speeds of single-source CT scanners have only improved slightly: from 500 to 330 milliseconds. Although these gains may appear small, they represent huge engineering accomplishments. This is because the "g-forces" on the detector and X-ray tube equipment that is rotating around the patient increase as the square of the rotational speed of the detector (see Table 16-1). Because of this, it is unlikely that future advances in rotational speeds will be obtained without considerable changes to detector and gantry designs.

An additional advance in coronary CT was the advent of multislice scanners. This is an essential step in enabling coronary CT for two reasons. First, it allowed the entire CT scan to take place in a single breath hold. Secondly, it allows for isotropic, 3D resolution.

Table 16-1

G-Forces on a Typical CT Scanner as a Function of Rotational Speed

Rotation Speed (s)	G-Forces
1	4
0.6	11
0.5	16
0.43	22
0.33	37

In general, the g-forces will increase as the square of the decrease in rotational speed.

Isotropy in coronary CT imaging is essential because of the often torturous route the coronaries make as they traverse the epicardium. In order to assess the presence of coronary plaques, resolution variations can change the appearance of lesions significantly. Comparisons of sensitivity and specificity in a coronary CTA (CCTA) multicenter trial demonstrated unacceptably high numbers of segments of the vessels that could not be evaluated[15,16] when using 16-slice scanners. However, when 64-slice systems are used, the number of segments that cannot be evaluated is significantly reduced. These differences are well appreciated and national accreditation guidelines have adopted 64 slices as the minimum standard for CCTA.[23]

Radiation Safety

Radiation safety in CT imaging is an absolute necessity because of the strength of the X-ray source and the frequency of testing. By comparison with radionuclide imaging, the energy flux from an X-ray tube is on the order of 0.1 J/s (depending on the scanner and its settings), compared to 2.5×10^{-5} J/s with a 30-mCi source of Tc-99m. The difference between the two is the length of exposure to the patient in seconds for an X-ray study and hours for a radionuclide study. For the staff who will be present for each study, every day, the cumulative exposure can be significant if proper radiation protection procedures are not followed.

Staff Protection

The fundamental concepts of radiation protection used in radionuclide imaging are appropriate for radiation protection in CT imaging: time, distance and shielding. In CT imaging, all of these tools are used to limit staff exposure. The most important of these is designing workflows that avoid having clinical staff in the imaging room while the scanner is producing X-rays. Workflows for CT imaging should be constructed so that staff can observe the patient at all times, whilst not being in the same room as the patient. This is accomplished using remote patient monitoring and remote injection systems. In the event of a problem in the scanner area, radiation sources is turned off prior to entry of clinical staff into the room. Staff should also stay in the control room during the study to maximize the distance away from the X-ray tube.

Radiation shielding using lead or leaded glass is very effective in attenuating X-ray photons. When compared with SPECT and PET tracers, there is a 10-fold reduction in radiation flux after a 1-mm slab of lead (as compared to sixfold reduction for 141-keV and only a 6% reduction for 511-keV photons; see Figure 16-5). Radiation shielding should be considered for installation on all walls that have work or patient areas on the other side. An exception might be if a wall was in contact with storage or outside.

Total patient exposure during a CT scan is determined by four parameters: (1) mAs, total electron flux in the X-ray tube; (2) kVp, maximal kinetic energy of the electron in the tube; (3) the distance the patient is passed through the scanner during exposure to the X-ray beam; and (4) the pitch, or speed in which the patient is moved through the scanner. Definitions and dosimetry relationships of CT radiation exposure can be found in Table 16-2.

In cardiac imaging, patient radiation dosage can be reduced through the use of ECG pulsing. This approach ramps up the mAs of the X-ray tube during the diastolic phase of the cardiac cycle and then lowers the tube current during other phases. Although this technique does result in a certain loss of functional data and can occasionally result in nondiagnostic studies if a "bad" beat occurs during the CT acquisition, it can represent a significant reduction in patient dosage, sometimes by 50% or more (Somatom, Siemens, Forchheim, Germany).[24,25]

DISPLAY OF CT DATA

Reconstruction and Filtering

The reconstruction of CT data is typically accomplished using a filtered backprojection (FBP)

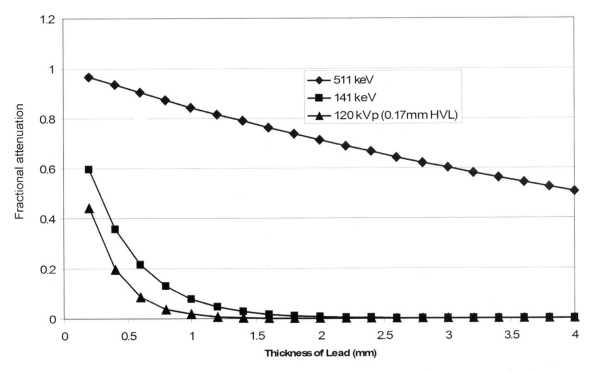

Figure 16-5.   Lead shielding is very effective in stopping the low-energy photons from an X-ray tube. There are differences in attenuation in lead depending on kVp and the filtering materials used.

reconstruction algorithm. This algorithm is based on the radon transform, which assumes that counts received at the detector are equal to the sum of all of the counts along the line of the detector.

For the measurement of attenuation, this model is remarkably accurate. If we look at the counts received at the jth projection, the attenuation equation can be reduced to the radon transform:

$$I = I_0 \exp\left(-\sum_{i \in N_{i,j}}^{N} \mu_i \Delta l\right)$$

or

$$\ln\left(\frac{I_0}{I}\right) = \sum_{i \in N_{i,j}}^{N} \mu_i \Delta l$$

where I is the counts received at jth detector pixel, I_0 is the counts that would be received without the patient in the field of view, μ_i is the attenuation at the ith image pixel, and $N_{i,j}$ is the set of image pixels between the jth detector pixel and the source. Commercial reconstruction programs also model system 3D geometry, scatter correction, beam hardening, and other camera-specific corrections.

Table 16-2

Relationship Between Radiation Dosage and Various CT Scanner

Parameter	Effect on Dosage
mAs	Linear increase
Length of scan	Linear increase
Pitch	Linear decrease
kVp	30% decrease/20 kVp reduction

Table 16-3

Representative HU Units for Various Tissue Types Imaged at 120 kVp

Lung	–900 HU to –500 HU
Lipid	–80 HU to –40 HU
Water	0 HU
Fibrous tissue and muscle	60–120 HU
Contrast-enhanced blood	200–600 HU
Coronary calcium	600–1000 HU
Bone	1000 HU

The quantity that is displayed in CT imaging is the Hounsfield unit (HU). This unit is based on a semiempirical linear scale where water attenuation is defined as 0 and air attenuation is defined as –1000. All other materials are determined by mapping their measured attenuation coefficient onto this scale (see Table 16-3 for representative HU for various materials). The useful attenuation range for CT data is different, depending on the organ being imaged. For example, lung fields are typically imaged with a range of 800 HU centered

on 40 HU. For CCTA, typical parameters center on 200 HU with a range of 600 (see Figure 16-6).

The most common display is the transaxial image display. This projection display format will be used in all interpretation schemes because it has the least amount of geometric and projection distortions. If lesions cannot be confirmed on the transaxial slices, they are unlikely to be real. Reconstruction of the transmission data is typically performed by a vendor-specific algorithm that models system 3D geometry, scatter correction, beam hardening, etc.

For Ca screening procedures, the scoring is performed on the image transaxial data. In these types of studies, it may not be necessary to use isotropic voxel dimensions (3 mm slice thickness with 0.75 mm in plane resolution is very common in coronary Ca screening procedures, (see Figure 16-7). For high resolution, 3D studies, such as CCTA, isotropic spatial resolution is crucial and slice thickness must match the in-plane pixel sizes.

The maximum intensity projection, or MIP, is another common display format. This technique

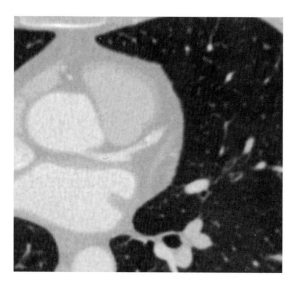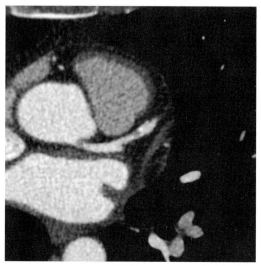

Figure 16-6. Windowing is used in displaying CT images. In the figure on the left, the entire dynamic range of the image is displayed. In the image on the right, the coronary lesion is better visualized using a standard 200 window center, 600 window width settings.

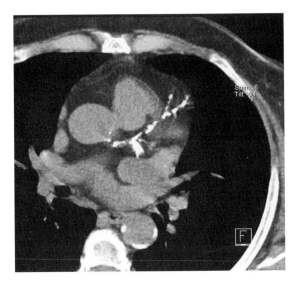

Figure 16-7. An example of extensive coronary calcium in an asymptomatic patient.

creates a planar 2D image from a finite slab of slices. To create the projection, the user will define a slab thickness, and the CT workstation will then determine an MIP from that slab by taking the maximum intensity value along a line of sight toward the user (see Figure 16-8). This has the effect of greatly improving the signal-to-noise ratio, whilst preserving the image contrast and boundary resolution (which would normally be sacrificed in a conventional blurring technique). A disadvantage of the MIP is that it can obscure real lesions depending on the viewing angle. If there is an area of high contrast between a soft lesion and the user, the MIP will take the values of the contrast, and the lesion will be lost.

Another important tool is the curved multiplanar reformat (curved MPR). In this view, the vessel will be projected onto a set of views that

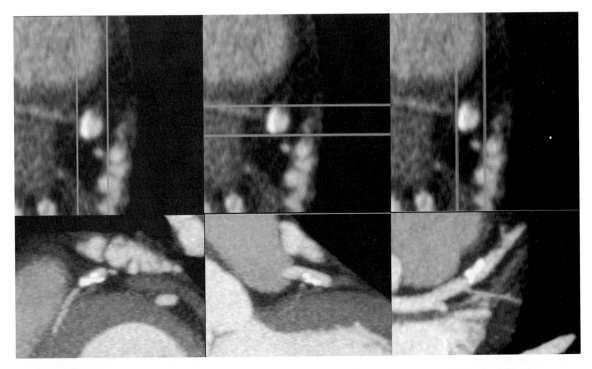

Figure 16-8. The appearance in a maximum intensity projection (MIP) of a lesion can be very different depending on the direction of the projection. The MIP is sensitive to hard lesions, such as calcium, and less sensitive to soft lesions. In these examples, looking left to right at the sagittal, coronal, and transverse projections, the lesion can appear as a partially occlusive mixed plaque to a hard plaque encircling the vessel.

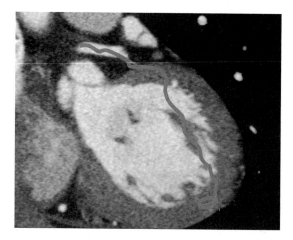

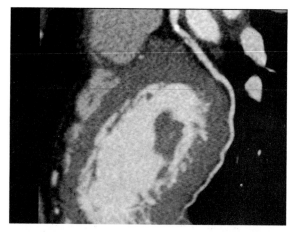

Figure 16-9. The curved MPR removes the tortuous curves in the vessel and projects the vessel onto a single 2D projection. Although this is a very convenient way of looking at the entire vessel, geometric distortions can create artifacts.

will create a virtual "stack" of cross sections of the vessel. First, a centerline is defined through the vessel (Figure 16-9). Then, by defining a set of orthogonal planes to the centerline, a stack of cross sections is created. In these views, lesion size and composition can be assessed quantitatively. However, the problem with the curved MPR is that the resampling can mask artifacts and create spatial distortions that resemble soft plaques[25] (see Figure 16-10).

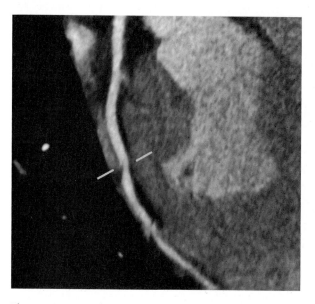

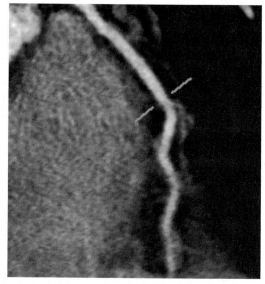

Figure 16-10. The figure on the left demonstrates a curved MPR artifact that completely disappears in a different projection.

QUALITY CONTROL

The quality control program for performing cardiac CT centers on confirming the proper working status of the scanner, identification of any imaging artifacts in patient imaging, and creating consistent readable images for the interpreting physician. Quality control of the scanner itself is accomplished daily by imaging a CT-specific phantom. This phantom is designed to rapidly assess the scanner for (see Figure 16-11)

1. image quality: high- and low-contrast measurements and resolution;
2. absolute CT number calibration (0 for water and −1000 for air);
3. image noise;
4. image uniformity; and
5. slice thickness.

These measurements are typically performed daily, and the results should be recorded and confirmed to be within the manufacturers' tolerances. Manufacturers will also check the system regularly for exposure calibration and laser light accuracy.

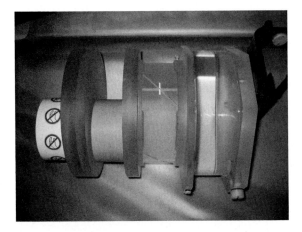

Figure 16-11. The QC phantom used in CT contains the elements for performing high- and low-contrast image quality, water value calibration, image noise and uniformity, and slice thickness.

The quality of patient studies is dependent on many factors beyond the performance of the imaging system. Breathing, heart rate, beam hardening, metal artifacts all can play a role in determining the quality of the final CT image. Breathing artifacts in cardiac CT can occur in CCTA studies that exceed a comfortable breath hold of a patient (typically 10 seconds). When this occurs, there can be a repeating effect in the data in which the same tissue may be seen twice in a single slice. This can easily be detected in a coronal view of the patient as a discontinuity in the surface of the mediastinum.

Beam hardening artifacts occur when the lower-energy photons of the X-ray beam are disproportionately removed and can be worse with metal or calcium. The resulting beam has higher average energy, giving it better penetrating power than the original beam. The result is lower attenuation values (or HU) and dark streaks through the image originating from near these dense structures. In chest CT studies, this is often caused by the sternum, large coronary calcifications, or breast shields (see Figure 16-12). Although not as common as in peripheral studies of the hips or head, beam hardening can limit the quantitative accuracy of studies. Beam hardening can be detected by changing the imaging display window to amplify image contrast in the transaxial views. Beam hardening effects can be reduced by using a higher kVp tube voltage and starting with a harder beam. An extreme example of beam hardening can occur with metal artifacts such as with pacemakers, implanted defibrillators, and surgical clips. In this case, all photons are removed from the beam, leaving no detected counts at the detector. This has the effect of introducing singularities into the reconstruction, which cause bright streaking appearances in the images.

COMMON PROCEDURES

The CT procedures that can be performed today play an important role in diagnosis of disease, risk management, evaluation of cardiac symptoms, and the postevaluation of interventional procedures.

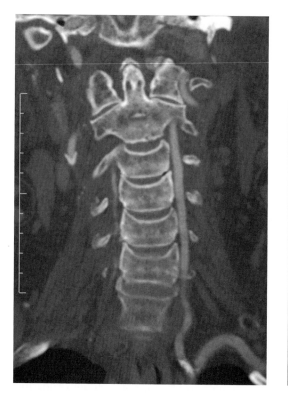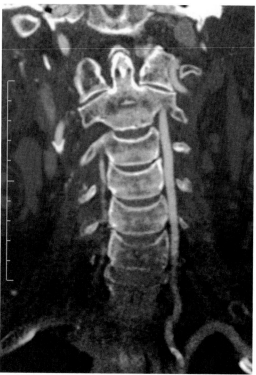

Figure 16-12.   In this carotid study, beam hardening from the shoulders causes a dark "banding" artifact in the image (80 kVp image on the right). By using a higher kVp setting, beam hardening can be reduced (140 kVp image on the left).

Ca Scoring

Coronary calcium screening is a non-contrast-enhanced CT imaging procedure used to detect the presence of significant calcium deposits in the coronary arteries and thoracic vasculature associated with atherosclerosis. Coronary calcium buildup is a natural process for patients with active atherosclerosis. It is thought that coronary calcium is the body's response to stabilize arterial plaques and reduce the likelihood of plaque rupture[26]; however, attempts to validate this model have not verified this hypothesis.[27–33] Despite the fact that coronary calcium is not a direct measurement of plaque vulnerability, long-term risk stratification can be achieved using this technique.[34,35]

Throughout the twentieth century, the nature and composition of atherosclerotic plaque were investigated, with the simplest model for plaque being based on a two-component model having lipid and fibrous components.[34–37] Calcium was also identified as a key component of these plaques.[38,39] Because of its opacity to X-rays, coronary calcium was recognized as an important surrogate for total plaque burden despite the lack of a causal relationship between plaque rupture and coronary calcium.[26,35] Coronary calcium assessment has been recognized by the American College of Cardiology and American Heart Association as having prognostic value.[40] Early studies of the prognostic value of coronary calcium assessment were performed using the EBCT scanners described above. These scanners were particularly well suited for coronary calcium assessment because of the low radiation exposure and extremely fast scanning times (50 milliseconds). This work was expanded to include multislice scanning.[41,42]

Quantitative assessment of coronary plaque was first proposed by Agatston et al.[6] in 1990. This risk model relied on the measurement of the degree of calcification (described as a weighting factor) and its volume determined from a thresholding procedure applied to the CT images. Specifically, for each slice the score of a particular lesion is given by

$$S = w \bullet A$$

where A is the area of the lesion and

$$w = \begin{cases} 1 \text{ for } 130 \ HU \leq CT^{\max} < 200 \ HU \\ 2 \text{ for } 200 \ HU \leq CT^{\max} < 300 \ HU \\ 3 \text{ for } 300 \ HU \leq CT^{\max} < 400 \ HU \\ 4 \text{ for } 400 \ HU \leq CT^{\max} \end{cases}$$

And $CT^{\max}$ is the maximum CT value (HU) of the lesion in that slice. The total Agatston score is the sum of all S values from all slices. This semiquantitative model for plaque burden has been widely accepted and applied, despite its shortcoming of not being a true physical measurement (such as coronary calcium mass in mg).

As of 2007, coronary calcification assessment in an asymptomatic, low-Framingham-risk population is not considered an appropriate indication, and, in moderate- and high-risk patients, it is considered uncertain.[20] However, many individuals and their physicians have recognized its value in the early detection of atherosclerosis and behavior modification for the management of risk factors. Most practitioners will discuss with their patients the value of Ca scoring when three or more cardiac risk factors are present. Common risk factors sited are

1. hypertension,
2. hyperlipidemia,
3. smoking, and
4. family history of CAD.

Patients who are also not well suited for coronary calcium scoring are those patients who have had a previous diagnosis of CAD, since the detection of significant calcification is almost certain and will add little to the overall evaluation of the patient.[20]

CORONARY CTA

CCTA provides a detailed assessment of obstructive coronary vascular occlusions in a noninvasive setting. In a large number of studies, comparable accuracies can be achieved with CCTA as with other noninvasive CAD assessment imaging tools, such as nuclear and stress echo. However, CCTA has opened a Pandora's box of questions about noninvasive imaging because, as CCTA imaging moved beyond 16- to 64-slice systems and toward dual-tube imaging to remove imaging artifacts, they have unmasked real atherosclerotic lesions and noncardiac findings of which little is known about their prognostic significance.

Because of this, most US insurance carriers have taken a "wait-and-see" stance on reimbursement for these imaging tests for many indications. As the prognostic data and recommendations for patient management strategies become available, reassessment of the reimbursement question for more broad indications is inevitable.

IMAGE ACQUISITION SETUP

CCTA is a rapid and efficient tool for imaging the coronary arteries. Current guidelines for CCTA are flexible, owing to the rapidly changing hardware and software environment. Despite this, minimum standards have been established. The Intersocietal Commission on Accreditation of Computed Tomography Laboratories (ICACTL) has taken the position that the data are not supportive of accreditation for CT machines with low slices and slower than 500 milliseconds rotation speed.[23]

As with any angiographic study, proper patient preparation and exclusions because of contraindications are crucial. Kidney tolerance of the contrast, location, and abundance of metallic objects in the thorax are all important considerations.

Iodine allergy, although common, may not represent an absolute contraindication. It is commonly accepted that patients with high heart rates should have their hear rate reduced to less than 60 bpm using β-blockers.[43,44] Use of nitrates can also improve vascular size, improving image quality.

ECG gating is essential in all CCTA studies to freeze the coronaries in time. This is accomplished at the time of least cardiac motion, typically diastole. The best diastolic phase can often be found at 75% of the RR interval; however, this is not an absolute rule for all patients. By examining reconstructions of 65%, 75%, and 85% of the RR interval, the interpreting physician can select "best diastolic phase." Another confounding problem with the selection of the best diastolic phase is that it may not be the same for all three vessels.[44]

Routinely, technologists provide the interpreting physician with at least three reconstructions, and the interpreter chooses the best phase for each vessel. These reconstructions should create a volume transaxial stack of CTA data with isotropic resolution in all three directions, cubic voxel size with less than 1 mm on each side, and adequate noise filtering. The physician should inspect all reconstructions and select the best reconstruction for each vessel (see Figure 16-13).

INTERPRETATION

The interpretation of CCTA studies is a four-step process:

1. Identification of obstructive coronary lesions
2. Identification of positive remodeling
3. Classification (soft, mixed, and calcified), counting, and quantification of overall atherosclerotic burden
4. Interpretation and reporting on significant noncardiac findings

The tools that the clinician uses to perform these tasks are 3D processing tools that are commonly found on CT interpretation workstations. The interpretation is performed typically using three different views of the coronary arteries (see Figure 16-14):

1. *A global, slice-by-slice examination of the raw transaxial cuts.* This is typically accomplished by paging through the images, top to bottom, for each vessel. This projection set is very helpful in differentiating between imaging artifact and true lesions.

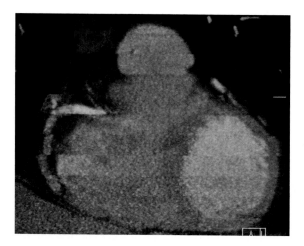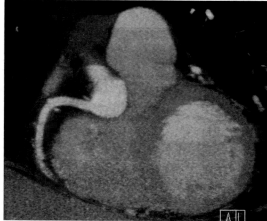

Figure 16-13. The coronary arteries move at different velocities during the cardiac cycle. In this example of the RCA reconstructed at 67% of the RR interval, there are numerous motion artifacts. However, when reconstructed at 77% of the RR interval, those artifacts are resolved.

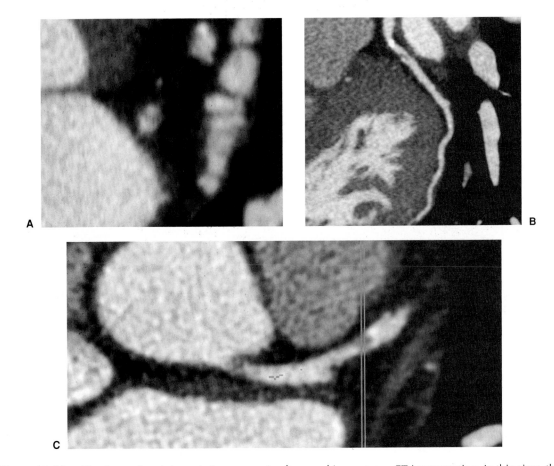

Figure 16-14.   The three-view interpretation screen is often used in coronary CT interpretation. In this view, the transaxial (A), curved MPR (B), and cross-sectional views (C) all can be assessed.

2. *Curved planar reformat*: In this view, the vessel is virtually straightened by the software program so that the entire vessel can be viewed in a single planar projection. The vessel is then rotated around the axis of rotation to search for artifactal narrowing.

3. *Cross-sectional images*: The cross-sectional view displays the vessel on a perpendicular plane to the direction of the vessel. This view can be very helpful in identifying and characterizing atherosclerotic plaque. This view can also be very deceptive. Side branches and mismatch between adjacent slice volumes can appear as lesions and should be confirmed through the other two views.

DIAGNOSTIC ACCURACY STUDIES

Several studies have been used to evaluate the accuracy of CCTA versus conventional interventional angiography. These results have consistently demonstrated very high accuracy rates for CCTA. Specifically, a meta-analysis of 29 published studies from 2002 to 2006, involving a total of 2024 patients using 16-slice or higher systems, demonstrated an 81% value for sensitivity and a 93%

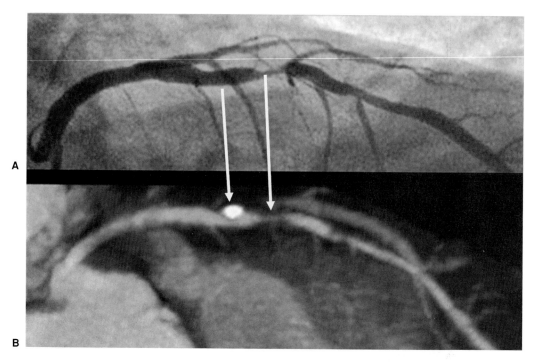

Figure 16-15. One of the limitations of conventional coronary angiography is that it is a planar technique that can only image the lumen. Because of this, it can miss many hard lesions and is not sensitive to high-risk soft-plaque remodeling.

specificity, when using interventional angiography as the gold standard.[45] Although these numbers did reflect a high diagnostic accuracy, the authors note that 10.6% of all segments were uninterpretable. One of the major limitations of these studies is a result of combining 16-slice detector results with 64-slice studies. In a single-center study, using 64-slice CTA and 67 patients, the sensitivity was elevated as 94% and the specificity was 99%, with no segments needing to be excluded from the analysis.[46] Although this study was small and single center, it illustrates the significant improvements in image quality that are achievable when going from 16- to 64-slice CTA of the coronaries.

In comparing invasive angiography with CCTA, it is important to note that traditional invasive angiography is a luminogram: a tracing of the lumen alone. CCTA is a volumetric image of the plaque itself and the lumen. Positive remodeling can give the impression of a very significant lesion with minimal change in the actual lumen size. Similarly, the effect of traditional invasive angiography projection can cause a lesion to be missed if the plaque is imaged in 2D, face on (see Figure 16-15). Fundamentally, traditional invasive angiography and CCTA image two different things. Traditional invasive angiography images the lumen; CCTA images both the lumen and the plaque.

Limitations

CCTA still suffers from two major limitations: (1) the low temporal resolution (~200 milliseconds) still introduces many artifacts in the image and (2) the radiation exposure is still excessively high to use the technique for serial imaging and routine management of atherosclerosis.

Improvement in both of these categories will be necessary for CTA to achieve widespread acceptance.

PERIPHERAL VASCULAR STUDIES

Peripheral artery disease management plays an important role in most cardiovascular practices. These vascular procedures are well understood for their value and are reimbursed by most medical insurance carriers.

The most common peripheral angiographic study is the peripheral runoff study. In this study, a bolus of contrast is injected into the patient and followed from when it exits the heart to the lower extremities. This technique requires that the scanner "chase" the contrast bolus into the lower extremities. To accomplish this, the CT scanner system must be able to cover sufficient volumes rapidly and not to "fall behind" in chasing the contrast bolus. This is typically accomplished using a 16-slice or higher CT scanner. Peripheral runoff studies have been demonstrated to be helpful in the evaluation of arterial injury from trauma,[47] detection of blockages,[48] and preoperative workup for stent placement.[48]

Another common peripheral study is the carotid CTA. These studies are typically ordered when a duplex echo has failed to accurately define the luminal narrowing (typically as a result of excessive calcification). In these studies, a bolus will be followed from the aortic arch to the Circle of Willis. Great attention will be paid to lesions in the carotid bifurcation. Increased blood velocity and shear will make the bifurcation particularly vulnerable to atherosclerotic buildup. In these studies, luminal narrowing is measured and the degree of calcification is recorded.

Other studies that can be performed are renal CTA, abdominal aortic aneurysm, iliac aneurysm, or stent patency. These studies should be a part of any cardiovascular CTA program, and partnerships between cardiologists and radiologists can be helpful in establishing these programs, and appropriate competency should be established before initiating these programs.[49]

FUTURE DIRECTIONS

Coronary Plaque Composition Using Dual-Energy CT

There is general agreement that some types of quantitative descriptor of coronary plaques will be essential for predicting patient outcomes and for learning whether medical therapies or lifestyle changes are modifying the morphology and/or the biology of plaques. Numerous studies as well as clinical experience show that identification and interventional treatment of luminal obstructive lesions fail to address a large cohort of patients who suffer adverse outcomes as a result of plaque rupture.[50,51] Specifically, vulnerable plaques are difficult to identify with conventional techniques because

1. their composition has a similar opacity to surrounding soft tissue, making them difficult to visualize using conventional X-ray-based techniques;
2. arterial remodeling can hide significant plaques in catheter-based examinations; and
3. the size of vulnerable lesions is often less than 2 mm, at least as evaluated using intraluminal-optimized techniques.

The American Heart Association has established a categorization of plaques:

- *Types I, II, and III*: Small, early-stage lesions, from a fatty streak to more lipid-rich lesions.
- *Type IV lesions*: Not necessarily stenotic, but may be vulnerable because of high lipid content with or without mural thrombus. May also result in acute coronary syndrome. May or may not have calcified deposits.
- *Type V lesions*: Distinct changes in geometry and greater occlusiveness and fibrotic type Vb (calcified) and Vc lesions (noncalcified).
- *Type VI*: Complicated lesions, with underlying components of types IV and V lesions.

The introduction of calcium into the development of the fibrotic cap remains an area of intense research, but it is believed that calcification may begin very early in the development of coronary plaques.[52–57] Calcium participation in the development of the fibrotic cap is thought to stabilize the plaque, although that has not been firmly established.[57,58] Also, it has been postulated that coronary calcium plays a crucial role in vessel wall remodeling.[59]

Dual-Energy Approaches to CTA

The first medical application of dual-energy X-ray imaging was in 1963 for the assessment of calcium loss in bones.[60] In its original application, two X-ray tubes set at different energies could be used to detect calcium loss in osteoporosis patients. Because these studies were conducted using planar techniques, they were nonquantitative. The first suggestion that a similar but quantitative technique could be applied to CT was made in 1976 by Ruegsegger et al.[61] As the technique evolved, it became apparent that the quantitative CT technique could be useful in identifying fat deposits in the liver,[62,63] pulmonary nodules,[64] and abdomen.[65] Most materials could be identified in this manner, so long as the object under consideration was significantly larger than the resolution kernel of the imaging system.[66,67]

Dual-tube, dual-energy CT scanners represent a significant advance in CT imaging by incorporating two high-speed X-ray tubes into a single gantry. Each X-ray tube can operate either in a dual-source mode (identical kVp and mAs) or in a semi-independent fashion (different kVp). In the dual-energy mode (differing kVp settings on the A and B systems), simultaneous measurements can be made of the patient at different energies.

The theoretical construction of a solution for imaging small coronary plaques is to model them as made of two very different materials: Lipid- and soft tissue-like structures and calcium deposits. Physically lipid/soft tissues and calcium have large differences in attenuation for the range of X-ray energies (80–140 kVp). Simultaneous dual-energy CT imaging is used to generate two perfectly registered, simultaneous transmission maps, enabling direct comparisons of the two kVp studies. By comparing differences between the two CT images, it is possible to determine the composition of the plaques (see Figure 16-16).

Low-Dose, Real-Time Imaging Using 256-Slice Imaging

With detector arrays progressively getting larger— 4-, 8-, 16-, 40-, 64-, and 256-slice systems—it would only seem logical that higher slice systems, such as a 256-slice CT system, could provide even greater improvements in image quality. But is bigger always better? In this case, it is. A 256-slice system could represent a significant advancement in coronary CT by reducing patient dosage, reducing image artifacts, and performing real-time CT imaging.

A major goal of CCTA imaging is to develop techniques that can be used for monitoring of patient therapy. However for CT to achieve this objective, it will be necessary to drastically reduce the patient's radiation exposure. One approach to accomplishing this is to use a scanner capable of imaging the entire myocardium in a single rotation. In this mode, a sequential "step-and-shoot" technique can be employed with a side step. This has the effect of only using radiation dosage during the arc that is used for the image. Estimates for this type of imaging for CCTA work will be in the range of 2 to 4 mSv.[68]

Real-time imaging also has the advantage of imaging patients with significant cardiac arrhythmias. This is enabled because the large format array does not rely on consistency in the position of the heart between rotations. This also will reduce stack misregistration artifacts commonly seen in 64-slice imaging (Figure 16-13).

CONCLUSION

Cardiovascular CT represents one of the most powerful additions to the tools that are available to practicing cardiologist for accurate, noninvasive

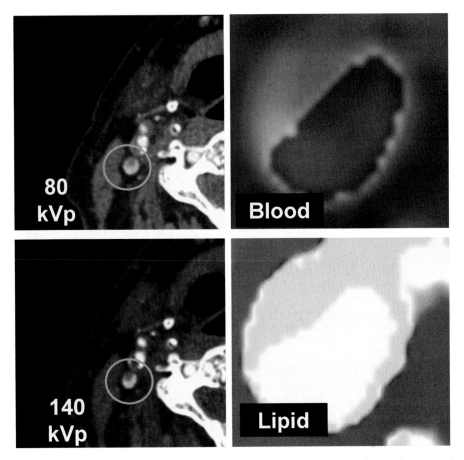

Figure 16-16.   Dual-energy CT image opens up the possibility of characterizing plaques based on the intrinsic signature different materials make on the different kVp images. In this image, the iodine in the blood can be segmented to locate lumen and the lipid in the plaque can also be identified. (See color insert.)

diagnosis of CAD, peripheral artery disease, and patient management. Advancements in the field also open up the possibility of using this technique for the assessment of plaque vulnerability and compositions.

Considerable work remains to allow for this modality to achieve its potential, including accurate outcomes data, to better define appropriate indications for this technique, reduced radiation exposure to take advantage of its capability of imaging patients earlier in the evolution of their atherosclerosis, and patient management models

that demonstrate to practitioners and payers the value of this modality.

REFERENCES

1. Roentgen WC. *Uber eine neue Art von Strahlen.* Wurzburg: Physik – medic; 1895.
2. Nobel Foundation. *Nobel Lectures, Physics 1901–1921.* Amsterdam: Elsevier Publishing Company; 1967.
3. Lindsten J, ed. *Nobel Lectures, Physiology or Medicine 1971–1980.* Singapore: World Scientific Publishing Co.; 1992.

4. Forssmann W. Sondierung des rechten Herzens. *Klin Wochenschr*. 1929;8:2085.

5. Nobel Foundation. *Nobel Lectures in Physiology or Medicine 1942–1962*. Singapore: World Scientific Publishing Co.; 1999.

6. Agatston AS, Janowitz WR, Hildner FJ, et al. Quantification of coronary artery calcium using ultrafast computed tomography. *J Am Coll Cardiol*. 1990;15:827–832.

7. Devries S, Wolfkiel C, Shah V, et al. Reproducibility of the measurement of coronary calcium with ultrafast computed tomography. *Am J Cardiol*. 1995;75:973–975.

8. Rumberger JA, Simons DB, Fitzpatrick LA, et al. Coronary artery calcium area by electron beam computed tomography and coronary atherosclerotic plaque area: A histopathologic correlative study. *Circulation*. 1995;92:2157–2162.

9. Shaw LJ, O'Rourke RA. The challenge of improving assessment in asymptomatic individuals: The additive prognostic value of electron beam tomography. *JACC*. 2000;36:1261–1264.

10. Ruping D, Shaoxiong Z, Bin L, et al. Electron-beam CT angiography with three-dimensional reconstruction in the evaluation of coronary artery bypass grafts. *Academic Radiology*. 1998;5:863–867.

11. Chernoff DM, Cameron RJ, Higginsa CB. Evaluation of electron beam angiography in healthy subjects. *AJR*. 1997;169:93–99.

12. Achenbach S, Giesler T, Ropers D, et al. Detection of coronary artery stenoses by contrast-enhanced, retrospectively electrocardiographically-gated, multislice spiral computed tomography. *Circulation*. 2001;103:2535–2538.

13. Budoff MJ, Achenbach S, Duerinckx A. Clinical utility of computed tomography and magnetic resonance techniques for noninvasive coronary angiography. *J Am Coll Cardiol*. 2003;42:1867–1878.

14. Deibler AR, Kuzo RS, Vohringer M, et al. Imaging of congenital coronary anomalies with multislice computed tomography. *Mayo Clin Proc*. 2004;79(8):1017–1023.

15. van der Zaag-Loonen HJ, Dikkers R, de Bock GH, Oudkerk M. The clinical value of a negative multi-detector computed tomographic angiography in patients suspected of coronary artery disease: A meta-analysis. *Eur Radiol*. 2006;16(12):2748–2756.

16. Sun Z, Jiang W. Diagnostic value of multislice computed tomography angiography in coronary artery disease: A meta-analysis. *Eur J Radiol*. 2006;60(2):279–286.

17. Leber AW, Johnson T, Becker A, et al. Diagnostic accuracy of dual-source multi-slice CT-coronary angiography in patients with an intermediate pretest likelihood for coronary artery disease. *Eur Heart J*. 2007;28(19):2354–2360.

18. Miller JM. Coronary Artery Evaluation using 64-Row Multidetector Computed Tomography Angiography (CORE-64): Results of a Multicenter, International Trial to Assess Diagnostic Accuracy Compared with conventional Coronary Angiography. American Heart Association Scientific Sessions 2007, Late Breaking Clinical Trials. Orlando, FL.

19. Budoff MJ, Shinbane, eds. *Cardiac CT Imaging: Diagnosis of Cardiovascular Disease*. Springer-Verlag; 2006.

20. Hendel RC, et al. ACCF/ACR/SCCT/SCMR/ASNC/ NASCI/SCAI/SIR 2006 appropriateness criteria for cardiac computed tomography and cardiac magnetic resonance imaging. *J Am Coll Cardiol*. 2006;48(7):1475–1497.

21. Lackner K, Thurn P. Computed tomography of the heart: ECG-gated and continuous scans. *Radiology*. 1981;140(2):413–420.

22. Harell GS, Guthaner DF, Beiman RS, et al. Stop-Action cardiac computed tomography. *Radiology*. 1977;123:515–517.

23. Intersocietal Commission for the Accreditation of Computed Tomography Laboratories. ICACTL Standard for Computer Tomography (CT) Operations. http://www.icactl.org/icactl/pdfs/ICACTLStds_ Part2Final07.pdf.

24. Jakobs TF, Becker CR, Ohnesorge B, et al. Multi-slice helical CT of the heart with retrospective ECG gating: Reduction of radiation exposure by ECG-controlled tube current modulation. *Eur Radiol*. 2002;12:1081–1086.

25. Circulation package from Siemens, OSIRIX.

26. Beckman JA, Ganz J, Creager MA, Ganz P, Kinlay S. Relationship of clinical presentation and calcification of culprit coronary artery stenoses. *Arterioscler Thromb Vasc Biol*. 2001;21:1618–1622.

27. Ross R. The pathogenesis of atherosclerosis: a perspective for the 1990s. *Nature*. 1993;362:801–809.

28. Stary HC. Composition and classification of human atherosclerotic lesions. *Virchows Arch A Pathol Anat Histopathol*. 1992;421:277–290.

29. Stary HC, Chandler AB, Dinsmore RE, et al. A definition of advanced types of atherosclerotic lesions and a histological classification of atherosclerosis. A report from the Committee on Vascular Lesions of the Council on Arteriosclerosis, American Heart Association. *Circulation*. 1995;92:1355–1374.

30. Tanenbaum SR, Kondos GT, Veselik KE, et al. Detection of calcific deposits in coronary arteries by ultrafast computed tomography and correlation with angiography. *Am J Cardiol*. 1989;63:870–872.

31. Falk E, Shah PK, Fuster V. Coronary plaque disruption. *Circulation*. 1995;92:657–671.

32. Fuster V, Lewis A. Conner Memorial lecture. Mechanisms leading to myocardial infarction: insights

from studies of vascular biology. *Circulation*. 1994;90:2126–2146.

33. Davies MJ. The composition of coronary artery plaque. *N Engl J Med*. 1993;69:377–381.

34. Agatston AS, Janowitz WR, Hildner FJ, et al. Quantification of coronary artery calcium using ultrafast computed tomography. *J Am Coll Cardiol*. 1990; 15:827–832.

35. Conroy RM, Pyorala K, Fitzgerald AP, et al. Estimation of ten-year risk of fatal cardiovascular disease in Europe: The SCORE project. *Eur Heart J*. 2003;24:987–1003.

36. Aschoff L. *Lectures on Pathology*. New York, NY: Paul B Hoeber; 1924.

37. Aschoff L. Introduction. In: Cowdry EV, ed. *Arteriosclerosis: A Survey of the Problem*. New York, NY: Macmillan Publishing Co; 1933:1–18.

38. Yu SY. Calcification processes in atherosclerosis. *Adv Exp Med Biol*. 1974;43:403–425.

39. Schmid K, McSharry WO, Pameijer CH, Binette JP. Chemical and physicochemical studies on the mineral deposits of the human atherosclerotic aorta. *Atherosclerosis*. 1980;37:199–210.

40. O'Roake RA, et al., American College of Cardiology/American Heart Association expert consensus document on electron-beam computed tomography for the diagnosis and prognosis of coronary artery disease. *J Am Coll Cardiol*. 2000;36:326–340.

41. Moser KW, Bateman TM, O'Keefe JH, McGhie AI. Interscan variability of coronary artery calcium quantification using an electrocardiographically pulsed spiral computed tomographic protocol. *Am J Cardiol*. 2004;93(9):1153–1155.

42. Becker CR, Kleffel T, Crispin A, et al. Coronary artery calcium measurement: agreement of multirow detector and electron beam CT. *AJR*. 2001;176:1295–1298.

43. Raff GL, Gallagher MJ, O'Neill WW, Goldstein JA. Diagnostic accuracy of non-invasive coronary angiography using 64 slice spiral computed tomography. *J Am Coll Cardiol*. 2005;46(3):552–557.

44. Leschka S, Wildermuth S, Boehm T, et al. Noninvasive coronary angiography with 64-section CT: Effect of average heart rate and heart rate variability on image quality. *Radiology*. 2006;241:378–385.

45. Hamon M, Giuseppe Biondi-Zoccai GL document, Malagutti P, et al. Diagnostic performance of multislice spiral computed tomography of coronary arteries as compared with conventional invasive coronary angiography: A meta analysis. *J Am Coll Cardiol*. 2006; 48:1896–1910.

46. Leschka S, Alkadhi H, Plass A, et al. Accuracy of MSCT coronary angiography with 64-slice technology: First experience. *Eur Heart J*. 2005;26(15): 1482–1487.

47. Soto JA, Munera F, Morales C, et al. Focal arterial injuries of the proximal extremities: Helical CT angiography as the initial method of diagnosis. *Radiology*. 2001;218:188–194.

48. Lawrence JA, Kim D, Kent KC, Stehling MK, Rosen MP, Raptopoulos V. Lower extremity spiral CT angiography versus catheter angiography. *Radiology*. 1995;194:903–908.

49. Kramer CM, et al. ACCF/AHA 2007 clinical competence statement on vascular imaging with computed tomography and magnetic resonance. *J Am Coll Cardiol*. 2007;50:1097–1114.

50. Okura H, Taguchi H, Kubo T, et al. Impact of arterial remodelling and plaque rupture on target and non-target lesion revascularisation after stent implantation in patients with acute coronary syndrome: An intravascular ultrasound study. *Heart*. 2007;93:1219–1225.

51. Hoffmann U, Moselewski F, Nieman K, et al. Noninvasive assessment of plaque morphology and composition in culprit and stable lesions in acute coronary syndrome and stable lesions in stable angina by multidetector computed tomography. *J Am Coll Cardiol*. 2006;47:1655–1662.

52. Taylor AJ, et al. 34th Bethesda Conference: Can atherosclerosis imaging techniques improve the detection of patients at risk for ischemic heart disease? *J Am Coll Cardiol*. 2003;41(11):1855-1917.

53. Vallabhajosula S, Fuster V. Atherosclerosis: Imaging techniques and the evolving role of nuclear medicine. *J Nucl Med*. 1997;38:1788–1796.

54. Boden W, et al. Optimal medical therapy with or without PCI for stable coronary disease. *NEJM*. March 26, 2007, online.

55. Jonasson L, Holm J, Skalli O, Bondjers G, Hansson GK. Regional accumulations of T cells, macrophages, and smooth muscle cells in the human atherosclerotic plaque. *Arteriosclerosis*. 1986;6:131–138.

56. Stary HC. Composition and classification of human atherosclerotic lesions. *Virchows Arch A Pathol Anat Histopathol*. 1992;421:277–290.

57. Lee RT, Grodzinsky AJ, Frank EH, Kamm RD, Schoen FJ. Structure-dependent dynamic mechanical behavior of fibrous caps from human atherosclerotic plaques. *Circulation*. 1991;83:1764–1770.

58. Cheng GC, Loree HM, Kamm RD, Fishbein MC, Lee RT. Distribution of circumferential stress in ruptured and stable atherosclerotic lesions: A structural analysis with histopathological correlation. *Circulation*. 1993;87: 1179–1187.

59. Gibbons GH, Dzau VJ. The emerging concept of vascular remodeling. *N Engl J Med*. 1994;330: 1431–1438.

60. Cameron JR, Sorenson J. Measurement of bone mineral in-vivo; an improved method. *Science*. 1963;142: 230–234.

61. Ruegsegger P, Elsasser U, Anliker M, et al. Quantification of bone mineralization using computed tomography. *Radiology*. 1976;121:93–97.

62. Raptopoulos V, Karellas A, Bernstein J, Reale FR, Constantinou C, Zawacki JK. Value of dual-energy CT in differentiating focal fatty infiltration of the liver from low-density masses. *AJR Am J Roentgenol*. 1991;157(4): 721–725.

63. Wang B, Gao Z, Zou Q, Li L. Quantitative diagnosis of fatty liver with dual-energy CT. An experimental study in rabbits. *Acta Radiol*. 2003;44(1):92–97.

64. Higashi Y, Nakamura H, Matsumoto T, Nakanishi T. Dual-energy computed tomographic diagnosis of pulmonary nodules. *J Thorac Imaging*. 1994;9(1): 31–34.

65. Lane JT, Mack-Shipman LR, Anderson JC, et al. Comparison of CT and dual-energy DEXA using a modified trunk compartment in the measurement of abdominal fat. *Endocrine*. 2005;27(3):295–299.

66. Johnson TR, Krauss B, Sedlmair M, et al. Material differentiation by dual energy CT: Initial experience. *Eur Radiol*. 2006 Dec 7 [Epub ahead of print].

67. Michael GJ. Tissue analysis using dual energy CT. *Australas Phys Eng Sci Med*. 1992;15(2):75–87.

68. Toshiba Medical Systems. http://madeforlife.toshiba.com/events/rsna_256/CTRP1056US.PDF.

SECTION 7

IMAGING VENTRICULAR FUNCTION

CHAPTER 17

Technical Aspects of Scintigraphic Evaluation of Ventricular Function

Kim A. Williams

INTRODUCTION

The noninvasive assessment of resting left ventricular (LV) performance has become an integral part of the evaluation of patients with known or suspected cardiac disease, having important diagnostic, therapeutic, and prognostic significance.[1–15] Scintigraphic measures of cardiac function historically included estimation of cardiac output, valvular regurgitant fractions, and shunt detection. The measurement of these parameters has been largely undertaken by echocardiographic techniques for the past two decades. However, the measurement of ejection fraction (EF) has consistently found clinical application in the evaluation of patients with known or suspected LV dysfunction, those postmyocardial infarction, and those with valvular disease, as well as monitoring the cardiotoxic effects of chemotherapeutic drugs. Also, exercise radionuclide angiography (RNA) has

been widely used to diagnose myocardial ischemia, often complementing myocardial perfusion imaging.

Currently there are five scintigraphic techniques that can be utilized clinically:

1. First-pass radionuclide angiocardiography (FPRNA);

2. Planar-gated equilibrium radionuclide angiography (ERNA), often called multiple-gated acquisition ("MUGA") or equilibrium radionuclide ventriculography (RNV);

3. Ambulatory blood pool monitoring (nuclear "VEST," or nuclear stethoscope);

4. Gated SPECT myocardial perfusion imaging (GSPECT); and

5. Gated SPECT equilibrium blood pool imaging (GBPS).

Technical Comparison of Radionuclide Methods

The evaluation of LV systolic function has become one of the most common applications of nuclear imaging, using FPRNA, ERNA, GSPECT, and, more recently, GBPS. From the standpoint of expertise in acquiring quality studies, ERNA has been the choice for blood pool imaging, rather than the less time-consuming FPRNA,[15–17] as a result of the relative ease of data acquisition, automated processing, and rapid interpretation. However, recently there has been renewed interest in FPRNA, at least in part because of the availability of Tc-99m-labeled perfusion tracers, which allow simultaneous evaluation of myocardial perfusion and ventricular function.[13,18–22] Still, the widespread application of FPRNA has been limited by the need for a high-count-rate-capable gamma camera, dependence on impeccable bolus technique, and the absence of valvular (especially tricuspid) incompetence for data quality.[23]

As perfusion imaging has grown, it is estimated that more than 90% of SPECT perfusion images are obtained with GSPECT. This "add-on" technique renders incremental diagnostic and prognostic data. For example, an LVEF of >45% or end-systolic volume <70 mL is associated with an excellent prognosis in patients with CAD, regardless of their attendant perfusion defect scores.[24]

The ambulatory version of blood pool monitoring with a nonimaging probe or portable device has been particularly useful for beat-to-beat assessment of LV function in atrial fibrillation, those in intensive-care settings, and those needing evaluation of function during various activities.[25] However, this technique has found limited clinical acceptance and utilization.

FPRNA has some distinct technical advantages over the other methods. These include (1) the acquisition of data in less than 30 seconds; (2) right ventricular function with less overlap of activity in other chambers[23]; (3) the use of multiple radiopharmaceuticals including bone, renal, and myocardial scintigraphic agents[13]; (4) a proven robust measurement of stress ventricular function at true peak exercise; and (5) the presence of a wealth of prognostic information available for management of patients with ischemic heart disease based on stratification by FPRNA exercise LVEFs.[5,7,9]

Despite these advantages, widespread use of FPRNA has been limited by the need for large bore intravenous access,[23] precise bolus technique,[22] and a high-count-rate-capable, often dedicated, gamma camera.

Widespread use of GBPS was long restricted by the lack of software for quantitation of EF on many computer systems, but this limitation has recently been solved for both right[26] and left ventricles with automated three-dimensional (3-D) analytic methods.[27,28] Similar to the planar technique, GBPS has been analyzed for Fourier amplitude and phase, rendering accurate 3-D assessment of the origin of ventricular tachycardia,[29] as in arrhythmogenic right ventricular dysplasia,[30] and rendering superior images for evaluation of LV and RV shape (topography).

QUALITY PERFORMANCE IN IMAGE ACQUISITION AND PROCESSING

FPRNA Acquisition

If ERNA is to be performed in addition to FPRNA, after placement of a large bore (14- or 16-gauge) antecubital intravenous line, 1.5 mg of stannous pyrophosphate is mixed with 30 mL of the patient's blood for approximately 60 seconds and is then infused. Resting FPRNA is performed after a 10-minute delay, to allow further red blood cell (RBC) uptake of stannous ions. Tc-99m pertechnetate (25–30 mCi, 925–1110 MBq), in a volume of less than 1 mL, is given by rapid flushing with at least 30 mL of normal saline through the indwelling catheter. This can be followed by planar or tomographic (SPECT) ERNA images. Examples of this combined RNA approach are shown in Figures 17-1 through 17-3.

For FPRNA, Tc-99m DTPA is often used if no ERNA are required. Perfusion agents, such as

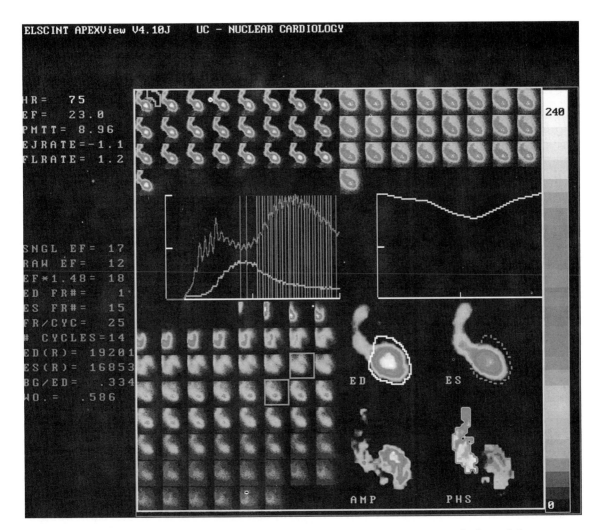

Figure 17-1. FPRNA (anterior projection) images are shown, with the serial images at the lower left, demonstrating tracer transit from the superior vena cava, to right atrium, to right ventricle to the pulmonary phase, left heart phase, and systemic circulation. Using regions of interest (ROIs) drawn over the LV and left lung (far upper left image, also blue and green), histograms are obtained (shown above serial images, in blue and green, respectively), which show overlapping RV counts with systoles (curve valleys) and diastoles (curve peaks) from which the cardiac cycles (CYC) are derived, which comprise the representative cycle. Each cardiac cycle is marked (red for diastole, green for systole). The pulmonary curve is used to compute the pulmonary mean transit time (PMTT). The length of the representative cycle in frames (FR) is used to derive the heart rate (HR). The images of the raw representative cycle are shown at upper right. This is subjected to the frame method of background subtraction (i.e., using the background to end-diastolic image ratio (BG/ED) and the washout factor (WO) needed to set the pulmonary area to zero counts), in order to derive the corrected representative cycle (upper left images) from which single ROI ejection fraction (SNGL EF), which is higher than the raw EF, but lower than the dual-ROI-derived EF, which is used to account for valve plane motion. The Fourier amplitude (AMP) and phase (PHS) images at the lower right demonstrate reduced inferior wall amplitude and delayed contraction of the inferior wall and apex, respectively. (See color insert.)

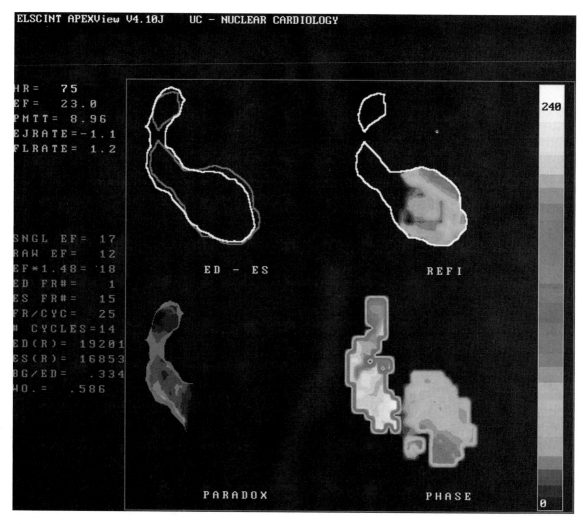

Figure 17-2. FPRNA (anterior projection) functional images are shown, with end-diastolic and end-systolic perimeter image at the upper left (ED–ES), a paradox image (lower left), regional ejection fraction index (REFI, upper right), and Fourier-phase images (lower right). The Fourier-phase image demonstrates delayed contraction of the inferior wall and apex. These functional images allow assessment of regional function without the use of visual interpretation of cine images. (See color insert.)

Tc-99m sestamibi or tetrofosmin may be utilized if perfusion images are desired, but not Tc-99m teboroxime, since it is trapped in the pulmonary parenchyma.[13]

Images are usually obtained using a single- or multicrystal high-count rate gamma camera fitted with a high-sensitivity parallel-hole collimator (e.g., SIM 400, Scinticor, Milwaukee, WI, or El-Gems CardiaL (formerly Elscint), Haifa, Israel). Images are acquired in the right anterior oblique or anterior projection using 25 (±4) frames per cardiac cycle.

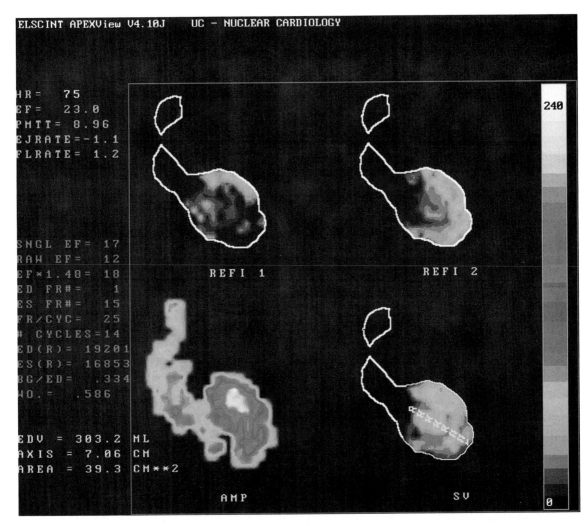

Figure 17-3.   Additional FPRNA (anterior projection) functional images are shown, with regional ejection fraction index for the first and second halves of systole (REFI1 and REFI2, upper frames), an alternative method of determining the presence of delayed contraction. Note that the inferior and apical regions have more ejection fraction in the latter half of systole, compared with the anterolateral wall. Fourier amplitude (AMP, lower left) and stroke volume (SV, ED minus ES, lower right) images are shown. The graphic extending from the valve plane to the apex on the SV image is used to compute the LV volume using the Sandler and Dodge equation for the anterior projection. (See color insert.)

FPRNA Analysis (Figures 17-1 through 17-3)

FPRNA data are analyzed using the frame method for LVEF and commercially available computer software.[13,16,17] This software creates a representative LV volume curve by summing frames of several (usually 5–10) cardiac cycles, which are aligned by matching their end diastoles (histogram peaks) and end systoles (histogram valleys) during the operator-defined levophase of tracer transit. The pulmonary frame background-corrected representative cycle is then interrogated with a fixed region of interest in order to obtain the final first-pass LV time–activity curve. This ROI is drawn over the LV as defined by a first harmonic Fourier transformation-phase image, which distinguishes clearly the LV from aortic counts. End diastole is taken as the first frame of the representative cycle. End systole is defined as the frame with the minimum counts in the histogram. Historically, the LVEF was taken as the end-diastolic counts minus the end-systolic counts, divided by the background subtracted end-diastolic counts.

A second ROI (end-diastolic) can be derived from a Fourier transformation amplitude image, with masking of the lower 10% of image intensity, which extends the ROI in a basal direction, usually 1 to 3 pixels, up to the amplitude signal of the aortic root. The remainder of this ROI is drawn to match the first region of interest (end systolic). The dual-ROI LVEF is determined as the end-diastolic ROI counts minus the end-systolic ROI counts, divided by the background subtracted end-diastolic ROI counts. Fourier-guided dual-ROI analysis of FPRNA results in a more accurate accounting for valve plane motion during the

cardiac cycle, giving EFs that are highly reproducible and similar in value to ERNA.[15]

ERNA Acquisition (Figures 17-4 and 17-5)

A detailed discussion of ERNA acquisition and processing is presented in Chapter 19. For purposes of comparing methods for assessing ventricular function, a brief discussion is included. As noted above for FPRNA with ERNA, 1.5 mg of stannous pyrophosphate can be mixed with 30 mL of the patient's blood for approximately 60 seconds and is then reinfused. In some patients, quality labeling of RBCs is more certain using the "in vitro" technique of adding Tc-99m pertechnetate (25–30 mCi, 925–1110 MBq) to 50 mL of blood, after reduction of the hemoglobin with stannous pyrophosphate.

ECG-gated planar equilibrium blood pool images are best acquired using high-resolution collimation. Images for LVEF calculation are obtained in the best-septal (shallow) left-anterior oblique view. This angle, usually 25 to 60 degrees, must be carefully set using a persistence mode prior to

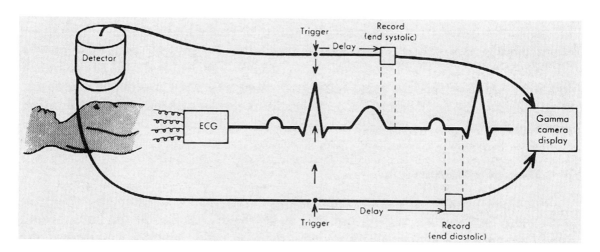

Figure 17-4.   Diagram from the original description of ECG-gated imaging, demonstrating the triggering and delays used to acquire end-systolic and end-diastolic frames from multiple cardiac cycles. (Reprinted with permission from Strauss et al.[42])

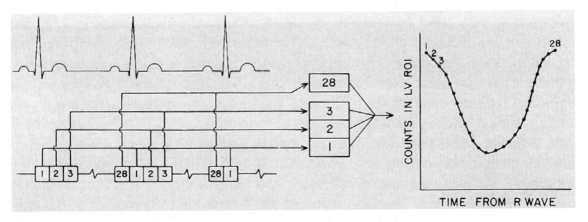

Figure 17-5.   Multiple-gated cardiac imaging is diagramed using ECG triggering to acquire 28 frames per cardiac cycle. This results in a time–activity curve that represents LV volume and can be used to calculate ejection fraction, as well as rates of ventricular emptying and filling. (Reprinted with permission from Zaret and Berger.[43])

acquisition. For regional wall motion assessment, the best-septal view plus and minus 45 degrees should be obtained ("anterior" and "lateral" views). Each planar-gated image should be acquired for 6 to 10 minutes duration, dividing each cardiac cycle into a minimum of 32 frames.

ERNA Processing (Figure 17-6)

For LVEF determination, automated variable ROI are usually generated on the planar-gated equilibrium blood pool data throughout the cardiac cycle, using the commercially available software. This method automatically identifies the LV master region of interest by Fourier phase imaging, typically requiring no operator intervention. Edge detection is typically performed using a combination of first and second derivatives of the count profiles. The first derivative edge (e.g., nadir of counts between the septum and lateral walls) is too loose and inclusive of background. The second derivative (e.g., the inflection point at which counts increase rapidly instead of slowly) is too tight around the chamber and excludes counts around the edges. Thus, most software methods use the 50% level between the thresholds obtained with the two derivative techniques. This is performed for each

individual frame, and the resulting time–activity histogram is representative of relative LV volume. This curve requires background correction, using an automated periventricular background ROI, which allows determination of the counts/pixel in the background. Thus, this ROI must routinely be carefully evaluated and adjusted if necessary to avoid inclusion of high-count structures (e.g., spleen and descending aorta), which could artifactually increase the LVEF.

VEST Acquisition and Analysis
(Figure 17-7)

The nuclear VEST is essentially a nonimaging form of ERNA, with the identical radiopharmaceutical administration, planar ERNA imaging for calibration, and planar imaging with the device place on the chest to confirm correct placement.

As shown in Figure 17-7, the alterations in blood pool counts on a beat-to-beat basis can be analyzed, regardless of rhythm and physiological conditions. However, care must be maintained to ensure that the position of the device is not appreciably altered by movement, e.g., changing from supine to sitting to standing, such that the accuracy of the measurement of function is maintained.

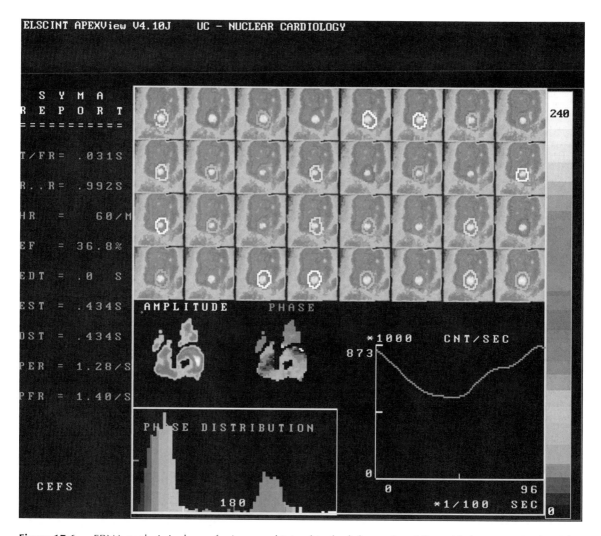

Figure 17-6. ERNA analysis is shown for images obtained in the left anterior oblique 45-degree projection. The 32 ECG-gated frames are analyzed using a guiding region of interest (ROI, in cyan, frame 1) obtained either manually or using Fourier-phase and amplitude images to automatically locate and outline the LV. Automated LV edge detection is performed using a combination of first and second derivatives of count profiles inside the guiding or master ROI. Background correction is performed based on the counts per pixel within a small periventricular ROI (in cyan, frame 16), drawn carefully to avoid the ventricle or the spleen. The counts within the 32 ROIs are shown after background correction in the lower right histogram. The first derivative of this ventricular volume curve is used to compute the peak filling and emptying rates (PFR and PER). The Fourier-phase and amplitude functional images demonstrate inferoapical and septal hypokinesis with late contraction, when compared with the RV and the basal lateral portion of the LV. (See color insert.)

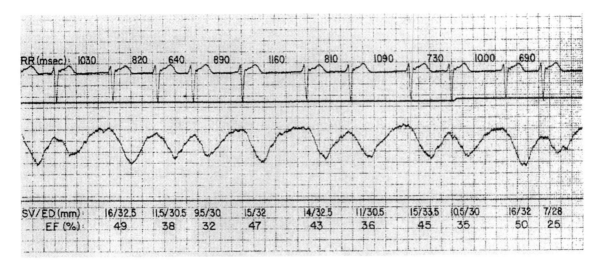

Figure 17-7. Data from a nonimaging equilibrium blood pool-measuring device, often called the "nuclear VEST," "nuclear stethoscope," or "nuclear probe," are shown. These beat-to-beat LVEF's results were obtained in a patient with atrial fibrillation, in which the EF tends to vary directly with the LV filling time. EF could be followed in a continuous fashion or the ECG trigger could be utilized to obtain a "gated" equilibrium LV ejection fraction. (From Schneider et al.[44])

GBPS Acquisition, Reconstruction, and Analysis (Figure 17-8)

ECG-gated projections for SPECT reconstruction are usually obtained using high-resolution collimation in a fashion similar to gated SPECT perfusion imaging, scanning from right anterior oblique-45-degree to left posterior oblique-45-degree projections. A total of 60 projections of 15 to 30 seconds duration at 3-degree steps should give adequate count density. At each projection either 8 or 16 frames per cardiac cycle should be acquired.

After collimator sensitivity and center of rotation correction, low-pass prefiltered projections are reconstructed into transaxial slices of the blood pool for each of the 8 or 16 frames of the cardiac cycle. Transaxial slices (e.g., 2-pixel thickness) are reconstructed using a Butterworth backprojection filter (e.g., a critical frequency of 0.5 and order of 14.0). The transaxial slice sets can then be reoriented in cardiac planes (i.e., short axis, horizontal long axis, and vertical long axis) for each of the eight frames of the cardiac cycle. Mid-ventricular

horizontal and vertical long-axis slices are obtained and analyzed for wall motion or EF. If 8 frames are acquired, the eight slices can be expanded to 16 frames by weighted frame interpolation and temporal filtering.

Because of the high contrast of SPECT, the blood pool images can be analyzed in automated fashion with one of several commercially available programs, which quickly process and display automated calculation of RV and LV EFs and volumes. Changes in volume are tracked from ED to ES for calculation of wall motion and regional thickening. These results are typically displayed in revolving 3-D images or simple polar map format. Additional information regarding GBPS may be cound in Chapter 19.

GSPECT Acquisition, Processing, and Analysis (Figures 17-9 and 17-10)

As one of the most commonly performed radionuclide methods for assessment of ventricular function is GSPECT, an entire chapter (Chapter 18)

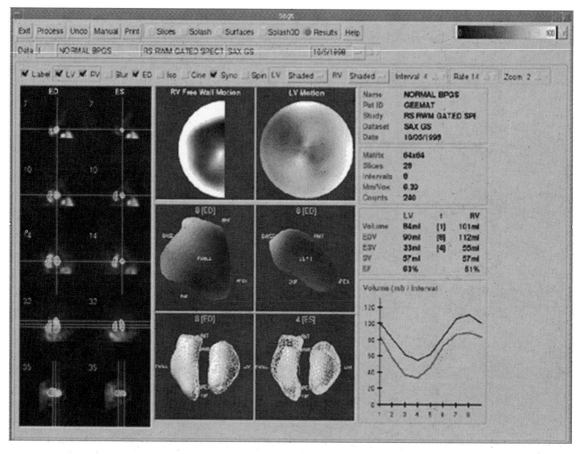

Figure 17-8. Gated SPECT blood pool images are shown analyzed with the commercially available QBS program (Cedars-Sinai) used for display and automated calculation of RV and LV ejection fraction and volume. Changes in volume are tracked from ED to ES, for calculation of wall motion and regional thickening, displayed in polar map format. Three-dimensional diagrams (above) and actual SPECT slices with fitted edges (below) are also shown. (Images courtesy of Dr. Guido Germano.) (See color insert.)

has been devoted to this method. Historically, GSPECT myocardial perfusion imaging has been most often performed with poststress ECG gating. It is now recognized that gated rest perfusion imaging can be performed, even in laboratories performing dual-isotope imaging with thallium-201,[31–33] provided that these studies are obtained with an adequate count density. This is beneficial, since reversible ischemia on stress perfusion images will alter the appreciation of regional wall motion and lower LVEF, likely caused by underrepresentation of the endocardium in images with substantial degrees of ischemia.[34]

During acquisition, careful attention must be paid to the presence of cardiac arrhythmias, since reconstruction of only portions of the cardiac cycle because of gating irregularities may result in degradation of the final perfusion images.[35] The projection images for SPECT reconstruction images are usually acquired using high-resolution collimation, although some systems employ high-quality general-purpose cast (rather than foil) collimators. A total of 180 degrees of projection images are usually obtained, scanning from right anterior oblique-45 degrees to left posterior oblique-45 degrees. A total of 60 projections of

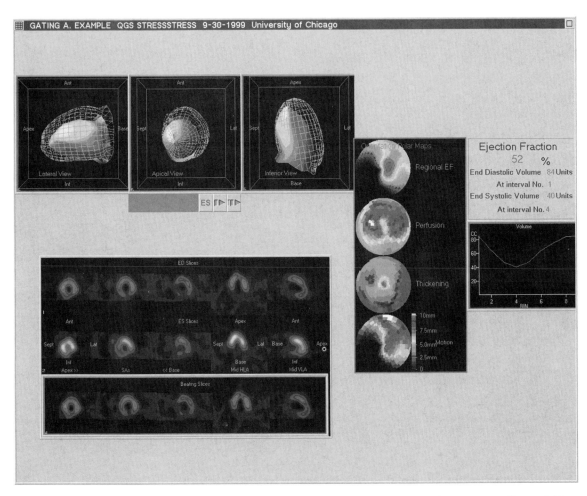

Figure 17-9.   Gated SPECT myocardial perfusion images are shown analyzed with the commercially available QGS program (Cedars-Sinai), as in Figure 17-8, but obtained with Tc-99-tetrofosmin. The images demonstrate hypoperfusion and hypokinesis with reduced thickening in the inferior wall. The apparent septal hypokinesis on the 3-D, regional EF and motion maps is an artifact as a result of previous median sternotomy with coronary artery bypass surgery and can be distinguished from ischemic dysfunction by the presence of normal systolic thickening of the septal myocardium. (See color insert.)

15- to 30-second duration at 3-degree steps will give adequate count density, for a usual total of 15 to 25-minute acquisition time, using less acquisition time with multiple-headed gamma cameras. At each projection, either 8 or 16 frames per cardiac cycle should be acquired.

For image processing, a wide range of SPECT reconstruction filters and settings have been utilized, depending on the tracer characteristics, the amount of myocardial tracer activity, the system and collimator characteristics, and the software used for analysis. After collimator sensitivity and center of rotation correction, low-pass prefiltered projections are reconstructed into transaxial slices for each of the 8 or 16 frames of the cardiac cycle for gated SPECT, or the single ungated or summed gated projection set. Transaxial slices are usually reconstructed using a Butterworth

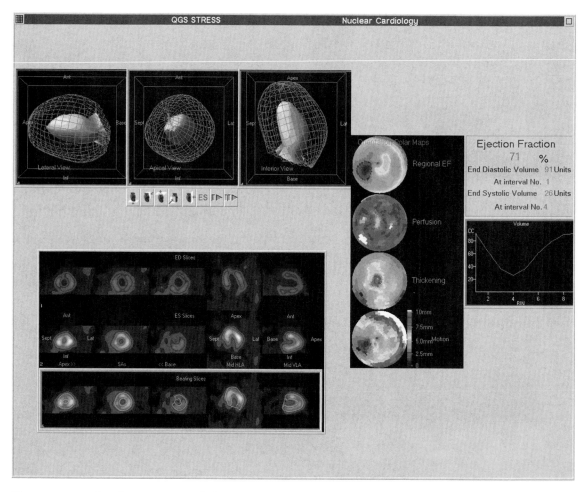

Figure 17-10. Gated SPECT myocardial perfusion images are shown analyzed with the commercially available QGS program (Cedars-Sinai) used for display and automated calculation of ejection fraction and volume. Changes in volume are tracked from ED to ES, for calculation of wall motion and regional thickening, displayed in polar map format. Three-dimensional diagrams (above) and actual SPECT slices with fitted edges (below) are also shown. These images were obtained with thallium-201 in a normal patient. (See color insert.)

backprojection filter (e.g., with a critical frequency of 0.35 and an order of 10.0). The transaxial slice sets are then reoriented in cardiac planes (i.e., short axis, horizontal long axis, and vertical long axis) for each of the eight frames of the cardiac cycle. Midventricular horizontal and vertical long-axis slices can be analyzed for regional wall motion or EF (see gated SPECT section below). If 8 frames are acquired, these eight slices can be expanded to 16

frames by weighted frame interpolation and temporal filtering for a smoother cinematic display.

Acquisition of SPECT data synchronized with the electrocardiographic R-wave is generally performed using 8 or 16 gating intervals and allows evaluation of both global (EF) and regional (myocardial wall motion and wall thickening) cardiac functions. These eight sets of projection images are routinely summed in order to obtain a single planar projection set ("ungated") for perfusion evaluation and comparison with nongated images.

The exponential increase in the use of gated SPECT perfusion has been fueled by the increased availability of automatic and semiautomatic algorithms for edge detection and the quantification of functional cardiac parameters.[36–38] This reflects not only the improved quality control and diagnostic accuracy of interpreting perfusion images in light of regional and global LV performance but also the incremental value of gated SPECT over perfusion imaging alone for prognosis.[39–41] For these reasons, a recent policy statement of the American Society of Nuclear Cardiology encouraged the use of gated SPECT with every perfusion study in which gating is feasible (http://www.asnc.org/policy/ecg-gating.htm).

As noted above, recent published experience from multiple sites indicates that gated thallium-201 SPECT imaging is possible.[31–33] However, thallium-201 images are poorer in counts and higher in scatter. Therefore, they require multiheaded gamma camera imaging, higher thallium-201 tracer doses, and smaller patients, in order to obtain adequate count density in the study. Alteration of backprojection filters (e.g., Butterworth critical frequency of 0.25) may be useful on some systems. At best, because of poorer ventricular cavity resolution, thallium-201-gated SPECT EFs and volumes may not be as reproducible as Tc-99m sestamibi.[32]

REFERENCES

1. Greenberg H, McMaster P, Dwyer EM; the Multicenter Postinfarction Research Group. Left ventricular dysfunction after acute myocardial infarction: The results of a prospective multicenter study. *J Am Coll Cardiol.* 1984;4:867–874.
2. Nesto RW, Cohn LH, Collins JJ Jr, Wynne J, Holman L, Cohn PF. Inotropic contractile reserve: A useful predictor of increased 5 year survival and improved post-operative left ventricular function in patients with coronary artery disease and reduced ejection fraction. *Am J Cardiol.* 1982;50:39–44.
3. Ritchie JL, Hallstrom AP, Troubaugh GB, Caldwell JH, Cobb LA. Out-of-hospital sudden coronary death: Rest

and exercise left ventricular function in survivors. *Am J Cardiol.* 1985;55:645–651.
4. Williams KA, Sherwood DF, Fisher KM. The frequency of asymptomatic and electrically silent exercise-induced regional myocardial ischemia during first-pass radionuclide angiography with upright bicycle ergometry. *J Nucl Med.* 1992;33:359–364.
5. Lee KL, Pryor DB, Pieper KS, et al. Prognostic value of radionuclide angiography in medically treated patients with coronary artery disease. A comparison with clinical and catheterization variables. *Circulation.* 1990;82: 1705–1717.
6. Muhlbaier LH, Pryor DB, Rankin JS, et al. Observational comparison of eventfree survival with medical and surgical therapy in patients with coronary artery disease. 20 years of follow-up. *Circulation.* 1992;86(5, Suppl): II198–II204.
7. Jones RH, Johnson SH, Bigelow C, et al. Exercise radionuclide angiocardiography predicts cardiac death in patients with coronary artery disease. *Circulation.* 1991;84(3, Suppl):I52–I58.
8. Johnson SH, Bigelow C, Lee KL, Pryor DB, Jones RH. Prediction of death and myocardial infarction by radionuclide angiocardiography in patients with suspected coronary artery disease. *Am J Cardiol.* 1991;67(11):919–926.
9. Pryor DB, Harrell FE Jr, Lee KL, et al. Prognostic indicators from radionuclide angiography in medically treated patients with coronary artery disease. *Am J Cardiol.* 1984;53(1):18–22.
10. Zhu WX, Gibbons RJ, Bailey KR, Gersh BJ. Predischarge exercise radionuclide angiography in predicting multivessel coronary artery disease and subsequent cardiac events after thrombolytic therapy for acute myocardial infarction. *Am J Cardiol.* 1994;74:554–559.
11. Jones RH, Borges-Neto S, Potts JM. Simultaneous measurement of myocardial perfusion and ventricular function during exercise from a single injection of Tc-99m sestamibi in coronary artery disease. *Am J Cardiol.* 1990;66:68E–71E.
12. Berman DS, Kiat H, Maddahi J. The new 99mTc myocardial perfusion imaging agents: 99mTc-sestamibi and 99mTc-teboroxime. *Circulation.* 1991;84(3, Suppl): I7–I21.
13. Williams KA, Taillon LA, Draho JM, Foisy MF. First-pass radionuclide angiographic studies of left ventricular function with Tc-99m-Teboroxime, Tc-99m-Sestamibi and Tc-99m-DTPA. *J Nucl Med.* 1993;35:394–399.
14. Williams KA, Taillon LA. Gated planar technetium-99m-sestamibi myocardial perfusion image inversion for quantitative scintigraphic assessment of left ventricular function. *J Nucl Cardiol.* 1995;2:285–295.
15. Williams KA, Bryant TA, Taillon LA. First-pass radionuclide angiographic analysis with two regions of interest: Improved "substitutability" for gated

equilibrium ejection fractions. *J Nucl Med.* 1998;39(11): 1857–1861.

16. Gal R, Grenier RP, Carpenter J, Schmidt DH, Port SC. High count rate first-pass radionuclide angiography using a digital gamma camera. *J Nucl Med.* 1986;27:198–206.

17. Gal R, Grenier RP, Schmidt DH, Port SC. Background correction in first-pass radionuclide angiography: Comparison of several approaches. *J Nucl Med.* 1986; 27:1480–1486.

18. Villanueva-Meyer J, Mena I, Narahara KA. Simultaneous assessment of left ventricular wall motion and myocardial perfusion with technetium-99m-methoxy isobutyl isonitrile at stress and rest in patients with angina: Comparison with thallium-201 SPECT. *J Nucl Med.* 1990;31:457–463.

19. Sporn V, Perez-Balino N, Holman BL, et al. Simultaneous measurement of ventricular function and myocardial perfusion using the technetium-99m isonitriles. *Clin Nucl Med.* 1988;13:77–81.

20. Bisi G, Sciagra R, Bull U, et al. Assessment of ventricular function with first-pass radionuclide angiography using technetium 99m hexakis-2-methoxyisobutylisonitrile: A European multicentre study. *Eur J Nucl Med.* 1991;18: 178–183.

21. Boucher CA, Wackers FJ, Zaret BL, Mena IG. Technetium-99m sestamibi myocardial imaging at rest for assessment of myocardial infarction and first-pass ejection fraction. Multicenter Cardiolite Study Group. *Am J Cardiol.* 1992;69:22–27.

22. Williams KA, Taillon LA. Left ventricular function in patients with coronary artery disease using gated tomographic myocardial perfusion images: Comparison with contrast ventriculography and first-pass radionuclide angiography. *J Am Coll Cardiol.* 1996;27:173–181.

23. Williams KA, Walley PE, Ryan JW. Detection and assessment of severity of tricuspid regurgitation using first-pass radionuclide angiography and comparison with pulsed Doppler echocardiography. *Am J Cardiol.* 1990; 66:333–339.

24. Sharir T, Germano G, Kavanagh PB, et al. Incremental prognostic value of post-stress left ventricular ejection fraction and volume by gated myocardial perfusion single photon emission computed tomography. *Circulation.* 1999;100:1035–1042.

25. Tamaki N, Strauss HW. Ambulatory ventricular function monitoring for serial assessments of cardiac function during exercise. *J Cardiol.* 1987;17:875–885.

26. Nichols K, Saouaf R, Ababneh AA, et al. Validation of SPECT equilibrium radionuclide angiographic right ventricular parameters by cardiac magnetic resonance imaging. *J Nucl Cardiol.* 2002;9(2):153–160.

27. De Bondt P, Nichols K, Vandenberghe S, et al. Validation of gated blood-pool SPECT cardiac measurements tested using a biventricular dynamic physical phantom. *J Nucl Med.* 2003;44:967–972.

28. Nichols K, Humayun N, De Bondt P, Vandenberghe S, Akinboboye OO, Bergmann SR. Model dependence of gated blood pool SPECT ventricular function measurements. *J Nucl Cardiol.* 2004;11:282–292.

29. Botvinick EH, O'Connell JW, Kadkade PP, et al. Potential added value of three-dimensional reconstruction and display of single photon emission computed tomographic gated blood pool images. *J Nucl Cardiol.* 1998;5:245–255.

30. Casset-Senon D, Babuty D, Alison D, et al. Delayed contraction area responsible for sustained ventricular tachycardia in an arrhythmogenic right ventricular cardiomyopathy: Demonstration by Fourier analysis of SPECT equilibrium radionuclide angiography. *J Nucl Cardiol.* 2000;7:539–542.

31. Maunoury C, Chen CC, Chua KB, Thompson CJ. Quantification of left ventricular function with thallium-201 and technetium-99m-sestamibi myocardial gated SPECT. *J Nucl Med.* 1997;38:958–961.

32. Lee DS, Ahn JY, Kim SK, et al. Limited performance of quantitative assessment of myocardial function by thallium-201 gated myocardial single-photon emission tomography. *Eur J Nucl Med.* 2000;27:185–191.

33. Germano G, Erel J, Kiat H, Kavanagh PB, Berman DS. Quantitative LVEF and qualitative regional function from gated thallium-201 perfusion SPECT. *J Nucl Med.* 1997;38:749–754.

34. Johnson LL, Verdesca SA, Aude WY, et al. Postischemic stunning can affect left ventricular ejection fraction and regional wall motion on post-stress gated sestamibi tomograms. *J Am Coll Cardiol.* 1997;30:1641–1648.

35. Nichols K, Yao SS, Kamran M, Faber TL, Cooke CD, DePuey EG. Clinical impact of arrhythmias on gated SPECT cardiac myocardial perfusion and function assessment. *J Nucl Cardiol.* 2001;8:19–30.

36. DePuey EG, Nichols K, Dobrinsky C. Left ventricular ejection fraction assessed from gated technetium-99m-sestamibi SPECT. *J Nucl Med.* 1993;34(11):1871–1876.

37. Germano G, Kiat H, Kavanagh PB, et al. Automatic quantification of ejection fraction from gated myocardial perfusion SPECT. *J Nucl Med.* 1995;36(11):2138–2147.

38. Smith WH, Kastner RJ, Calnon DA, Segalla D, Beller GA, Watson DD. Quantitative gated single photon emission computed tomography imaging: A counts-based method for display and measurement of regional and global ventricular systolic function. *J Nucl Cardiol.* 1997;4(6):451–463.

39. DePuey EG, Rozanski AR. Using gated technetium-99m sestamibi SPECT to characterize fixed myocardial defects as infarct or artifact. *J Nucl Med.* 1995;36:952–955.

40. Taillefer R, DePuey EG, Udelson JE, Beller GA, Latour Y, Reeves F. Comparative diagnostic accuracy of Tl-201 and Tc-99m sestamibi SPECT imaging (perfusion and ECG-gated SPECT) in detecting coronary artery disease in women. *J Am Coll Cardiol.* 1997;29:69–77.

41. Smanio PEP, Watson DD, Segalla DL, Vinson EL, Smith WH, Beller GA. Value of gating of technetium 99m sestamibi single-photon emission computed tomographic imaging. *J Am Coll Cardiol.* 1997;30:1687–1692.

42. Strauss HW, Zaret BL, Hurley PJ, et al. A scintiphotographic method for measuring left ventricular ejection fraction in man without cardiac catheterization. *Am J Cardiol.* 1971;28:575–580.

43. Zaret B, Berger H. Techniques of nuclear cardiology. In: Hurst JW, ed. *The Heart.* New York: McGraw-Hill; 1981.

44. Schneider J, Berger HJ, Sands MJ, Lachman AB, Zaret BL. Beat-to-beat left ventricular performance in atrial fibrillation: Radionuclide assessment with the computerized nuclear probe. *Am J Cardiol.* 1983;51:1189–1195.

CHAPTER 18

ECG-Gated SPECT Imaging

James A. Arrighi

OVERVIEW OF GATED SPECT

Physiologic Principles

The assessment of global and regional left ventricular performance is a key element in evaluating patients with cardiac disease. Ventricular performance may be assessed using a number of different parameters, including cardiac output (the volume of blood flow per minute), cardiac index (cardiac output corrected for body surface area), and ejection fraction. Measurement of ejection fraction is the most common noninvasively obtained parameter for assessment of ventricular performance. Left ventricular ejection fraction (LVEF) is influenced by the major determinants of ventricular performance: contractility, heart rate, and loading conditions. These may be affected by physiologic state (e.g., rest, exercise, and systemic stress) and/or disease processes. The prognostic importance of LVEF is well established[1] (Figure 18-1).

Two basic parameters of left ventricular function are important to consider when describing ventricular function and the effect of disease on the heart. *Global* left ventricular function refers to the overall performance of the ventricle as a pump. Global function can be expressed as LVEF, which is defined physiologically as the difference between end-diastolic and end-systolic volumes, divided by the end-diastolic volume. Thus, calculation of LVEF requires accurate estimation of these volumes. The left ventricular volume curves that are generated by gated SPECT programs should be consistent with physiologic volume curves, with clear definition of end systole and end diastole. *Regional* left ventricular function is also important to assess, since regional dysfunction may occur before global function (LVEF) is affected. Regional function is usually evaluated qualitatively after review of cine images but may also be analyzed by quantitative measurements.[2] Evaluation of regional function requires images of sufficient spatial and temporal resolution so as to allow assessment of wall motion and/or thickening. Assessment of both global and regional function

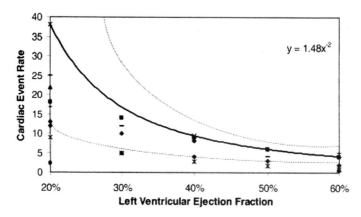

Figure 18-1.   Relationship of cardiac event rate and left ventricular ejection fraction with poststress gated SPECT, based on analysis of cumulative evidence from published studies. The line of best fit (solid line) is based on a power regression function (95% CI, dotted lines) optimizing explanatory variation. (From Shaw and Iskandrian.[1])

is necessary for a complete evaluation of cardiac function.

Overview of Technical Principles

The principal aspect of the technique is utilization of ECG gating, in order to generate a series of images that represent phases in the cardiac cycle throughout systole and diastole. In essence, images that are acquired and reviewed for the assessment of perfusion may actually be the summed images of 8 to 16 images that are collected during various phases of the cardiac cycle (Figure 18-2), allowing for the construction of a series of images that represent the temporal phases of the cardiac cycle.

Once images throughout the cardiac cycle are generated, estimates of left ventricular volume are performed using algorithms designed to delineate the endomyocardial border and the valve plane. Analysis of the change in volume of the ventricle over the cardiac cycle allows calculation of LVEF. The accuracy of this calculation depends on a number of factors, including the adequacy of the ECG gating signal, the lack of heart rate variability, overall counts, acquisition and filtering parameters, the performance characteristics of the program, and the presence of artifacts or extracardiac activity. A thorough understanding of the quantitative pro-

gram being used, as well as the recommended acquisition parameters and normal limits, is essential to maintain the quality and accuracy of the technique.

In addition to the quantitative analysis, cine display of the gated images allows qualitative assessment of global and regional function. Discordance between the reader's qualitative assessment of ventricular function and the calculated LVEF suggests possible errors in acquisition or analysis and warrant investigation. Assessment of regional wall motion and thickening usually is made based on qualitative review of these images; quantitative analysis of regional function has not been validated fully.

ACQUSITION OF GATED SPECT IMAGES

Patient Preparation

In addition to the usual setup and quality control procedures used for all cardiac SPECT perfusion studies, gated SPECT requires an adequate ECG signal, with a clearly identifiable R-wave. Three ECG leads are used by most systems, positioned over the left and right clavicles, and in the right lower abdomen. Technologists should review the tracing before positioning the patient and, if possible, include a sample ECG strip in the patient

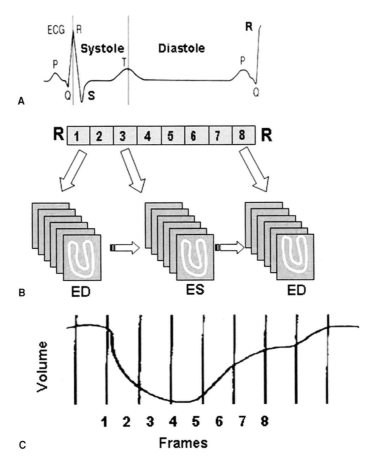

Figure 18-2.   Principle of ECG-gated SPECT acquisition. The R-R interval on ECG is divided into eight frames (**A**). Images are acquired over multiple cardiac cycles for each projection in order to generate frames that represent each eighth of the cardiac cycle, including end diastole (ED) and end systole (ES) (**B**). After automated definition of myocardial borders, left ventricular volumes are calculated for each frame, in order to generate the volume curve from which ejection fraction is calculated (**C**). (From Paul and Nabi.[38])

record. If the ECG signal is inadequate, or if significant arrhythmias are present, ungated SPECT should be performed. If gated SPECT is attempted with a marginal ECG signal or borderline arrhythmia, the interpreting physician should be informed so as to be alert for potential gating artifacts.

Image Acquisition: Dose

The selection of radiopharmaceutical and doses generally are chosen for reasons independent

of gating, such as physician preference, patient weight, and indication for study. For same-day technetium-based protocols (i.e., low dose–high dose), the high-dose study is best for gating, as a result of its higher counts. The low-dose study may be gated as well if it is high quality with adequate counts, particularly in relatively thinner patients. For 2-day technetium-based protocols (high dose–high dose), either or both studies may be gated. For typical dual-isotope protocols (rest thallium–stress technetium), the technetium study is gated. Thallium scintigraphy may also be gated (see subsequent section below).

Acquisition Parameters

Gated SPECT acquisition divides the imaging data from each projection into 8 or 16 frames, which represent equal time intervals of the cardiac cycle. The general acquisition parameters of imaging are similar for gated or nongated SPECT. Although practitioners may sometimes alter these parameters in order to increase image quality (usually meaning longer acquisitions to improve counts), it is never appropriate to change these parameters at the expense of the static perfusion images.

General Acquisition Parameters   Acquisition protocols for SPECT studies are outlined in the imaging guidelines published by the American Society of Nuclear Cardiology.[3] In general, for technetium studies, a "step-and-shoot" or "continuous" mode for 64 projections over a 180-degree orbit (from 45-degree right anterior oblique to 45-degree left posterior oblique) is preferred. The time per projection is 20 to 25 seconds; increasing this time may result in improved counts, but at the expense of total imaging times that exceed 30 minutes. For dual-isotope studies, the technetium images are gated, and the resting thallium images usually are not gated. Gated stress-redistribution thallium imaging is discussed later in this chapter.

Acquisition Parameters Specific to Gating   There are three major parameters that must be considered, which are specific to the gated portion of the SPECT study: acquisition mode, R-R interval acceptance window, and frame rate. The factors that influence the setting of these parameters are software capabilities, dose of radiopharmaceutical, and physician preference.

Acquisition Mode   Acquisitions may be performed in one of three modes, the first of which is the most common: fixed R-R interval, variable R-R interval, and list modes. In fixed R-R interval mode, the acceptance window is set at the beginning of the acquisition and remains fixed throughout the study. The initial setting of this interval is set after an analysis of the average R-R interval just prior to the start of acquisition. If the heart rate changes significantly during the acquisition, the gated portion of the SPECT study will be compromised. Variable R-R interval mode is similar, but the R-R interval is periodically sampled and updated *during* the acquisition. This allows the system to adjust for some degree of change in heart rate that may occur during the study. Finally, in list mode acquisition, data are collected with time data (relative to the ECG), i.e., the computer stores where and *when* all counts occurred. The advantage of list mode is that data can be reformatted retrospectively, and limits for R-R interval can be varied. Although this method is very effective, it requires a relatively large amount of computer memory and more processing time compared to standard frame mode acquisition.

R-R Interval Acceptance Window   Once the mean R-R interval is selected, the acceptance window defines the amount of deviation from this interval that is acceptable, expressed as a percentage of the R-R interval. Data within the limits of acceptance are stored, and data that fall outside of these limits are rejected. For example, a heart rate of 60 beats per minute translates into an R-R interval of 1000 milliseconds. A 40% window accepts beats from 20% below to 20% above the 1000 millisecond interval (i.e., R-R intervals from 800 to 1200 milliseconds are accepted). A 100% window accepts beats ±50% of the R-R interval, and an infinite or "open" window accepts all beats.

The appropriate window depends, in part, on the system utilized for acquisition (Figure 18-3). The primacy of the ungated SPECT perfusion images remains: it is preferred that all, or nearly all, counts be stored and used for the ungated images. Therefore, unless the camera system has a data buffer mechanism to capture rejected beats, the widest possible acceptance window (usually 100%) should be used as a default. If the heart rate varies considerably during the study, the gated images may be compromised, and the study should be

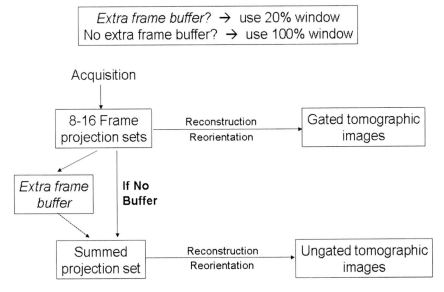

Figure 18-3.   Setting the R-R interval acceptance window. Eight- to 16-frame gated SPECT projection sets are reconstructed into gated tomographic images, for analysis of left ventricular function. Image sets are also summed for reconstruction of ungated images, for analysis of perfusion. If an extra frame buffer is available, window can be narrowed to 20%; beats rejected for gated images will be stored in the buffer and used for ungated images. In the absence of an extra frame buffer, a wide window (100%) is used, so that no frames are lost in the ungated images. (Adapted from Germano and Berman[39] by permission of Oxford University Press, Inc.)

read as an ungated study. Some systems have a data buffer, in which counts that are rejected for the gated study can be stored and used for reconstruction of the ungated images. In these systems, it is appropriate to set a narrower acceptance window (20%–30%), since the nongated images will not be compromised even in the setting of many rejected beats.

Frame Rate   The most common frame rate is eight frames per cardiac cycle.[3–5] This frame rate allows determination of LVEF and regional wall thickening with acceptable accuracy. Increasing the frame rate to 16 frames per cycle may be possible in many patients with relatively high counts and may increase the accuracy of the LVEF calculation, but at a higher risk of a poor-quality (low-count) study. Of note, when a frame rate of eight frames per second is used, the lower limit of normal LVEF may be reduced because of the lack of temporal resolution.

The use of gated SPECT for the assessment of diastolic function is feasible but requires the increased temporal resolution of a 16-frame study (Figure 18-4).[6] Generation of an accurate LV volume curve is necessary, and peak filling rate can then be calculated in a manner analogous to the method used for gated blood pool imaging.

IMAGE PROCESSING

General Processing Parameters

The first steps in image processing are related to reconstruction of the raw data into tomographic images. These steps are applied to both gated and ungated images and include filtering, image reconstruction, and reorientation of tomographic slices.

Filtering   The goal of effective filtering is to reduce the inherent "noise" in the image, making it more uniform or "smooth" and balancing this

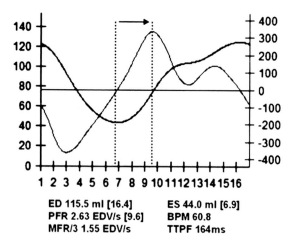

ED 115.5 ml [16.4]   ES 44.0 ml [6.9]
PFR 2.63 EDV/s [9.6]   BPM 60.8
MFR/3 1.55 EDV/s   TTPF 164ms

Figure 18-4. Left ventricular volume and filling curves derived from a 16-frame gated SPECT study. The increased temporal resolution of a 16-frame study allows accurate determination of peak filling rate, in the portion of the curve between the dashed vertical lines. ED, end diastole; ES, end systole; PFR, peak filling rate (in end-diastolic volumes per second, EDV/s); BPM, beats per minute; MFR/3, mean filling rate over the first third of diastole; TTPF, time to peak filling rate. (From Akincioglu et al.[6])

with the preservation of spatial resolution. In an image, high-frequency signals correspond to sharp details, such as the transition between a structure with intense radiotracer uptake adjacent to a structure with little uptake. Smaller structures also are represented by high-frequency signals. Lower frequencies represent areas of uniform uptake, in relatively larger structures. Filters act by reducing certain frequencies and/or enhancing selected frequencies, so as to achieve the optimal balance between noise and spatial resolution.

The most common filters used are passive filters, meaning that they filter out selected frequencies according to a defined filter function. Low-pass filters reduce higher-frequency signals, thus reducing image noise. High-pass filters reduce lower frequencies, thus increasing spatial resolution. In general, low-pass filters are applied to the raw data before reconstruction, since reduction of noise is the goal at this point. Low-pass

filters include Butterworth, Hanning, Hamming, and Parzen filters. A Butterworth filter is the most popular in most laboratories and is defined by a cutoff frequency and order. The cutoff frequency is the frequency at which the signal is attenuated by 50%. A higher-frequency cutoff filters out less noise, and a lower-frequency cutoff filters more. The order of the Butterworth filter defines the slope of the transition from no filtering to maximal filtering function.

Although an understanding of filtering and filter options is essential, it should be stressed that camera and software manufacturers generally have set default parameters on their systems. These defaults are usually based on the trials that have validated the particular hardware or software, and thus the quantitative parameters such as defect size, LVEF, etc., are based on standardized acquisition and filtering parameters. Deviation from these defaults may be done on a case-by-case basis, but with the understanding that the quantitative parameters generated by the software may be affected.

In general, it is recommended that the filter used for the gated, unsummed slices has a lower cutoff (i.e., more smoothing) than the filter used for the nongated, summed SPECT slices. Butterworth cutoff frequencies in the 0.25 to 0.45 range are typically used for the gated slices, whereas cutoff frequencies for summed slices are usually in the 0.5 to 0.65 range.

Gated SPECT Quantification

The process of quantifying the gated SPECT images in order to produce parameters of left ventricular size and function is largely automated in current software. A number of techniques have been developed to define the left ventricular cavity, construct a three-dimensional image of the ventricular cavity for each frame, and thus determine left ventricular volume and ejection fraction.[7–10] Several programs are commercially available, including the Cedars-Sinai Quantitative Gated SPECT (QGS), 4DM-SPECT developed at the University of Michigan, the Emory Cardiac Toolbox, and the Wackers-Lui Cardiac Quantification (WLCQ) program from Yale. The precise methodology by which each program defines myocardial borders is beyond the scope of this chapter. Since the normal limits for LVEF may vary by program and acquisition parameters (particularly frame rate), the user should be familiar with the documentation provided by the software manufacturer.

Validation of gated SPECT for calculation of LVEF from these programs has included comparisons to first pass,[7,11] gated blood pool imaging,[12–14] echocardiography,[14] magnetic resonance imaging,[4,15–17] and contrast ventriculography.[18] Overall, when compared to "gold-standard" measurements such as gated blood pool imaging and/or cardiac MRI, correlation coefficients are above 0.7 for all programs.[4,7,10,11,14–16,19] These methods are reproducible both on repeated measures and between difference observers.[7,19,20]

Although these software packages have been validated to variable degrees, the absolute measurements of LVEF and ventricular volumes may differ from one program to another. Therefore, it is important to know the normal values for the program being used. To illustrate this point, a study by Nichols and colleagues compared calculated left ventricular volumes and ejection fraction in 246 patients, using the Cedars-Sinai-developed program (QGS) and the Emory program (Emory Cardiac Toolbox).[21] As expected, the correlation between the two methods was excellent ($r = 0.90$ for LVEF) (Figure 18-5). The absolute LVEF

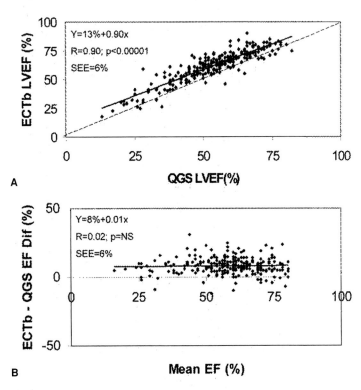

Figure 18-5. Linear regression curves for Emory Cardiac Toolbox (ECTb) versus Cedars-Sinai Quantitative Gated SPECT (QGS) left ventricular ejection fraction (LVEF) **(A)** and Bland–Altman curves of differences versus means for both methods **(B)**. *Solid lines* are linear least-squares fits, and the *dashed line* is the line of identity. (From Nichols et al.[21])

calculation, however, was significantly lower for QGS than for the Emory program ($53 \pm 13\%$ vs. $61 \pm 13\%$, $p < 0.0001$). Likewise, end-systolic and end-diastolic volumes were also lower with QGS. Similarly, in an additional group of 50 patients at low likelihood for coronary disease, the lower limit of normal LVEF was 44% for QGS and 51% for the Emory program. These differences were unaffected by differences in camera manufacturer or data acquisition protocols. In a similar study, Nakajima and colleagues compared four programs directly to equilibrium-gated blood pool imaging (QGS, Emory Cardiac Toolbox, 4DM-SPECT, and pFAST, a program more commonly used in Japan).[19] The overall correlation of each program to gated blood pool imaging was excellent (correlation coefficients from 0.69 to 0.84). There were differences, however, in the calculations of LVEF among the programs. Specifically, when compared to gated blood pool imaging, LVEF was 5% units higher with QGS, 2% higher for pFAST, 6% higher for 4DM-SPECT, and 10% higher for Emory Cardiac Toolbox. These studies highlight the importance of knowing the limits associated with specific software packages.

Methodological Limitations and Differences

A number of limitations should be considered in the interpretation of gated SPECT imaging data. Some programs may be more susceptible to certain errors, but many limitations are common to most programs in widespread use. First, the calculated LVEF measured in 8-frame studies may be 3% to 4% units lower than that obtained by 16-frame methods.[7] Thus, the lower limit of normal may be in the 45% to 47% range, unless a correction factor has been applied. The limits of normal will be defined by the software manufacturer. Second, gated SPECT may underestimate left ventricular volumes, particularly in patients with small ventricles.[22] This often leads to erroneously high LVEF measurements in such patients. Finally, the programs may not perform well in the setting

of high extracardiac counts adjacent to the heart (liver and intestine), which may lead to inaccurate definition of the myocardial boundaries.[23]

Quality Control and Artifacts in Gated SPECT

Gated images are reviewed in a cine loop for qualitative assessment of overall function, regional function, and image quality. Actual gated slices should be reviewed without contours, and with contours to check for accuracy of the automated determination of myocardial borders. This step is critical in determining whether the study is limited for technical reasons, such as poor counts, gating problems, or failure of the software algorithms.

The artifacts that are most specific to gated SPECT studies are caused by problems in the actual ECG gating of the images. This may be caused by an inadequate gate signal, or physiologic variation in the R-R interval. Additional sources of artifact include patient motion, extracardiac activity, and overall poor counts.

Gating problems may be physiologic, because of marked variability in heart rate, or technical, because of inadequate ECG signal. Problems with gating are most pronounced on the later frames in the cardiac cycle (i.e., frames 7 and 8) and may lead to inaccurate left ventricular time–activity curves and cine images. These late frames may be corrupted in one of two ways. In some cases, the last few frames may appear dark, as a result of few counts in that frame. In programs in which each frame is normalized to itself, the last few frames may appear very noisy, because of amplification of a low-count image.

When the cine image is viewed, these gating artifacts tend to appear as "flashing" artifact, since one or two frames in the cine loop have either low counts or high noise. The reconstructed tomographic images in these frames may have streaks across the entire image as well, caused by reconstruction of count-poor data.[24] Any suggestion of artifact in these cine loop images should raise concern that the quantitative gated SPECT data may be corrupted.

The actual impact of gating errors is quite variable. Two separate studies by Nichols and colleagues suggest that the effect of arrhythmias on gated SPECT studies is most evident in erroneous calculations of wall thickening and that mean ventricular volumes and LVEF are relatively unaffected,[25,26] as the mean LVEF, end-diastolic volume, and end-systolic volume changed by less than 5%.[26] However, gating problems may cause inaccurate calculation of volumes and LVEF, sometimes producing left ventricular time–activity curves that are flat and cine loops that appear grossly hypokinetic.[27] In the study by Nichols et al., although mean LVEF for all patients was relatively unaffected by arrhythmias, the maximal observed change in individual cases was 18% to 28%.[26] Unusual patterns of the left ventricular volume curve (e.g., unusually flat curves and curves with oddly placed peaks) are clues to potential problems with the LVEF calculation.[27]

Extracardiac activity immediately adjacent to the heart may affect cardiac images in several ways. The reconstruction process may create artifactual defects in the area of the myocardium adjacent to the extracardiac hot spot because of the effects of filtering.[28] Alternatively, spillover of activity may occur from the extracardiac structure into the myocardium, which may mask defects or blur the definition of the myocardial borders. In both cases, the likelihood of failure of the automated process to define the myocardial borders is increased. Analysis of the contours applied to the reconstructed tomographic slices will identify such errors. Some programs allow manual processing, allowing the user to manually constrain the regions of interest to try to correct this problem.

Count-poor images and uncorrectable motion artifacts affect both the summed static slices and the gated images and may significantly affect image quality and thus the diagnostic accuracy of the study. The effect is variable, but reconstruction of count-poor data may lead to streak artifacts, noisy images, and inhomogeneity of myocardial counts.

Motion artifacts of even less than 1 cm may cause blurring, and greater degree of motions may cause severe distortion of the ventricle[29] and may likewise cause artifactual defects and blurring.

GATED SPECT WITH THALLIUM-201

Gated thallium SPECT protocols are not well defined, and common programs in use for automated calculation of LVEF were validated using technetium-based agents. As such, the normal limits in the documentation of these programs may not apply to thallium-gated SPECT. In order to optimize thallium studies, it is probably necessary to image longer per stop (30–40 seconds), and/or decrease the number of projections from 64 to 32, in order to increase counts per projection.[3,30] Adjustments to filtering, i.e., lowering the cutoff frequency for more smoothing of thallium images, should also be considered.[30] Several reports have indicated that compared to technetium-gated SPECT, thallium images are more likely to be poor quality and may have more variability if reported LVEF, left ventricular volumes, and regional wall motion scores.[31,32] Although overall correlation of LVEF in groups of patients appears to be good, one should expect some increased variability in measures, potentially inaccurate volumes, and increased difficulty in assessing regional wall motion with thallium.

Despite the potential concerns of gating with thallium-201, a number of groups have reported good correlation between LVEF obtained by gated thallium SPECT compared to LVEF obtained with Tc-99m sestamibi SPECT or equilibrium radionuclide angiography.[30,33–35] A few studies also suggest the added prognostic value for gated thallium SPECT. Matsuo and colleagues reported that two parameters on gated thallium studies were associated with cardiac events: LVEF <45% and poststress depression compared to rest LVEF.[36] Another report stated that the use of a combination of perfusion and regional wall motion data from gated thallium SPECT increased the sensitivity for detection of CAD from 27%, using perfusion alone, to 51%.[37]

FUTURE DIRECTIONS

The development of gated SPECT imaging has been one of the most important advances in diagnostic imaging of the last decade. The additional information from gated images allowed the simultaneous assessment of perfusion and function in one diagnostic study. It allowed accurate measurement of ventricular function, improved prognostic power, and a significant improvement in diagnostic accuracy. Development of more sensitive imaging systems, capable of acquiring more counts in less time, may improve the accuracy of gated SPECT and allow increased temporal resolution. Techniques should be developed to standardize automated scoring of regional function and more accurately determine volumes. Finally, tracers with improved target-to-background ratio should be developed, for more accurate determination of myocardial boundaries. With appropriate attention to detail, quality control, and future refinements, gated SPECT imaging will remain a useful diagnostic tool for many years to come.

REFERENCES

1. Shaw LJ, Iskandrian AE. Prognostic value of gated myocardial perfusion SPECT. *J Nucl Cardiol*. 2004; 11:171.
2. Sharir T, Berman DS, Waechter PB, et al. Quantitative analysis of regional motion and thickening by gated SPECT perfusion images: Normal heterogeneity and criteria for abnormality. *J Nucl Med*. 2001;42:1630.
3. Hansen CL, Goldstein RA, Berman DS, et al. Imaging guidelines for nuclear cardiology procedures: Myocardial perfusion and function single photon emission computed tomography. *J Nucl Cardiol*. 2006;13:e97.
4. Faber TL, Vansant JP, Pettigrew RI, et al. Evaluation of left ventricular endocardial volumes and ejection fractions computed from gated perfusion SPECT with magnetic resonance imaging: Comparison of two methods. *J Nucl Cardiol*. 2001;8:646.
5. Cooke CD, Garcia EV, Cullom SJ, Faber TL, Pettigrew RI. Determining the accuracy of calculating systolic wall thickening using fast Fourier transform approximation: A simulation study based on canine and patient data. *J Nucl Med*. 1994;35:1185.
6. Akincioglu C, Berman DS, Nishina H, et al. Assessment of diastolic function using 16-frame Tc99m-sestamibi gated myocardial perfusion SPECT: Normal values. *J Nucl Med*. 2005;46:1102.
7. Germano G, Kiat H, Kavanaugh PB, et al. Automatic quantification of ejection fraction from gated myocardial perfusion SPECT. *J Nucl Med*. 1995;36:2138.
8. Germano G, Kavanaugh PB, Su HT, et al. Automatic reorientation of three-dimensional, transaxial myocardial perfusion SPECT images. *J Nucl Med*. 1995;36:1107.
9. Faber T, Cook C, Folks R, et al. Left ventricular function and perfusion from gated SPECT perfusion images: An integrated method. *J Nucl Med* 1999;40:650.
10. Liu Y, Sinusas AJ, Khaimov D, Gebuza BI, Wackers FJT. New hybrid count- and geometry-based method for quantification of left ventricular volumes and ejection fraction from ECG-gated SPECT: Methodology and validation. *J Nucl Cardiol* 2005;12:55.
11. Vallejo E, Dione DP, Sinusas AJ, et al. Assessment of left ventricular ejection fraction with quantitative gated SPECT: Accuracy and correlation with first-pass radionuclide angiography. *J Nucl Cardiol*. 2000;7:461.
12. Everaert H, Bossuyt A, Franken PR. Left ventricular ejection fraction and volumes from gated single photon emission tomographic myocardial perfusion images: Comparison between two algorithms working in three-dimensional space. *J Nucl Cardiol*. 1997;4:472.
13. Calnon DA, Kastner RJ, Smith WH, et al. Validation of a new counts-based single photon emission computed tomography method for quantifying left ventricular systolic function: Comparison with equilibrium radionuclide angiography. *J Nucl Cardiol*. 1997;4: 464.
14. Chua T, Lin LC, Thiang TH, et al. Accuracy of the automated assessment of left ventricular function with gated perfusion SPECT in the presence of perfusion defects and left ventricular dysfunction: Correlation with equilibrium radionuclide ventriculography and echocardiography. *J Nucl Cardiol*. 2000;7:301.
15. Bax JJ, Lamb H, Dibbets P, et al. Comparison of gated single-photon emission computed tomography with magnetic resonance imaging for evaluation of left ventricular function in ischemic cardiomyopathy. *Am J Cardiol*. 2000;86:1299.
16. Tadamura E, Kudoh T, Motooka M, et al. Assessment of regional and global left ventricular function by reinjection Tl-201 and rest Tc-99m sestamibi ECG-gated SPECT: Comparison with three-dimensional magnetic resonance imaging. *J Am Coll Cardiol*. 1999;33:991.
17. Mochizuki T, Murase K, Tanake H, et al. Assessment of left ventricular volume utilizing ECG-gated SPECT with technetium-99m-MIBI and technetium-99m-tetrofosmin. *J Nucl Med*. 1997;38:53.

18. Williams KA, Taillon LA. Left ventricular function in patients with coronary artery disease assessed by gated tomographic myocardial perfusion images. Comparison with assessment by contrast ventriculography and first-pass radionuclide angiography. *J Am Coll Cardiol.* 1996;27:173.

19. Nakajima K, Higuchi T, Taki J, et al. Accuracy of ventricular volume and ejection fraction measured by gated myocardial SPECT: Comparison of 4 software programs. *J Nucl Med.* 2001;42:1571.

20. Hyun IY, Kwan J, Park KS, et al. Reproducibility of Tl-201 and Tc-99m sestamibi gated myocardial perfusion SPECT measurement of myocardial function. *J Nucl Cardiol.* 2001;8:182.

21. Nichols K, Santana CA, Folks R, et al. Comparison between EBTb and QGS for assessment of left ventricular function from gated myocardial perfusion SPECT. *J Nucl Cardiol.* 2002;9:285.

22. Nakajima K, Taki J, Higuchi T, et al. Gated SPECT quantification of small hearts: Mathematical simulation and clinical application. *Eur J Nucl Med.* 2000;27:1372.

23. Achtert A, King MA, Dahlberg ST, Pretorius PH, LaCroix KJ, Tsui BMW. An investigation of the estimation of ejection fractions and cardiac volumes by a quantitative gated SPECT software package in simulated gated SPECT images. *J Nucl Cardiol.* 1998;5:144.

24. Cullom SJ, Case JA, Bateman TM. Electrocardio-graphically gated myocardial perfusion SPECT: Technical principles and quality control considerations. *J Nucl Cardiol.* 1998;5:418.

25. Nichols K, Dorbala S, DePuey E, Yao SS, Sharma A, Rozanski A. Influence of arrhythmias on gated SPECT myocardial perfusion and function quantification. *J Nucl Med.* 1999;40:924.

26. Nichols K, Yao SS, Kamran M, Faber TL, Cooke D, DePuey EG. Clinical impact of arrhythmias on gated SPECT cardiac myocardial perfusion and function assessment. *J Nucl Cardiol.* 2001;8:19.

27. Kasai T, DePuey EG, Shah AA, Merla VC. Impact of gating errors with electrocardiography gated myocardial perfusion SPECT. *J Nucl Cardiol.* 2003;10:709.

28. Nichols K, DePuey EG, Rozanski A. Automation of gated tomographic left ventricular ejection fraction. *J Nucl Cardiol.* 1996;3:475.

29. Djaballah W, Muller MA, Bertrand AC, et al. Gated SPECT assessment of left ventricular function is sensitive to small patient motions and to low rates of triggering errors: A comparison with equilibrium radionuclide angiography. *J Nucl Cardiol.* 2005;12:78.

30. Germano G, Erel J, Kiat H, Kavanaugh PB, Berman DS. Quantitative LVEF and qualitative regional function from gated thallium-201 perfusion SPECT. *J Nucl Med.* 1997;38:749.

31. Hyun IY, Kwan J, Park KS, Lee WH. Reproducibility of Tl-201 and Tc-99m sestamibi gated myocardial perfusion SPECT measurement of myocardial function. *J Nucl Cardiol.* 2001;8:182.

32. DePuey EG, Parmett S, Ghesani M, Rozanski A, Nichols K, Salensky H. Comparison of Tc-99m sestamibi and Tl-201 gated perfusion SPECT. *J Nucl Cardiol.* 1999;6:278.

33. He ZX, Cwajg E, Preslar JS, Mahmarian JJ, Verani MS. Accuracy of left ventricular ejection fraction determined by gated myocardial perfusion SPECT with Tl-201 and Tc-99m sestamibi: Comparison with first-pass radionuclide angiography. *J Nucl Cardiol.* 1999;6:412.

34. Maunoury C, Chen CC, Chua KB, Thompson CJ. Quantification of left ventricular function with thallium-201 and technetium-99m-sestamibi myocardial gated SPECT. *J Nucl Med.* 1997;38:958.

35. Maunoury C, Antonietti T, Sebahoun S, Barritault L. Assessment of left ventricular function by 201Tl SPECT using left ventricular cavity-to-myocardium count ratio. *Nucl Med Commun.* 2001;22:281.

36. Matsuo S, Matsumoto T, Nakae I, et al. Prognostic value of ECG-gated thallium-201 single photon emission tomography in patients with coronary artery disease. *Ann Nucl Med.* 2004;18:617.

37. Shirai N, Yamagishi H, Yoshiyama M, et al. Incremental value of assessment of regional wall motion for detection of multivessel coronary artery disease in exercise (201)Tl gated myocardial perfusion imaging. *J Nucl Med.* 2002;43:443.

38. Paul AK, Nabi HA. Gated myocardial perfusion SPECT: Basic principles, technical aspects, and clinical applications. *J Nucl Med Tech.* 2004;32:179.

39. Germano G, Berman D. Gated SPECT. In: Iskandrian AS, Verani MS, eds. *Nuclear Cardiac Imaging: Principles and Applications.* 3rd ed. New York: Oxford University Press; 2002:121–136.

CHAPTER 19

Planar and SPECT Equilibrium Radionuclide Angiography

James A. Arrighi
Brian G. Abbott
Frans J. Th. Wackers

EQUILIBRIUM RADIONUCLIDE ANGIOGRAPHY

As noted in Chapter 17, equilibrium radionuclide angiography (ERNA) is a reliable and accurate technique for assessing left ventricular function. The major potential advantages of ERNA, which is usually performed using planar imaging, over other more commonly used techniques for assessment of ventricular function, such as echocardiography, are its accuracy, reproducibility, and relative simplicity. Because this is a count-based technique, ERNA analysis does not rely on geometric assumptions for calculation of ejection fraction (EF). ERNA using tomographic imaging (gated blood pool SPECT [GBPS]) is a promising technique that may have advantages over standard planar ERNA, such as three-dimensional (3-D) reconstruction and improved separation and effective resolution of cardiac structures. Emerging techniques such as 3-D echocardiography, ECG-gated magnetic resonance imaging (MRI), and

ECG-gated CT may offer alternative volume-based methods for assessment of ventricular function but are not used commonly in routine clinical practice.

RADIOPHARMACEUTICALS AND RADIOLABELING

ERNA or GBPS is performed using Tc-99m-labeled autologous RBCs. The three available methods to radiolabel erythrocytes are the *in vivo*, *modified in vivo*, and *in vitro* techniques. Each of these methods uses the stannous ion (in the form of stannous pyrophosphate) as a reducing agent to facilitate the binding of Tc-99m pertechnetate to hemoglobin. The in vitro technique is a multistep procedure for erythrocyte labeling, which involves withdrawal of blood, reduction of hemoglobin, and Tc-99m labeling in a test tube, and subsequent intravenous reinjection of labeled blood into the body. This method results in the highest labeling efficiency (>97%). Commercial kits are available

301

that simplify this procedure. Other acceptable methods are the in vivo and modified in vivo techniques.[1] Both methods utilize an intravenous injection of 10 to 20 μg/kg of cold stannous pyrophosphate administered 15 to 30 minutes prior to RBC erythrocyte labeling. For the in vivo technique, this is followed by the direct intravenous administration of 20 to 30 mCi (740–1110 MBq) of Tc-99m pertechnetate. For the modified in vivo technique, the patient's blood is drawn into a syringe containing the anticoagulant acid-citrate-dextrose or heparin and then incubated with 20 to 30 mCi of Tc-99m pertechnetate at room temperature for at least 10 minutes before reinjection.[2] The labeling efficiency for the in vivo method is 60% to 70%, and approaches 90% for the modified in vivo technique.[3,4] Imaging is usually performed 20 minutes after injection. All of these techniques are acceptable according to current imaging guidelines published by the American Society of Nuclear Cardiology.[5]

Some clinical situations may lead to inefficient erythrocyte labeling. These include diseases affecting the red blood cells (including anemia, hematologic malignancies, sickle cell disease, and hemolytic disorders), immune disorders, and certain drugs (heparin, methyldopa, hydralazine, doxorubicin, quinidine, digoxin, prazosin, antibiotics, and anti-inflammatory agents).[6] In typical practice, inadequate labeling is most commonly caused by poor technique. Common technical problems include inadequate reduction of RBCs and injection of Tc-99m pertechnetate through a heparinized intravenous line. Therefore, when possible, the Tc-99m pertechnetate should be administered through direct intravenous injection.

IMAGE ACQUISITON AND PROCESSING

Planar Imaging

Currently, planar ERNA is used more commonly than GBPS. Images are typically acquired using a small field of view gamma camera, or a larger field of view camera with appropriate zoom factor (1.2–2.2). A parallel-hole, all-purpose, or high-resolution collimator produces good resolution with acceptable imaging times. For adequate counting statistics, images usually are acquired for preset counts of approximately 200,000 to 250,000 counts per image frame, corresponding to a 5- to 10-minute acquisition time. Count densities within the left ventricle of at least 20,000 to 40,000 counts/cm^3 are optimal.[5] Planar images are acquired in at least three views: anterior, 45-degree left anterior oblique, and left lateral (Figure 19-1). A 30-degree left posterior oblique may also be obtained to optimize assessment of inferior wall motion. The left anterior oblique view gives the best separation of the left and right ventricles and is used for quantification of left ventricular function.

For exercise studies, higher frame rates are usually used, with a high-sensitivity or low-energy all-purpose collimator. Images are obtained during the final 2 to 3 minutes of supine or semierect bicycle stress, in the left anterior oblique view.

Image acquisition is gated to the patient's ECG, allowing for the summation of data over multiple cardiac cycles. The triggering signal for the computer usually is the R wave of the patient's ECG, which then sends a signal to start an acquisition sequence. If the ECG signal is weak or complicated by artifact, subsequent image interpretation will be inaccurate and may lead to erroneous (usually low) measurements of ventricular function.

Framing Requirements The minimum framing rate for resting ERNA is 16 frames/cycle (approximately 50 ms/frame). If quantitative assessment of regional EF or diastolic filling is desired, it is preferable to increase the temporal resolution (e.g., to 32 frames/cycle or 25–30 ms/frame). For exercise studies, because of increased heart rate, the higher framing rate is required.

Arrhythmia Filtering Since the ventricular time–activity curve is generated from multiple cardiac cycles, accuracy is optimal when R-R interval is stable during the time of acquisition. For

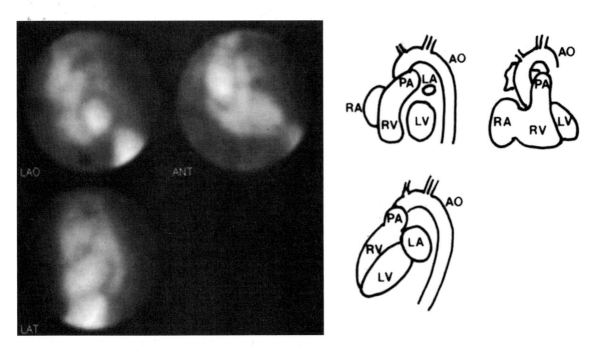

Figure 19-1.   Standard views of equilibrium radionuclide angiocardiography: anterior (Ant), left anterior oblique (LAO), and left lateral (LL). End-diastolic frames are represented in the left column, end-systolic frames in the middle column. Diagrammatic representation of frames in the right column. RA, right atrium; RV, right ventricle; LA, left atrium; LV, left ventricle; PA, main pulmonary artery; AO, aorta.

assessment of systolic function, the study will not be adversely affected if irregular beats account for <10% to <15% of total. If irregular beats are frequent, arrhythmia filtering is required.

Several methods can be used for arrhythmia filtering. In frame mode acquisition, irregular beats are rejected by either postbeat filtration or dynamic beat filtration. With the postbeat filtration method, detection of an R-R interval that falls outside of a prespecified limit results in rejection of all subsequent beats until the R-R interval returns to an acceptable value. With dynamic beat filtration, incoming beat-by-beat data are stored in a temporary computer buffer, and only beats falling within the prespecified R-R interval limit are retained in the permanent study file, allowing more complete rejection of irregular beats. Studies may also be acquired in list mode. In list mode acquisition, data are collected with time data (relative to the ECG) and the study is not processed until acquisition is completed. The advantage of list mode is that data can be reformatted retrospectively, and limits for R-R interval can be varied.

Atrial fibrillation may adversely affect EF calculation, particularly if R-R intervals vary widely. Physiologically, the beat-to-beat variability observed in atrial fibrillation causes corresponding variability in beat-to-beat EF.[7] ERNA may still be used for assessment of ventricular performance in patients with adequate rate control, and the calculated left ventricular ejection fraction (LVEF) represents the average EF for the period of acquisition.

Gated Blood Pool SPECT

The shift from planar to SPECT imaging as the chief modality for myocardial perfusion imaging has renewed interest in the concept of performing radionuclide ventriculography of cardiac structure and function using the more technically advanced SPECT systems. With appropriate software, acquisition can be performed with standard equipment and procedures with only minor modifications. A dual-headed system is preferred to increase count density and reduce acquisition time. Typically, a 90-degree head configuration is employed to obtain projections more than a 180-degree circular arc from 45-degree RPO to 45-degree LPO (360 degrees may be used for triple-head cameras) using a parallel-hole high-resolution collimator. Similar to perfusion studies, 64 projections of 20 to 30 seconds per stop are typically sufficient and can be performed in approximately 15 minutes.[5] ECG gating should be performed preferably with a frame rate of at least 16 frames per cardiac cycle. Count statistics are critical with GBPS, and the ability to effectively filter arrhythmias is limited. Arrhythmia filtering is similar to that for planar ERNA. Careful assessment for the presence of gating and arrhythmia artifacts is essential for quality control.

A key advantage of GBPS is that, following image acquisition, the reconstructed images may be analyzed from a variety of orientations. Therefore, ideal ventricular separation may be selected after acquisition, eliminating the potential problem that is associated in planar ERNA. Additionally, the 3-D nature of GBPS allows for a variety of image orientations to permit maximum cardiac chamber visualization.

VISUAL ASSESSMENT OF IMAGES

All studies should be viewed qualitatively, in conjunction with the quantitative data. Images are displayed as an endless cinematic loop of the cardiac cycle. Images should be viewed in a systematic fashion:

1. *Image quality.* Images are assessed for target-to-background ratio, adequacy of RBC labeling, and potential gating problems (image "flickering"). An ECG strip should be inspected to look for potential problems in gating.

2. *Characterization of cardiac structures.* Each view should be inspected for a complete assessment of chamber size (Figure 19-1). If both rest and stress studies are performed, it is recommended that both studies are displayed simultaneously for direct visual comparison.

For planar ERNA, the following views are evaluated:

Anterior view—right ventricular size and function (inferior and apical regions are best visualized), right atrial size, and pulmonary outflow track size.
LAO view—assess septal separation of ventricles and right and left ventricular size and function (septal, apical, and lateral walls of left ventricle).
Left lateral view—left ventricular function (anterior, apical, and inferior walls), left atrial size.

For GBPS, reconstruction facilitates a selective, unobstructed view of each of the cardiac chambers, permitting a more comprehensive assessment of regional wall motion and EF, particularly when cine-looped images of the cardiac chambers are displayed in surface-shaded or volume-rendered 3-D reconstructions. Typical software programs allow the right and left ventricles to be displayed in a 3-D format, which may be manipulated, allowing for an almost limitless number of views (Figure 19-2).

3. *Regional wall motion.* Left ventricular wall motion is assessed on all views and graded as either normal, hypokinetic, akinetic, or dyskinetic (systolic expansion). Specific attention is given to the regional nature of wall motion abnormalities. *Paradoxical* septal motion can be caused by the presence of left bundle branch block, ventricular pacing, prior cardiac surgery, and, occasionally, septal myocardial infraction. Right ventricular wall motion is difficult to assess completely with planar ERNA, as a result of considerable overlap with other cardiac structures on equilibrium studies.

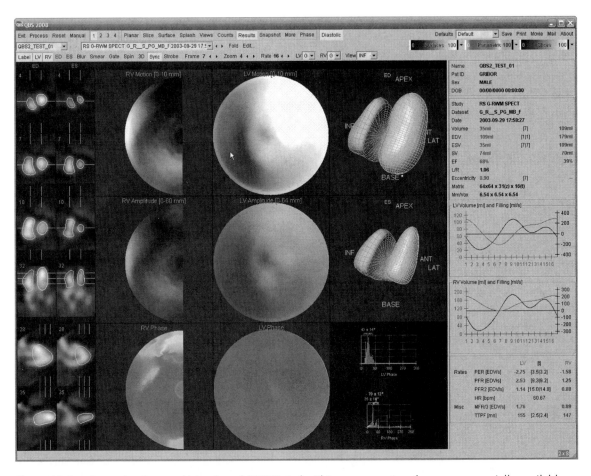

Figure 19-2. Example of a gated blood pool SPECT study. This screen capture from a commercially available program (QBS, Cedars-Sinai) shows representative tomographic views on the left side of the figure and volumetric, 3-D reconstructions on the right side of the figure (left ventricle in red and right ventricle in blue). Left and right ventricular volume curves and calculated ejection fractions are shown at the far right. (Courtesy of G. Germano, PhD.) (See color insert.)

The inferoapical segment of the right ventricle is best visualized on the anterior view. With GBPS, both ventricles can be assessed completely using the display software.

4. *Extracardiac uptake.* Normally, there is some activity in the liver, spleen, and stomach. The proximity of the spleen to the left ventricle should be noted, as it may affect background measurements in subsequent quantitative analysis. Increased activity in the stomach area is most likely gastric mucosa and indicates poor RBC labeling and may affect overall study quality. Ventricular hypertrophy, pericardial effusion, or a prominent pericardial fat pad may cause a prominent photopenic zone surrounding the heart.

Potential Value of GBPS

As noted earlier in this chapter, an increasing number of reports have demonstrated the clinical superiority of SPECT ERNA versus planar imaging for determining regional ventricular wall motion irregularities and abnormalities of the heart structures, particularly the great vessels and the right ventricle, owing to the enhanced spatial separation of the cardiac chambers.[8–13] Scoring systems for segmental wall motion have been developed to identify the segments in relation to territories supplied by the coronary arteries.[12,14,15]

QUANTITATIVE ASSESSMENT OF IMAGES

The EF is clinically the most important quantitative parameter obtained from planar ERNA. LVEF is calculated from left ventricular count changes during the cardiac cycle in the planar LAO image. A region of interest is drawn around the left ventricle using manual or automatic edge detection programs (Figure 19-3). Regions can be drawn on all frames, or at end diastole and end systole.

Whatever method is used, the regions should be assessed visually to ensure that only the left ventricle is included. Background subtraction is performed using a region of interest 1 to 3 pixels lateral to the posterolateral left ventricular blood pool. The background region should not incorporate excessive extracardiac activity, such as the spleen. Normally, background count activity accounts for approximately 50% of activity within the ventricular region of interest; if elevated, the calculated EF may be spuriously elevated.

After background subtraction, a time–activity curve is generated, which closely parallels an angiographic time–volume curve (Figure 19-3). The curve should have an appropriate shape, i.e., with a well-defined systolic trough and no significant drop-off of counts in last diastolic frames. It may be useful to filter the curves using Fourier analysis, which reduces statistical fluctuations.

Overall, the calculation of LVEF by planar ERNA is highly reproducible and accurate (Figure 19-4). This technique has been validated against contrast ventriculography and correlates well with such measurements over a wide range of EFs.[16,17] For most commercially available software

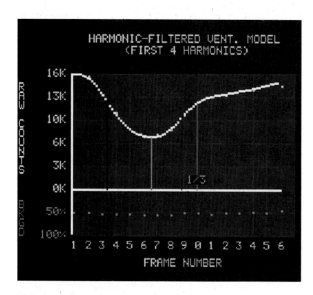
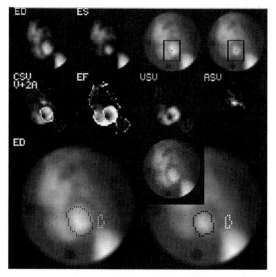

Figure 19-3. Time–activity curve in patient with normal left ventricular function (left panel). Separate regions of interest were drawn on end-diastolic (ED) and end-systolic (ES) frames, with adjacent background region of interest (right panel).

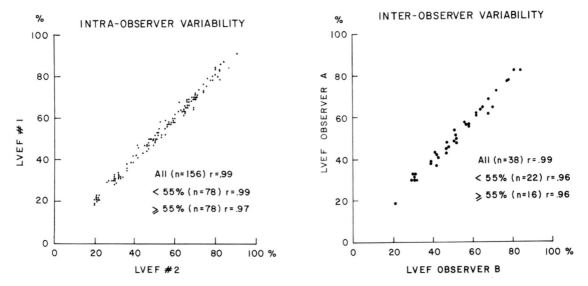

Figure 19-4.   Intra- and interobserver variability of left ventricular ejection fraction (LVEF) calculation by equilibrium radionuclide angiocardiography, demonstrating the excellent consistency of the method. (From Wackers FJTh, Berger HJ, Johnstone DE, et al. Multiple gated cardiac blood pool imaging for left ventricular ejection fraction: Validation of the technique and assessment of variability. *Am J Cardiol* 1979;43:1159.)

packages, the lower limit, if normal, for LVEF is approximately 50%. This may vary slightly from laboratory to laboratory, depending on the software used for data acquisition and analysis. Variability of LVEF should be determined on a regular basis in each individual laboratory and should not exceed approximately 4% for resting studies.

SPECT ERNA

LVEF can be determined from GBPS on the basis of count changes in the end-diastolic and end-systolic regions of interest, similar to the methodology for planar RNA. GBPS methods of determining LVEF may produce *consistently higher values* compared to those obtained via planar ERNA methods, partly because of the ability of SPECT ERNA to effectively exclude left atrial count activity from the LV region of interest.

Right Ventricular Function

The assessment of right ventricular function may be important in a number of clinical situations, including patients with pulmonary disease, congen-ital heart disease, heart failure, and valvular disease. Its unusual shape, however, complicates the calculation of EF using planar equilibrium techniques, since it is difficult to avoid overlap with other cardiac structures in any single view. Because of the contamination of right ventricular counts with right atrial counts, right ventricular EF by standard ROI methods on planar equilibrium studies underestimates EF as compared to that measured by the first-pass technique. Although some groups have reported reasonable accuracy with planar ERNA studies,[18–20] the first-pass technique remains the method of choice for assessment of right ventricular function. The lower limit of normal for RVEF in most laboratories is 40% to 45%.

A number of studies have shown that SPECT ERNA provides right ventricular volumes and EFs that correlate well with both planar-first pass RNA and calculations by gated MRI and gated CT.[21–23] For example, Nichols and colleagues compared SPECT ERNA to gated-MRI in patients with pulmonary hypertension or tetralogy of Fallot, over a wide range of right ventricular function.[21] The correlation between the two techniques was excellent: mean right ventricular EF, end-diastolic volume, and end-systolic volume did not differ. Interobserver variability showed no significant differences in repeated measures.

Left Ventricular Diastolic Function

Quantitative parameters of left ventricular filling are derived from the time–activity curve. Several parameters of left ventricular filling can be obtained from the time–activity curve (Figures 19-5 and 19-6). The most commonly used parameter is peak filling rate (PFR), which represents the maximum value of the first derivative of the time–activity curve. It is expressed in units of end-diastolic volumes (or sometimes stroke volumes)

per second. Since PFR normally declines with age, normal cutoff values are difficult to define. In general, normal PFR for middle-aged and elderly persons is greater than 2 to 2.5 end-diastolic volumes per second. The time to peak filling rate (TPFR) is the time of PFR relative to end systole, expressed in milliseconds (normal >180 milliseconds). The filling fraction method separates diastole into several time intervals and determines the percentage of stroke volume at one third, one half, and two thirds of diastole. The atrial contribution to filling can be assessed by quantification of the time spent and/or increase in ventricular volume (counts) that is caused by atrial systole. Regional assessment of diastolic filling is possible by sectoring the left ventricle and examining regional time-activity curves.[24]

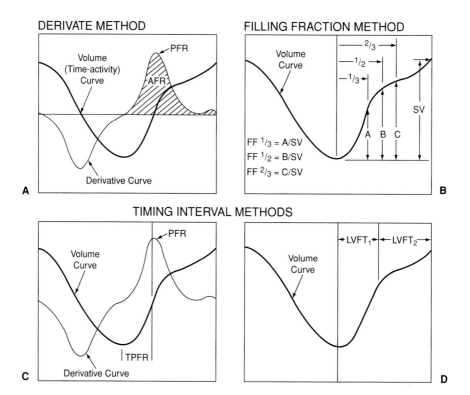

Figure 19-5. Parameters of diastolic function on equilibrium radionuclide angiocardiography. (**A**) Peak filling rate (PFR) method, (**B**) filling fraction method, (**C**) time to peak filling rate (TPFR) method, and (**D**) measurement of atrial contribution to filling (LVFT2 equals time spent in atrial filling period).

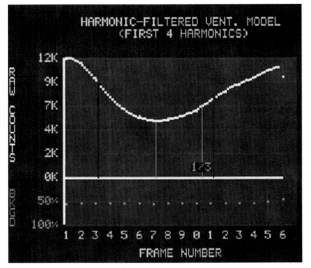

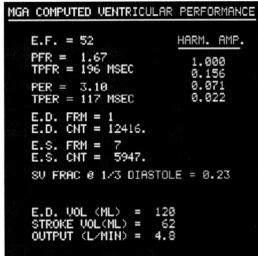

Figure 19-6. Example of time–activity curve with a reduction in peak filling rate. Note that the slope of the diastolic portion of the curve is flat compared to that in Figure 19-3. Although left ventricular ejection fraction is normal at 52%, peak filling rate is reduced at 1.67 end-diastolic volumes per second.

Functional and Parametric Images

Data from the ERNA and GBPS may be reconstructed in a manner that displays physiologic or parametric (mathematical) parameters in an image format. The *stroke–volume image* is a graphical representation of the difference in regional relative volume changes from end diastole to end systole on a pixel-by-pixel basis. Regional wall motion abnormalities appear as areas of reduced activity. The *EF image*, similar to stroke volume image, may also be used to assess regional ventricular function. It is obtained by dividing the stroke volume image by the end-diastolic images, resulting in a pixel-by-pixel representation of the EF equation. In a normal ventricle, the typical stroke volume or EF image appears more intense at the periphery and less intense in the center of the image, reflecting the fact that most of the volume changes occur in the outer zone and less in the center of the ventricle. The *paradox image*, which represents the difference between end-systolic and end-diastolic counts (the converse of the stroke–volume image), reflects regions in which blood volume increases during systole, such as the atria and dyskinetic left ventricular segments.

Phase analysis refers to a parametric analysis technique of each pixel of the image of a gated blood pool study. Each pixel can be considered as having its own time–activity curve, which then can be fitted with its first harmonic Fourier transform (a symmetrical cosine curve). The *amplitude image* reflects the regional volume of ejection for each pixel but is computed from the entire cardiac cycle rather than just from end-diastolic and end-systolic images. Thus, the amplitude image is independent of the timing of ejection relative to global end systole and represents maximum ejection (amplitude) at *any* point in the cardiac cycle. Therefore, both the atria and the ventricles are visualized in a normal image. The *phase image* is a graphical representation of the timing of maximal ejection on a pixel-by-pixel basis and thus reflects synchrony of ventricular contraction. In general, the sequence of activation of the left ventricle is fairly uniform, and thus the normal phase image is fairly uniform in intensity, reflecting no major phase delays. Nonuniformity of the phase image identifies abnormal sequences of ventricular activation, as may occur in conduction disturbances, contraction abnormalities, or pre-excitation.

SUMMARY

ERNA is a highly accurate and reproducible technique for assessing left ventricular function. Its reproducibility makes it particularly well suited for clinical situations in which the serial monitoring of ventricular function is important. Future applications of gated blood pool imaging will likely include GBPS, which may provide improved accuracy for assessing ventricular function and synchrony of contraction.

REFERENCES

1. Callahan RJ, Froelich JW, McKusick KA, Leppo J, Strauss HW. A modified method for the in vivo labeling of red blood cells with tc-99m: Concise communication. *J Nucl Med*. 1982;23:315.
2. Hegge FN, Hamilton GW, Larson SM, Ritchie JL, Richards P. Cardiac chamber imaging: A comparison of red blood cells labeled with tc-99m in vitro and in vivo. *J Nucl Med*. 1978;19:129.
3. Kuehne R, Reuter E. High RBC labeling efficiency by controlling pretinning with the modified in vivo/in vitro labeling method. *J Nucl Med Technol*. 1999;27:222.
4. Hicks RJ, Wood B, Kalff V, Anderson ST, Kelly MJ. Normalization of left ventricular ejection fraction following resection of pheochromocytoma in a patient with dilated cardiomyopathy. *Clin Nucl Med*. 1991;16:413.
5. Corbett JR, Akinboboye OO, Bacharach SL, et al. Equilibrium radionuclide angiocardiography (imaging guidelines for nuclear cardiology procedures). *J Nucl Cardiol*. 2006;13:e56.
6. Zanelli G. Effect of certain drugs used in the treatment of cardiovascular disease on the "in vitro" labeling of red blood cells with tc-99m. *Nucl Med Commun*. 1982;3:155.
7. Wallis JW, Juni JE, Wu L. Gated cardiac blood pool studies in atrial fibrillation: Role of cycle length windowing. *Eur J Nucl Med*. 1991;18:23.
8. Groch MW, DePuey EG, Belzberg AC, et al. Planar imaging versus gated blood-pool spect for the assessment of ventricular performance: A multicenter study. *J Nucl Med*. 2001;42:1773.
9. Botvinick EH, O'Connell JW, Kadkade PP, et al. Potential added value of three-dimensional reconstruction and display of single photon emission computed tomographic gated blood pool images. *J Nucl Cardiol*. 1998;5:245.
10. Groch MW, Marshall RC, Erwin WD, Schippers DJ, Barnett CA, Leidholdt EM Jr. Quantitative gated blood pool spect for the assessment of coronary artery disease at rest. *J Nucl Cardiol*. 1998;5:567.
11. Fischman AJ, Moore RH, Gill JB, Strauss HW. Gated blood pool tomography: A technology whose time has come. *Semin Nucl Med*. 1989;19:13.
12. Corbett JR, Jansen DE, Lewis SE, et al. Tomographic gated blood pool radionuclide ventriculography: Analysis of wall motion and left ventricular volumes in patients with coronary artery disease. *J Am Coll Cardiol*. 1985;6:349.
13. Canclini S, Terzi A, Rossini P, et al. Gated blood pool tomography for the evaluation of global and regional left ventricular function in comparison to planar techniques and echocardiography. *Ital Heart J*. 2001;2:42.
14. Gill JB, Moore RH, Tamaki N, et al. Multigated blood-pool tomography: New method for the assessment of left ventricular function. *J Nucl Med*. 1986;27:1916.
15. McGhie AL, Faber TL, Willerson JT, Corbett JR. Evaluation of left ventricular aneurysm after acute myocardial infarction using tomographic radionuclide ventriculography. *Am J Cardiol*. 1995;75:720.
16. Folland ED, Hamilton GW, Larson SM, Kennedy JW, Williams DL, Ritchie JL. The radionuclide ejection fraction: A comparison of three radionuclide techniques with contrast angiography. *J Nucl Med*. 1977;18:1159.
17. Berman DS, Salel AF, DeNardo GL, Bogren HG, Mason DT. Clinical assessment of left ventricular regional contraction patterns and ejection fraction by high-resolution gated scintigraphy. *J Nucl Med*. 1975;16:865.
18. Tobinick E, Schelbert HR, Henning H, et al. Right ventricular ejection fraction in patients with acute anterior and inferior myocardial infarction assessed by radionuclide angiography. *Circulation*. 1978;57:1078.
19. Maddahi J, Berman DS, Matsuoka DT, et al. A new technique for assessing right ventricular ejection fraction using rapid multiple-gated equilibrium cardiac blood pool scintigraphy. Description, validation and findings in chronic coronary artery disease. *Circulation*. 1979;60:581.
20. Konstam MA, Kahn PC, Curran BH, Idoine J, Wynne J, Holman BL. Equilibrium (gated) radionuclide ejection fraction measurement in the pressure or volume overloaded right ventricle. Comparison of three methods. *Chest*. 1984;86:681.
21. Nichols K, Saouaf R, Ababneh AA, et al. Validation of spect equilibrium radionuclide angiographic right

ventricular parameters by cardiac magnetic resonance imaging. *J Nucl Cardiol.* 2002;9:153.

22. Daou D, Van Kriekinge SD, Coaguila C, et al. Automatic quantification of right ventricular function with gated blood pool SPECT. *J Nucl Cardiol.* 2004;11: 293.

23. Clements IP, Brinkman B, Mullan BP, O'Connor MK, Breen JF, McGregor CGA. Operator-interactive method for simultaneous measurement of left and right ventricular volumes and ejection fraction by tomographic electrocardiography-gated blood pool radionuclide ventriculography. *J Nucl Cardiol.* 2006;13:50.

24. Bonow RO, Dilsizian V, Rosing DR, Maron BJ, Bacharach SL, Green MV. Verapamil-induced improvement in left ventricular diastolic filling and increased exercise tolerance in patients with hypertrophic cardiomyopathy: Short- and long-term effects. *Circulation.* 1985;72:853.

SECTION 8

RADIATION SAFETY AND REGULATORY ISSUES

CHAPTER 20

Radiation Safety

Jennifer Prekeges

Radiation safety is one of the least glamorous aspects of nuclear medicine. But it should not be overlooked. Issues of radiation exposure have impacts on both the technologist and the patient that should be considered. In addition, disregard of radiation safety is a sure way to draw a critical report from radiation inspectors. This chapter will start by discussing units and instruments used for radiation measurement and then discuss radiation safety from the standpoint of the technologist and the patient. Principles of radiation protection, radiation dosimetry, and radiobiology will be touched on. We will also identify the additional radiation safety aspects to consider when positron emission tomography (PET) is used. By the end of this chapter, the reader should have an understanding of both principles and applications as they pertain to radiation safety in nuclear cardiology laboratories.

UNITS OF RADIATION MEASUREMENT

The multiplicity of units used to measure radioactivity, radiation fields, and radiation dose complicates the discussion of radiation safety. Additional complexity is added because, in this field, the United States has not moved very far along the road to Systems International (SI) units. In many clinical settings, radiation safety is in the purview of the technologist and/or a consulting health physicist. But the clinician should, nonetheless, have at least a modicum of familiarity with these terms, and so they are presented here in a fairly simplistic fashion. Those who wish for a more in-depth understanding are referred to the references at the end of the chapter.

Units of Radioactivity

The activity of a radioactive material is defined as the number of radioactive disintegrations occurring per second (dps) in a given sample. The non-SI unit, Curie, is still commonly used in the United States:

$$1 \text{ Ci} = 3.7 \times 10^{10} \text{ dps} \qquad (20.1)$$

Most of the rest of the world uses the SI unit, Becquerel:

$$1 \text{ Bq} = 1 \text{ dps} \qquad (20.2)$$

These values are used to designate the dosage of a radiopharmaceutical to be given to a patient. The Curie is a much larger value and the Becquerel a much smaller value that the numbers routinely used in nuclear medicine, so standard factor-of-1000 prefixes (milli-, micro-, kilo-, etc.) are employed. In clinical nuclear cardiology practice, a fairly limited activity range of 1 to 50 mCi (37 MBq–1.85 GBq) is used.

Radiation Field Strength

Radiation emissions (gamma rays and beta and alpha particles) cause ionizations of the atoms and molecules they interact with. The presence of a radioactive material (or other source of radiation) and the strength of the resulting radiation field are easily measured using simple gas-filled detectors such as Geiger counters, which will be discussed in the next section. These instruments report out the number of ionizations occurring within the chamber, and the applicable units have a form that reflects that measurement. The original unit is the Roentgen (R)[1]:

$$1 R = \frac{1 \text{ electrostatic unit of ionization}}{\text{cubic centimeter of air}}$$
$$= \frac{2.08 \times 10^9 \text{ ion pairs created}}{\text{g air}} \qquad (20.3)$$

For the most part, it makes the most sense to report radiation field strength in a rate format, such that the instruments are calibrated in milliRoentgen per hour (mR/h). There is also an SI unit for radiation field strength:

$$1 \times \text{unit} = \frac{1 \text{ joule of ionization energy}}{\text{kg air}}$$
$$= 3881 \text{ R} \qquad (20.4)$$

This unit is so large that it is rarely used.

The Roentgen is a very useful unit of measurement from the standpoint of radiation safety. But it has two significant drawbacks. First, it is defined only for photon radiation (X-ray and gamma rays). Second, it is defined only for an environment of air, which has a markedly different composition than tissue. For these reasons, the Roentgen cannot be used to discuss the amount of radiation energy absorbed in a technologist standing near a radiation source, for example. For this task we need a different unit.

Radiation Absorbed Dose

The Rad is a much more universally applicable unit, in that it can be used for any kind of radiation and any type of material. It is defined thus:

$$1 \text{ rad} = \frac{100 \text{ ergs of radiation energy absorbed}}{1 \text{ g of any material}} \qquad (20.5)$$

The corresponding SI unit, Gray, is widely used:

$$1 \text{ Gy} = \frac{100 \text{ joules}}{\text{kg}} = 100 \text{ rads} \qquad (20.6)$$

Radiation-absorbed dose is the proper unit to use when discussing the radiation dose to a particular organ from a nuclear medicine examination, or a radiation therapy treatment dose.

A conversion calculation from Roentgens (in air) to rads (in water-equivalent tissue) yields a value of 0.95.[1] We can thus make an approximate equality between radiation field strength (as measured by a Geiger counter or ionization survey meter) and the radiation-absorbed dose to an individual exposed to that radiation field. Keep in mind that this approximate equality does not hold true when materials other than water or water-equivalent materials are concerned, because the conversion is based on the electron density of the material in question vs. that of the air.

The universal applicability of rad is offset by the inability to measure it directly. Radiation-absorbed dose can only be measured directly by implanting calorimeters into the organ(s) of interest, clearly not a method amenable to routine use. Radiation-absorbed doses are commonly estimated using a variety of methods, depending on the specific circumstances. For radiopharmaceuticals, a committee of the Society of Nuclear Medicine, called the Medical Internal Radiation Dose or MIRD committee, has developed procedures for calculating the radiation dose to a given organ from a specific radiopharmaceutical. (The complete details of this calculation can be found in Ref. 2.)

Dose Equivalent

Another difficulty with the rad as a radiation unit is that it does not adequately express the biological effects of radiation. We know, for example, that alpha particles are significantly more damaging in tissues than gamma rays or beta particles. So 1 rad of gamma radiation is much less harmful than 1 rad of alpha particle radiation. In order to adequately express this difference, another unit, rem (for Roentgen-equivalent man), was developed. This unit multiplies the radiation-absorbed dose in rads by a quality factor (QF) that accounts for the level of harm of the type of radiation in question:

Dose equivalent in rem = (dose in rad)(QF)
(20.7)

Beta particles, gamma rays, and X-rays have a QF of 1, so, in most medical applications, the dose equivalent is numerically equal to the radiation-absorbed dose. Alpha particles are assigned a QF of 20, indicating that they are 20 times as damaging as beta particles or X-rays. The equivalent unit of biological effect in the SI schema is the Sievert:

$$Sv = (\text{dose in Gy})(QF) \quad (20.8)$$

Since 1 Gray is equal to 100 rads, 1 Sievert is equal to 100 rem. The Sievert is commonly used around the world. The units of dose equivalent are used to report out monthly readings from radiation badge measurements.

Effective Dose Equivalent

Finally, when considering radiation dose to patients and technologists, we must remember that a radiopharmaceutical that is injected or ingested will not be distributed evenly throughout the body but will, rather, collect in specific organs based on its chemical characteristics. Further, we know that some organs of the body are more radiosensitive than others. The effective dose equivalent (EDE) calculation multiplies the dose to each organ by its organ-specific weighting factor.[3] The weighted doses are summed to determine the EDE, which can then be compared to whole-body radiation exposure. The EDE is used to compare radiation doses to patients from radiopharmaceuticals with doses incurred in radiologic procedures. A similar calculation (using slightly different weighting factors) should be performed when an occupationally exposed radiation worker is internally contaminated with a radionuclide or radiopharmaceutical. The EDE in the occupational situation is added to the radiation badge reading, so that it is included as part of the accumulated radiation exposure.

RADIATION SAFETY INSTRUMENTS

The work horses of radiation safety all belong to a class of instruments called gas-filled detectors. They are simplistic but quite effective, and their operation is easy to grasp.[4,5] Two metal plates are charged with the maximum amount of charge these will hold, one positive and one negative (Figure 20-1). Air or some other gas between the plates prevents the recombination of the positive and negative charges; the two charged plates and the gas in between constitute a simple electronic capacitor. If a high-energy photon interacts with a molecule of the gas, it will ionize that molecule, producing a free electron that can migrate toward the positively charged plate (the anode). The resulting decrease in the plate's charge is measured by the electronics attached to the capacitor. We will discuss three types of gas-filled detectors that are commonly used in nuclear medicine: the dose calibrator, the ionization survey meter, and the Geiger counter.

Dose Calibrator

This instrument is used to measure the activity of radioactive materials. The gas chamber is in the

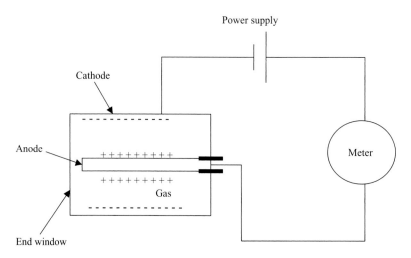

Figure 20-1.   Diagram of a gas-filled detector. Gas-filled detectors are very simple electronic instruments based on the operation of a capacitor. A source of electrical potential drives electrons onto one plate of the capacitor, leaving the other plate with a similar positive charge. Radiation interacting in the gas space creates electrons and positively charged ions, which are attracted to the anode and cathode, respectively. They neutralize some of the charge at the two plates. As the electrical supply works to restore the original charge, the amount neutralized can be measured by the meter, as either current or voltage.

form of a cylinder with a space in the center (Figure 20-2). A syringe or vial containing a radioactive sample is put into the space. Photons from the sample cross through the inner lining of the gas chamber and cause ionizations in the gas. The electrons migrate toward the anode and the positive ions toward the cathode. The electronics of the dose calibrator strive to keep the anode and cathode fully charged; neutralization of charge by electrons and positive ions, therefore, causes current to flow through the circuitry. This current is easily measured and with proper calibration converted to units of mCi or MBq.

Commercial dose calibrators are easy to use and very durable. Most nuclear medicine technologists consider them essential to their work (although Nuclear Regulatory Commission (NRC) guidelines no longer require a dose calibrator if all doses are received from a centralized radiopharmacy and are given only to the patients for whom they are intended). Dose calibrators have only two common sources of error. One is radioactive contamination of the chamber into which the syringe

is placed. A syringe measure in a contaminated dose calibrator will have a higher activity reading than what is actually in the syringe, but the amount of excess decreases as the contamination decays. This situation is easily remedied by cleaning to remove the contamination.

The other source of error is selection of the wrong isotope selector button. Because each radionuclide produces differing numbers of photons with different energies, the calibration factor (conversion from measured current to activity) is unique to a particular radionuclide. This calibration factor is essentially a multiplier, applied by the selection of the corresponding isotope selector button. If the wrong button is chosen, the wrong calibration factor is applied, and the activity reading is incorrect.

Ionization Survey Meter

This instrument is used to measure ambient radiation levels. It is essentially a gas-filled box with a central anode wire and the box itself serving as the

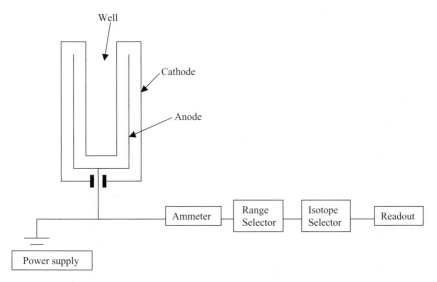

Figure 20-2.   Dose calibrator. A dose calibrator is used to measure the activity of a radiopharmaceutical. Its operation follows that of the gas-filled detector illustrated in Figure 20-1. The source container is placed into the well of the dose calibrator. Radiation emissions from the source pass through the chamber walls and cause ionizations in the gas between the anode and the cathode, neutralizing the charge resident on them. The current required to restore the anode and cathode to their maximum charge is measured and converted to activity units (Curies or Becquerels) according to a conversion factor that is specific to the radionuclide being measured.

cathode. Like the dose calibrator, the electronics of the ionization survey meter work to keep the anode and cathode fully charged. Ionizations produced by a source of X-rays or gamma rays cause current to flow, and this current can be directly converted to units of mR/h, using Eq. (20.1) above. The ionization survey meter is commonly used to measure ambient radiation levels, for example at the technologist workstation, from a patient being imaged.

Geiger Counter

The operation of a Geiger counter differs in a significant way from the first two instruments discussed. The capacitor design is similar, but the potential difference between the anode and the cathode is much higher. When a photon ionizes a gas molecule, the electron is pulled so strongly toward the anode that it has enough kinetic energy to cause more ionizations as it travels. Those secondary electrons likewise ionize additional gas molecules. The final result of a single photon in-

teraction is an avalanche of ionizations, resulting in a large electrical pulse within the chamber. The other major difference between dose calibrators and ionization survey meters, on the one hand, and Geiger counters on the other, is that whereas the former measure the current required to keep the anode and the cathode fully charged, the Geiger counter treats each avalanche of ionizations as a single pulse.

The Geiger counter, thus, has the ability to detect individual gamma rays, at least up to the limiting rate determined by its dead time. The units used on a Geiger counter are counts per minute (cpm), with each count representing one pulse, which in turn is assumed to represent one gamma ray having one initial interaction in the gas chamber. Many Geiger counters are also calibrated in mR/h, based on this assumption. They can be used both for surveys of the ambient radiation levels (in mR/h) and for detection of radioactive contamination (in cpm, which can, in turn, be converted to activity units of dps).

Geiger counters, thus, are very similar to ionization survey meters, but a couple of points of difference between them should be kept in mind. Ionization survey meters do not register very low radiation levels very well, so these should not be used for detection of contamination. These provide an excellent response to higher levels of radiation, at all gamma-ray energies. Geiger counters, on the other hand, give a much higher response to gamma rays in the 100 to 200 keV energy range, as opposed to higher-energy photons. This energy dependence should be kept in mind when switching from Tc-99m-based radiopharmaceuticals to positron radiopharmaceuticals.

Quality Control of Gas-Filled Detectors

Just as gamma cameras must be tested on a regular basis, these simple gas-filled detectors also require verification of proper performance. But since these instruments are far less complex than gamma cameras, their quality control tests are correspondingly simpler. The daily quality control test is an operation test.[1] It uses a radioactive check source to verify that the instrument is responding to radiation and that the value reported by the instrument is similar to what it was the day before. It is typically called a constancy test. The most common choice of a radionuclide source for this test is Cs-137. Its long half-life (30 years) means that a reading of a particular source will be the same from day to day. Once a year, the detectors must be recalibrated to be sure that they are reporting correct values. The daily checks are done by a nuclear medicine technologist; the annual recalibration generally requires a health physicist or other consultant.

Scintillation Detector

A second instrument used for radiation monitoring purposes is the scintillation detector, configured as either a well counter or a probe. Scintillation detectors used in nuclear medicine employ a scintillation crystal made of sodium iodide.

Gamma radiation absorbed in the sodium iodide crystal causes many electrons in the crystal's band structure to be raised from their ground state (the valence band) to an excited state (the conduction band), from where they return to the ground state with the accompanying emission of scintillation photons. The number of scintillation photons is registered as an electronic pulse by a photomultiplier tube and is directly related to the energy of the gamma ray that generated them. After proper calibration, the energy of each gamma ray can be determined, and a spectrum of energies from a particular radiation source can be evaluated.

Scintillation detectors have two qualities that make them the instrument of choice for radiation measurements that involve accurate determination of small amounts of radioactive substances. First, the scintillation crystal is solid rather than gaseous, such that gamma rays up to approximately 200 keV are highly likely to interact with its molecules. Second, the ability to determine the energy of each gamma ray allows the discrimination of the substance of interest from scattered and extraneous gamma rays. Thus, a scintillation detector is preferred for determination of radioactive contamination on a swab wiped across a countertop (a wipe test) or for determination of ingested radioactive iodine in the thyroid gland (a bioassay).

Scintillation detectors also require verification of proper performance. A daily calibration procedure confirms that the detector is correctly measuring the gamma rays of interest. The counting efficiency determines the correct conversion of the measured counts per minute to disintegrations per second, or activity; this value should be checked at least annually.

RADIATION SAFETY CONSIDERATIONS FOR THE TECHNOLOGIST

Nuclear medicine technologists are occupationally exposed radiation workers, similar to radiologic technologists, radiation therapists, and other users of ionizing radiation. Their radiation exposure is monitored by wearing a radiation badge to track whole-body radiation exposure and a ring badge to track hand exposure because of the manipulation of radioactive materials. The radiation exposure that nuclear medicine technologists receive is significantly different from that of other occupationally exposed radiation workers in one respect: in nuclear medicine, it is the patient who is the source of the radiation. Unlike X-ray, where technologists are exposed only when the X-ray machine is on, nuclear medicine technologists are exposed whenever they are around their patients. This fact necessitates different ways of thinking about radiation protection.

The three concepts of radiation protection are time, distance, and shielding (often abbreviated TDS). Radiation exposure is incurred when an individual spends time in the vicinity of a radiation source. Radiation exposure can be decreased by moving farther away from the source and/or spending less time near the source. When time and distance are not viable ways of decreasing radiation exposure, placing some shielding (commonly composed of lead or tungsten, both of which are excellent at absorbing high-energy photons) between the radiation source and the exposed individual can effectively reduce radiation exposure.

A convenient way to measure the effectiveness of a particular shielding material is to determine its half-value layer (HVL), which tells the thickness of the shielding material required to attenuate half of a beam of gamma rays of a given energy. The HVL values for Tc-99m and annihilation photons (Table 20-1) illustrate the fact that a shield's ability to absorb gamma rays is greatly dependent on the energy of the gamma rays.

Table 20-1

Half-Value Layers of Lead for Commonly Used Radionuclides

Gamma Ray Energy (keV)	HVL (mm)	Ref.
140	0.25	6, p. 92
511	4.0	7, p. 308

These considerations play out in a variety of ways in a nuclear medicine department. Imaging rooms should be designed so that a technologist sitting at the workstation will not be overexposed while watching patient studies. If the size of the imaging room must be constrained, then it is appropriate to include shielding between the gamma camera and the workstation. A leaded glass window may be necessary to facilitate observation of the patient. A health physicist can be helpful in dealing with these issues.

A second consideration is storage of radioactive materials. Whether radiopharmaceuticals are obtained in bulk quantities or individual doses, they must be shielded in a container (a "pig") made of lead or tungsten. They are stored, usually behind more shielding, in a room called the "hot lab." It also contains the dose calibrator and other radiation detection instruments, the check sources used to verify the operational status of these instruments, and radioactive waste. Since used syringes are both radioactively contaminated and potentially biohazardous, they are placed into a sharps container and stored until the radiation level reaches the level of background. The sharps container may then be disposed of in the usual way. If radionuclides of different half-lives are used (e.g., Tc-99m, $t_{1/2} = 6$ hours vs. Tl-201, $t_{1/2} = 73$ hours), the syringes and other waste should be segregated according to half-life, to facilitate disposal.

Patient care becomes a radiation safety consideration in nuclear medicine. Nuclear medicine technologists generally get more radiation exposure than radiologic technologists, and those who get the most radiation exposure are the technologists who take the best care of their patients. While radiation exposure in the course of doing nuclear medicine procedures is not something to be feared, one should always be aware of radiation exposure and how it can be reduced in any given situation. In particular, technologists should not use the hot laboratory as a place to congregate between studies. Another example of good practice is to explain the test being done, obtain patient history, and ask and answer questions, all before administering the radiopharmaceutical.

Nuclear medicine technologists can receive significant radiation exposure caused by the need to handle radioactive materials. This exposure can be greatly reduced through the use of syringe and vial shields, which are composed of lead, leaded glass, or tungsten, and are made to hold vials and syringes of specific sizes. One example of effective use of a syringe shield is during the treadmill injection of an exercise myocardial perfusion study. The technologist may need to hold the syringe for a minute or more while waiting for the patient to reach maximal exercise. A syringe shield stored at the location of the treadmill will be readily available for this situation.

A new aspect of nuclear medicine that raises radiation safety concerns is the use of radionuclide sources for attenuation correction in conjunction with myocardial perfusion imaging. These sources generally have high activities (50–500 mCi) and generate a radiation exposure rate that is considerably greater than background.[7] Technologists need to be aware of the additional radiation exposure they receive from these sources and to limit their time in close proximity to them.

Nuclear medicine technologists are occupationally exposed radiation workers and are subject to regulations put forth by the NRC. They wear both a body radiation detection badge and a ring containing a thermoluminescent dosimeter. The NRC sets both absolute and recommended limits on radiation exposure as measured by these devices (Table 20-2). The hand limits are much higher than the whole-body limits, because the hands do not contain important internal organs.

Table 20-2

Limits for Occupational Radiation Exposure

	NRC Annual Limits (rem/y)	ALARA Recommended Limits (rem/y)
Whole body	5	0.5
Extremities	50	5

ALARA, as low as reasonably achievable.

The ALARA (as low as reasonably achievable) limits are recommended target values, designed to keep the risk associated with occupational radiation exposure well below any level of concern.

Technologists generally change their radiation badges monthly, and the reports of radiation exposure should be reviewed no less often than quarterly. The NRC has an escalating series of responses, culminating in removal of an individual from radiation exposure if the badge reading is in excess of the quarterly limit (1.25 rem/quarter for the whole body and 12.5 rem/quarter for the hands). Such an action can have drastic consequences, and for this reason technologists are encouraged to pay attention to their radiation protection practices at all times.

RADIATION SAFETY FROM THE STANDPOINT OF THE PATIENT

All patients having nuclear medicine procedures are exposed to radioactivity. The amount of this exposure is limited by the dosage of radiopharmaceutical used, which in turn is set such that the radiation dose is similar to that received from common X-ray procedures. As noted above, radiation dosimetry from internally administered radiopharmaceuticals is most commonly estimated. The important thing to understand is that these are truly only estimates and do not take into account individual physiologic variability. These should be considered ballpark estimates only. Table 20-3 gives some representative values for several myocardial imaging agents and provides several relevant comparisons. While the thought of becoming radioactive is disconcerting to many patients, it should be emphasized that the equivalent doses are low compared to radiation levels that are known to cause harm. The position of the Health Physics Society is that below 5 to 10 rem (50–100 mSv), "risks of health effects are either too small to be observed or are nonexistent."[13]

The technologist should feel comfortable in drawing a comparison between nuclear medicine procedures and other types of radiologic procedures. He or she must also be able to explain

Table 20-3

Radiation Dose Estimates for Nuclear Cardiology Procedures and Comparisons

Radiopharmaceutical	Effective Dose Equiv. (mSv/MBq)	Dosage Range (MBq)	Effective Dose (mSv)	Effective Dose (rem)	Ref.
Tl-201	1.6×10^{-1}	75–150	12–24	1.2–2.4	8
Tc-99m sestamibi	1.4×10^{-2}	750–1100	12–15	1.2–1.5	8
Tc-99m tetrofosmin	8.0×10^{-3}	750–1100	6–9	0.6–0.9	9
Rb-82	1.2×10^{-2}	1100–1850	13–22	1.3–2.2	8
F-18 FDG	3.0×10^{-2}	370–740	11–22	1.1–2.2	8
Comparisons					
Occupational exposure limit			50	5.0	1
Average annual background exposure in the USA			3	0.3	1
Lumbar spine X-ray			1.3	0.13	1
Coronary catheterization			12	1.2	10
Coronary angioplasty			22	2.2	10
Attenuation scan, Gd-153			0.014	0.0014	11
Attenuation scan, Ga-68			0.154	0.0154	11
Attenuation scan, low-level CT scan			4	0.4	12
Attenuation scan, high-quality CT scan			5.4	0.54	11

how radiation exposure differs for nuclear medicine studies compared to radiologic examinations. Whereas an X-ray machine exposes only the part of the body within its field, a radiopharmaceutical exposes the whole body once it is injected. It leaves the body by excretion processes and becomes nonradioactive by radionuclide decay. Physical decay and biological excretion are independent processes that can be combined mathematically into the effective half-life:

$$T_E = \frac{T_P \, T_B}{T_B + T_P} \qquad (20.9)$$

where T_E is the effective half-life, T_P the physical half-life, and T_B the biological half-life of the pharmaceutical. The effective half-life is included in the calculation of organ dosimetry in the MIRD method. Note that T_B can be decreased by accelerating excretion processes after administration of the radiopharmaceutical. Excretion through the kidneys can be increased by encouraging hydration. Lipophilic radiopharmaceuticals such as sestamibi are excreted by the gall bladder into the small intestine; consumption of a fatty meal will cause the gall bladder to contract and expel its (ra-

dioactive) contents. More complete bowel preparation is required for some nuclear medicine procedures.

An additional source of radiation exposure for nuclear cardiology patients is from radiation sources used for attenuation correction. Many systems use sources such as Gd-153, which increase exposure by only a small amount relative to what the patient receives from the radiopharmaceutical. But a newer trend is the use of computed tomography to provide attenuation information. This increases patient radiation considerably. Even a "low-level" CT scan almost doubles the radiation dose to the patient from a myocardial perfusion study (Table 20-3).

RADIATION PROTECTION IN PET

The annihilation photons produced by PET radionuclides pose more significant radiation protection concerns. From the patient standpoint, these radionuclides are beta-emitters, meaning that the energy of the positron itself will be completely absorbed in the patient's body. This leads to higher radiation-absorbed doses in PET studies (Table 20-3). These doses are still considerably lower than the radiation dose received from a CT scan. The annihilation photons mostly escape the patient but, because of their high energy, travel farther and are detected at a much greater distance than the gamma rays emitted from non-PET radionuclides.

Imaging with PET radiopharmaceuticals, thus, requires additional considerations for department design. The PET suite will need to be considerably bigger than a gamma camera room, both because the scanner itself is larger and because the room needs to provide some of the distance needed for radiation protection purposes. The technologist workstation needs to be a separate area, behind leaded glass, while still allowing full view of the patient. An intercom and/or a closed-circuit camera may be needed to observe and communicate with the patient during the study's performance. Location of other nuclear medicine equipment, particularly gamma cameras, must be considered. Annihilation photons are energetic enough to pass through gamma camera collimators and the aluminum housing of the camera head, a factor that needs to be considered when configuring a department to include a PET scanner. A distance of 11 m is recommended between gamma cameras and the PET patient waiting areas.[14]

The location of the patient waiting room should also be rethought when PET is used. Radionuclides used in PET, such as F-18, have relatively short half-lives. Patients are therefore "hotter" in general, compared to non-PET nuclear medicine patients. For example, a patient receiving 10 mCi F-18 FDG will produce a radiation field of greater than 1 mR/h at 1 m distance.[6] It may be reasonable to put the PET patients in a different room. Some have also recommended separate bathroom facilities. Further, a PET patient walking by a gamma camera acquiring an image can produce a noticeable increase in counting rate. So the routing of patients also needs to be thought out.

Shielding used for PET radionuclides must be much thicker than that used for non-PET radionu-clides. The syringe shields and lead pigs used for PET are thick and heavy, and hot lab shielding must also be increased, including extra shielding around the dose calibrator chamber. (A visit to a cyclotron facility producing PET radiopharmaceuticals is recommended. Radiation safety precautions in these facilities are extensive and will impress the technologist with their importance.) Table 20-1 compares the HVLs of lead for 140-keV and 511-keV gamma rays. Sixteen times as much lead is needed to shield annihilation photons as is required for the same amount of protection with Tc-99m gamma rays. Tungsten provides approximately 1.4 times the shielding power of lead of equal thickness.[15]

Finally, the technologist needs to be continuously cognizant of radiation protection in PET. By anecdotal evidence, PET technologists are exposed at a level two or more times that of their non-PET colleagues (G. Segal, T. Lewellen, personal communications). PET technologists may, in fact, reach the ALARA limit of 0.5 rem/y whole-body exposure. Radiation exposure and badge readings should be carefully monitored, and pregnant technologists should take additional precautions.

Much of the additional radiation exposure to PET technologists is incurred in the process of performing injections. The technologist should complete all communication with the patient, including patient history and answering all questions, before administering the radiopharmaceutical. During administration, the shielded radiopharmaceutical syringe should be positioned such that the shield affords maximal protection. After injection, communication should be limited as much as possible while maintaining appropriate patient comfort and safety.

REGULATION OF THE NUCLEAR MEDICINE LABORATORY

Nuclear medicine practitioners must obey a large body of rules, all of which are based on three essential principles. The principle of accountability requires that radioactive materials be tracked from receipt to disposal. The principle of notification means that all persons should be made aware of the presence of a radiation hazard. And the principle of protection is aimed at keeping radiation exposure to both technologists and members of the general public as low as possible. Both the written regulations and the standards of practice in nuclear medicine stem from the application of these three principles.

The practice of nuclear medicine is regulated by the NRC, which issues licenses to users of radioactive materials, including medical users. With the license comes the right of the NRC to inspect the laboratory, and to require compliance with its regulations. In approximately half of the United States, the NRC has granted that power to state governments, such that the state issues the radioactive materials licenses, and, in turn, are audited by the NRC. In these states, called agreement states, the regulations are promulgated by the state Office of Radiation Protection and must be in substantial agreement with the federal regulations.

A key aspect of a radioactive materials license is the list of authorized users. An authorized user is an individual who meets the training requirements for use of radioactive materials, as specified by NRC regulations. Each authorized user is listed by name on the license. In nuclear medicine, the physician(s) directing the laboratory must be specifically authorized by the license; technologists are not authorized users but, rather, work under the direction of the authorized user. One's radioactive materials license must, therefore, be amended each time an authorized user is added or removed.

The license also names the radiation safety officer or RSO, who holds overall responsibility for the institution's license and radiation safety program. This person verifies that the institution is in compliance with its license and files license amendments. He or she also reviews radiation badge readings and recommends changes in practice to decrease radiation exposure. The RSO is usually a physician who has documented additional training and experience that meet NRC requirements.

It is possible for a technologist to serve as the RSO. Large research institutions have a full-time RSO; smaller institutions often use the service of a consulting health physicist to assist the RSO. No matter what the situation, it is important that the radioactive materials license be kept current and that the RSO communicates with the NRC/state inspectors.

Although those have been "slimmed down" recently, NRC regulations for medical licensees are extensive. In addition to the regulations themselves, the NRC publishes regulatory guides to assist licensees in preparing the license. Up-to-date versions of both documents are most easily accessed via the Internet.[16,17] In addition, various publications are designed to provide further guidance in regard to license preparation and meeting the regulations (Ref. 1, pp. 185–209).[18]

A number of common-sense rules are designed to lessen the likelihood of anyone other than the patients getting radioactive materials into their bodies. The hot laboratory must be secured to prohibit access by unauthorized persons. Food and drink are prohibited in areas where radioactive materials are used or stored, as is cosmetics application. Technologists should always wear gloves when handling radioactive syringes. Bench tops and other surfaces can be covered with absorbent paper, so that if contamination is found, it can easily be removed. Lab coats should be worn for the same reason. Surveys and wipe tests identify high radiation levels and contamination, respectively, allowing the technologist to clean or stay away from the area, as appropriate. Packages containing radioactive materials must be labeled and shipped according to Department of Transportation regulations and should be opened according to NRC-specified procedures. Signs identifying areas of radioactive materials use or high radiation levels are required, so that workers and the general public are properly notified of the presence of these hazards. Following simple guidelines like these can greatly decrease the risk of working with radioactive materials.

As noted above, the NRC has recently decreased the number of regulations pertaining to medical licensees, based on the level of risk involved in each activity. Some aspects of nuclear medicine, such as the practice of radionuclide therapy, have been given greater emphasis. Other aspects have been removed from the regulations themselves but are still considered "standard practice" and should be included in license applications. An example of this is the requirement to do radiation surveys and wipe tests for removable contamination. Whereas formerly a weekly wipe test to measure removable contamination was required, current NRC regulations simply state that "surveys [be] reasonable . . . . to evaluate the magnitude and extent of radionuclide levels, concentrations or quantities of radioactive materials and the potential radiological hazards."[17] The important principles behind the weekly wipe test are (1) that technologists should be aware of radiation levels and take steps to decrease their exposure and (2) that technologists should not be contaminating work surfaces with radioactive materials. Thus, the NRC has lessened the regulatory burden in both areas, knowing that good practice requires that the activities themselves continue.

The nuclear medicine practitioner should also bear in mind the role of the Food and Drug Administration (FDA). This US government agency regulates the drug industry, an umbrella that covers radiopharmaceuticals. A number of radiopharmaceuticals were "grandfathered" through the approval process, but those developed since 1975 have gone through a stringent (and expensive) approval process. For this reason, the costs of newer radiopharmaceuticals such as sestamibi and tetrofosmin are considerably higher than those of older radiopharmaceuticals such as thallium-201, even though the latter is more costly to produce. The use of a not-yet-approved radiopharmaceutical requires the user to obey specific rules that include obtaining the patient's consent and tracking of any adverse reactions.

CONCLUSION

Nuclear medicine is a dynamic modality that contributes significantly to medical diagnosis, but it does carry risks attendant to working with radioactive materials, as well as those attendant working in radiation areas. Good practice requires diligent attention to regulations and guidelines in addition to an understanding of the principles of radiation protection. While many in-depth references can be found, this chapter has attempted to provide a succinct overview of the topic to serve as a guide.

REFERENCES

1. Kowalsky RT, Falen SW. *Radiopharmaceuticals in Nuclear Pharmacy and Nuclear Medicine.* 2nd ed. Washington, DC: American Pharmacists Association; 2004, pp. 71, 72, 185–207, 442.
2. Loevinger R, Budinger TF, Watson EE. *MIRD Primer for Absorbed Dose Calculations.* Rev. ed. Reston, VA: Society of Nuclear Medicine; 1991.
3. Cherry SR, Sorenson JA, Phelps ME. *Physics in Nuclear Medicine.* 3rd ed. Philadelphia: Saunders; 2003, pp. 416–417.
4. Prekeges JL. *Instrumentation in Nuclear Medicine.* Sandbury, MA: Jones & Bartlett Publishers; in press.
5. Lombardi MH. *Radiation Safety in Nuclear Medicine.* Boca Raton, FL: CRC Press; 1999.
6. Christian PE, Bernier DR, Langan JK. *Nuclear Medicine and PET: Technology and Techniques.* 5th ed. St. Louis: Mosby; 2004, p. 308.
7. Miles J, Cullom SJ, Case JA. An introduction to attenuation correction. *J Nucl Cardiol.* 1999;6:449–457.
8. CDE Dosimetry Services, Inc. www.internaldosimetry.com/freedosestimates/adult/index.html. Accessed September 22, 2007.
9. Higley B, Smith FW, Gemmell HG, et al. Technetium-99m-1,2-bis[bis(2-ethoxyethyl)phosphino]ethane: human biodistribution, dosimetry, and safety of a new myocardial perfusion imaging agent. *J Nucl Med.* 1993;34:30–38.
10. Hall EJ. *Radiobiology for the Radiologist.* 5th ed. Philadelphia: Lippincott Williams and Wilkins; 2000.
11. Zaidi H, Hasegawa B. Determination of the attenuation map in emission tomography. *J Nucl Med.* 2003; 44:291–315.
12. Patton JA, Delbeke D, Sandler MP. Image fusion using an integrated, dual-head coincidence camera with X-ray tube-based attenuation maps. *J Nucl Med* 2000;41: 1364–1368.
13. Health Physics Society. Health Physics Society position paper: Radiation risk in perspective, adopted in revised version 8/04. http://hps.org/documents/radiation risk.pdf. Accessed September 12, 2005.

14. Society of Nuclear Medicine. Positron emission tomography education for technologists. Symposium attended 7/9–7/11/04.

15. Dell MA. Radiation safety review for 511-keV emitters in nuclear medicine. *J Nucl Med Technol.* 1997;25:12–17.

16. Code of Federal Regulations, Parts 20 and 35, www.nrc.gov/reading-rm/doc-collections/cfr/. Accessed September 12, 2005.

17. Nuclear Regulatory Commission. Program-specific guidance about medical use licenses, Final Report (NUREG-1556, vol. 9). http://www.nrc.gov/reading-rm/doc-collections/nuregs/staff/sr1556/v9/. Accessed September 12, 2005.

18. Siegel JA. *Guide for Diagnostic Nuclear Medicine.* Reston, VA: Society of Nuclear Medicine; 2001.

Index

Note: Page number with *f* indicates figure and *t* indicates table.